THE GREAT
PLAGUE

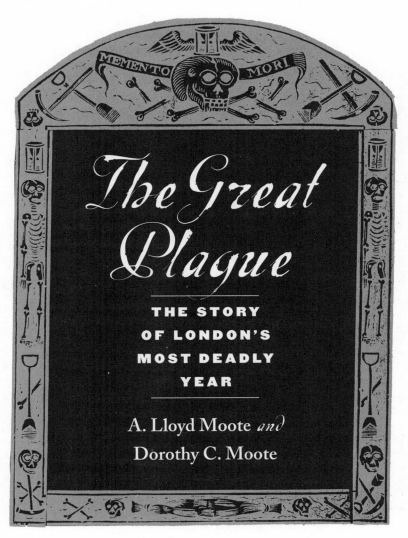

The Great Plague

THE STORY OF LONDON'S MOST DEADLY YEAR

A. Lloyd Moote *and* Dorothy C. Moote

THE JOHNS HOPKINS UNIVERSITY PRESS
Baltimore & London

The Johns Hopkins University Press
2715 North Charles Street
Baltimore, Maryland 21218-4363
www.press.jhu.edu

Library of Congress Cataloging-in-Publication Data
Moote, A. Lloyd (Alanson Lloyd)
The great plague : the story of London's most deadly year /
A. Lloyd Moote and Dorothy C. Moote
p. cm.
Includes bibliographical references and index.
ISBN 0-8018-7783-0 (hc)
1. Plague—England—London—History—17th century.
I. Moote, Dorothy C. II. Title.
RC178.G72L665 2003
362.1'969232'09421—dc21   2003006237

A catalog record for this book is available
from the British Library.

Maps by Adrienne Brook Gruver

In memory of Mary Frances
and for
Nancy, Karen, Salley,
Katherine, Peter, Daphne,
and Bob

What eye would not weep to see soe many habitacions uninhabited, ye poor sick not visited, ye hungry not fed, ye grave not satisfied. Death stares us continually in ye face in every infected person [that] passeth by us, in every coffin which is dayly and hourly carried along ye streets.

—JOHN TILLISON, September 14, 1665

CONTENTS

ILLUSTRATIONS

FIGURES

MAPS

TABLES

PREFACE

In 1994 we attended a conference on contagious diseases at the Wellcome Institute for the History of Medicine in London (now the Wellcome Centre for the History of Medicine at University College, London). A presenter questioned why people are drawn to writing about plague. She guessed that they had a macabre fascination with a disease that "reads like a gothic drama." We could respond only that plague is the touchstone or template for gothic drama. Anxiety, fear, horror—it's all there. The writer has to show great restraint not to describe the reality with purple prose. The quest to understand how people coped then and now is compelling. What follows is the story of a plague epidemic and of individual responses to it.

Our interest in plague goes back to the 1980s, when Dorothy was researching the reemergence of old diseases and the appearance of new diseases in the greater Los Angeles area. In 1981, public health authorities in New York, Los Angeles, and San Francisco were challenged by case after case of an illness with a wide range of symptoms and an unknown cause. Later that year the syndrome was identified as an immune deficiency disease, AIDS. That same year, in one of the outer suburbs of Los Angeles, an epidemic broke out among squirrels. This was an enzootic of plague, once the most dreaded disease of humans. Dorothy went to the area to talk with officials in charge of eradicating the disease from the animal population and preventing it from transferring to humans. This inspired her to study two short-lived epidemics of plague among early-twentieth-century residents of Los Angeles and San Francisco. (The latter outbreak, which infected 280 persons and resulted in 172 fatalities, has been chronicled by Marilyn Chase in *The Barbary Plague*.)[1]

Lloyd joined in to research far more serious epidemic outbreaks. Initially, we envisaged a multidisease study, beginning with the Black Death in the fourteenth century and ending with AIDS in the twentieth century. A publisher friend, Keith Ashfield, suggested that we write on a specific epidemic of one disease: "Why not the Great Plague of London in 1665?" The suggestion was challenging and exciting. The Great Plague of 1665 has instant recognition as a twin disaster with the Great Fire of London the following year, and much about the Great Plague remains unexplored or incompletely reported.

Human beings are compelled to make sense of catastrophes, whether they arise from human frailty or natural causes. Alarmed by dire reports of 30,000 to 40,000 deaths from an earthquake in Portugal in 1755, Voltaire wrote plaintively:

> Oh wretched man earth-fated to be cursed;
> Abyss of plagues, and miseries the worst![2]

Our goal was to find out how people lived through one of these catastrophes, to explore the resources on which they drew. How did they resolve the dilemma of whether to stay on at the risk of their lives or leave work and home for an uncertain reception by country people frightened of catching the plague from them? We wondered how those who stayed maintained a semblance of normalcy in the midst of death, dearth, and disorder. Had they received material help or discovered a wellspring of faith and endurance?

We have combined two professional backgrounds to explore these themes. Dorothy was a microbiologist who worked in public health and university laboratories and then taught in a medical magnet high school. She used a historical perspective to teach developments in biology, especially microbiology. Lloyd began as a political historian of seventeenth-century Europe and, over time, was drawn into the new social and cultural history. After retiring from teaching in 1993, we set out to see what the archives and published sources offered on the human side of the tragedy of the Great Plague. Professional friends offered encouragement and leads to out-of-the-way sources. Friends who are specialists of neither history nor medicine added their own enthusiasm for this undertaking. They found our subject timely and share a concern about how we all might react if a similar threat reached our shores.

Today, as anxieties persist over the menace of AIDS, biological warfare, and hemorrhagic fevers boiling up in Africa, the need to understand calamity reemerges.[3] Our age has inherited a rather hazy vision of past epidemics. The microbial revolution of the nineteenth century demystified infectious diseases by anointing their causes with scientific names like "bacteria," "protozoa," and "virus." Then antibiotics appeared, seemingly defending us as with a magic bullet. We late moderns like to believe that our medically privileged society is walled off from the pestilential past.

Earlier societies lived with a vivid memory of past epidemic disasters passed on through oral histories and reminders in prose, poetry, and vivid works of art. When any new plague struck, the cache of responses lodged in that collective memory provided tools for coping emotionally and practically.

AIDS has made us more conscious of past pestilences as we assess the devastation facing sub-Saharan Africa, which may eventually lose half its population younger than sixteen years. Yet this new affliction does not constitute a return to a dark age of indiscriminate disease and death. A major epidemic, spinning out of control, could not happen in the materially and scientifically advanced parts of today's globe, we keep telling ourselves even as we confront the new disease of SARS (severe acute respiratory syndrome), which mysteriously surfaced in southern China in November 2002.

The specter of biological terrorism following the attacks of September 11, 2001, on the World Trade Center and the Pentagon has brought us closer to the fears that haunted earlier generations. When powdery anthrax in letters sent by an unknown assailant made its erratic appearance through the U.S. mails, many panicked. Then, as public authorities sealed off areas and chemically treated letters and packages, the numbers of persons infected dropped, along with public concern. Anthrax cannot kill tens of thousands of persons, let alone hundreds of thousands, as have some previous epidemic disasters.

Traveling into such uncharted waters is the stuff on which fiction can be fashioned—or, more precisely, the fusion of historical fiction and science fiction. We know of two outstanding modern works on the plague: Connie Willis's *Doomsday Book* and Michael Crichton's *Timeline*. Both marvelous creations transport us back in time from our microbe-conscious world into that of the fourteenth century, using science-fiction technology.[4] The reader relates immediately to the people in these stories, just as Daniel Defoe's readers did in London in 1722. Defoe passed off his *Journal of the Plague Year* as a newly discovered "eyewitness" account from the Great Plague of London in 1665. Using fictional people but drawing on historical documents that are missing in science-fiction accounts, he described the fears and struggles in this time of great mortality more compellingly than historians have done.

Still, if we wish to learn from the past about confronting a deadly, runaway malady, why not let the persons who faced the catastrophe tell their stories in their own language and with their own understanding? We have focused our medical and historical lenses on how those who lived through the Great Plague experienced it in its totality—medically, politically, socially, economically, and religiously. With that aim, we have reserved any mention of our own age's biomedical and cultural understanding of plague to the end of this book, after our protagonists have had their say.

Plague epidemics of the past have been examined from just about every vantage point except individual experiences.[5] The sources for the individual approach do exist, as James Amelang notes in his edition of a tanner's account of a plague epidemic in Barcelona in 1651.[6] Personal accounts of London's Great Plague in 1665 are especially numerous and detailed. We knew of the published ones before we entered the archives; we were surprised by the additional narratives we found there.

Dorothy's concern, as a scientist trained to search for evidence with a microscope, was how to keep up with Lloyd, who seemed to work through manuscripts like a spymaster. Her first hurdle was to manage handwritten letters, diaries, or parish accounts and not doze after hours deciphering a nearly illegible script. Mastering early modern handwriting took weeks of staring at alphabetic samples and comparing these to the documents' *R*s, *E*s, *H*s, *G*s, double *F*s and *S*s. Also challenging were abbreviations, such as psh for parish and Lordship as Lo^PP. Another test was the seventeenth-century meaning of words such as *jealousy*—"I am jealous of you going out at night alone," meaning I am fearful for you. Spelling had not yet been standardized, and a writer might use several variations for a single word in the same letter. "Murtherd" in the street appeared for murdered; "lanthorn" was our lantern. English words from the German were in transition; an *ie* word like our *field* could be "feild." Causes of death were varied and imaginative: "killed by a planet" meant that the astrological signs were not right, or death might come by "surprise." Our favorite word usage was Samuel Pepys' account of eyeing the bounty from a captured Dutch ship at sea and estimating what the prize would be. When in port the prize was found to be greater than the estimate, it was a sur-prise. When we began to dream at night of seventeenth-century writing and words, we realized that we'd begun the process of interpreting the seventeenth-century hand. It is a carefully guarded secret among historians that archival work can be exhilarating, especially if it involves a topic as compelling as the dreaded plague.

We have drawn on more than twenty archives in Greater London, Essex, East Sussex, Hertfordshire, Oxford, and the United States. Each proved to harbor unexpected plague accounts. Dorothy began research in the old British Library at the British Museum by checking inventive adaptations of Defoe's *Journal of the Plague Year*. She wanted to look for Defoe's literary thumbprints to avoid recounting fictional tales of the Great Plague. Eight small volumes, all tied with ribbons because of dilapidated binding, arrived at her desk, precipitating her first rush of excitement with detective work on historical sources.

The anonymous accounts Dorothy had requested began with phrases like this: "As Told by a Citizen who continued all the while in *London,* never made public before." More than one historian of plague has picked up such a tract and been so taken by the drama that it became one of the "true stories" of that scholar's account of the Great Plague. Dorothy fell victim to such an account in another library. The story was of a grocer who had food delivered secretly to his door at night and who would send forth a blast of gunpowder as the food was transferred through a trap door (to decontaminate the food). The occupants were allowed out in the back garden at night to take in the fresh night air, which (it was hoped) was not miasmatic. After hours of Dorothy's transcribing, an archivist suggested that this story had the marks of the master storyteller Daniel Defoe. So much for avoiding pitfalls!

Another memorable moment came in the manuscripts room at London's Guildhall Library. Wishing to give a human face to those who had died of plague, Dorothy requested the parish death register of Saint Giles Cripplegate for 1665. There were four reasons for wanting these records. First, Saint Giles was an immense parish of twenty thousand inhabitants, larger than all but a handful of provincial cities and with fatalities in 1665 claiming half its residents. Second, its bulging register sometimes listed the street, lane, or alley after a plague victim's name, so we could use the register to develop a simplified epidemiological map. Third, sometimes the register listed the occupation of the deceased, which gave a window onto which occupations proved the most hazardous. Last, no one has done a detailed account of this huge parish.

A large rectangular volume arrived, and Dorothy began with a page listing all the parish's burials for the first three months of 1665. Beside many of the names, the parish clerk had added the cause of death, whereas many parishes in London listed only plague (often with a *p*). As one goes through the pages until May, the numbers of the dead slowly increase, with a variety of causes listed several times. The number of pages for the summer months increases dramatically until August, when 101 pages are needed to list all the fatalities, by then mostly of plague. A sense of the immensity of the calamity, with row after row of victims' names neatly inscribed, began to overtake us. Few discoveries in the archives since then have affected either of us as strongly.

There were other exceptional discoveries in the archives. Lloyd wanted to know what happened to business when plague sent the poor to their death and the wealthy to country havens. As far as we could tell, no historian had been able to track merchants trying to carry on. As Lloyd looked through the card catalogues at the Guildhall Library, he discovered plaguetime ledgers, business correspondence, and a rare merchant-family journal. As he read through George Boddington's remembrances of growing up, he turned a page to see, in bold letters at the top of a two-page entry: "Then was the Year of the Great Plague." He stood up, overcome with excitement.

In 1994 the Wellcome Institute for the History of Medicine's library purchased, at a handsome price, a letter from a London businessman writing in 1665 to his brother in the country about the threat to the brother's son if he stayed on in the capital as an apprentice during this plague season. The businessman assured his brother that his care for the boy would be as if he were his own son. Chris Hilton, associate curator of Western manuscripts, shared this newly arrived letter with us. The account is now part of our story of living through the Great Plague.

We can only begin to describe some of the bountiful archives that are available in London. At the top of the list is the Muniments' Room of Westminster Abbey, where ancient chests are kept bound with three to eight or more straps, each with its own lock and key; each key must be kept by a single person, and all keyholders must be present for the opening of a chest. Manuscripts and other special records were kept here over the centuries. In the room below, reached by a flight of stairs, are dozens of floor-to-ceiling, freestanding, timeworn wooden bookshelves, crammed with bound volumes. Commanding the entire room is an imposing oil painting of Charles II, England's ruler during the Great Plague. The manuscript room above is entered by a spiral staircase in a back corner and an old door some twenty-five feet above the floor. Here, helpful archivists, amused by Dorothy's American astonishment at the antiquity of the surroundings, opened Saint Margaret Westminster's invaluable records of the Great Plague.

After a harvest festival at Saint Mary at Hill church one Sunday, we by chance met Iain and Jane Radford. They took us around to numerous Christopher Wren churches, ending with All Hallows on the Wall by the Tower of London. The crypt was on view that day, with the original register opened to reveal the parish fatalities during the Great Plague—providential for our work as well as our relationship with these two delightful people. Iain was so enthusiastic about our project that he gave us the plague statistics for Barnes, an upstream provisioning town for London, and (with a smile) loaned us an unpublished history of the surrounding countryside during the Great Plague—a secondary source that only a few local historians knew about.

Our immersion in the Great Plague actually began at Colchester in Essex, where we rented a flat arranged by Lloyd's friend Ludmilla Jordinova, who encouraged us to begin with a smaller community that had lost nearly half its population in 1665 and 1666. As we settled in and contemplated where to begin, Lloyd remarked that it felt as though we were two parachuters, coming down in the dead of night without even a map. The local record office had good holdings, and Jane Bedford and Paul Coverly showed us parish accounts and government documents that revealed how the cloth-making trade, small merchants, and parish poor-relief workers came to grips with overwhelming loss of life and put together a network of relief that was astonishing. Lloyd remembers the days growing into weeks as he worked his way through the town's massive assembly book, its notations becoming smaller and smaller as a harried scribe crammed them onto the bottom of the page. One day Lloyd wondered whether he was clearly transcribing payments to the "dogg and catt killer" and another sum for the man who put red crosses on shut-up doors of infected households. Jane Bedford came to Lloyd's aid, assuring him that he was deciphering the crabbed hand correctly.

Our time in Colchester was made especially meaningful by the hospitality and warm acceptance given us by members of Saint Peter's parish, especially Maureen Hull, Mary Eldridge, and the vicar, Robin Wilson, who made us feel less like foreigners and brought us into a small but important part of English life. As Lloyd and the Christmas choir sang "In the Bleak Midwinter," Dorothy sensed the presence of former parishioners who had endured that incredibly cold December in 1665, when the living must have wondered why they had been spared and whether God would ever "stay his hand," releasing them from death's grasp.

We remained in Colchester for six months, going into London several days a week toward the end of this first research period. In London we were welcomed into our "second home" away from home with the Wellcome Institute and Library's wonderful academic family. We returned to England on four more research trips and always received the most generous hospitality any researcher could imagine from Sally Bragg, Roy Porter, and others at what is now the Wellcome Centre for the History of Medicine at University College, London.

Throughout our research and subsequent writing, we have sought to be faithful to what is known about our protagonists and to infer only what can reasonably be elicited from the sources. While hailing Defoe for his vivid imagining of the Great Plague, we have offered you these real characters, fitting their stories into the staggering events of that dreadful year of the Great Plague.

THE GREAT
PLAGUE

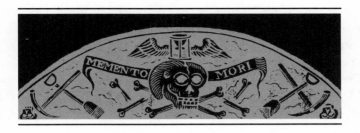

Prologue

They were all there at the beginning. In the heart of old London, Dr. Nathaniel Hodges was busily treating his patients with medical therapies that dated back to ancient times. A short walk away, at the Golden Fleece in the shadow of Saint Paul's cathedral, Sir William Turner tended to his stock of fine imported silks when he wasn't called to the Guildhall along with his fellow aldermen to discuss city policy with the lord mayor. An ambitious young member of the Royal Navy Board, Samuel Pepys, could be seen almost any day hailing a coach in the city and dashing through a gate in the ancient wall to the royal palace of Whitehall in the best part of suburban Westminster. Nearby were the newly developed Piazza of Covent Garden and its church, whose new minister, the Reverend Symon Patrick, preached to some of the most socially prominent and wealthy residents of the metropolis. In a much poorer part of the suburbs, in the parish of Saint Giles in the Fields, the apothecary William Boghurst offered his powders, pills, and a regimen of medical therapies in his office at the White Hart, which doubled as the Boghurst family's home.[1]

These five men were concerned for the welfare of their metropolis, with its half-million permanent citizens, seasonal residents, and visitors—close to one-tenth of the English population. Their world did not end at the outside borders of Greater London's one hundred thirty parishes, however, for the fortunes of King Charles II's capital were linked inexorably with the other nine-tenths of the country's population. Perishable fruit and fresh vegetables arrived from nearby villages, and grain for baking bread and brewing ale came from twenty or thirty miles away in the Home Counties that surrounded the capital. Drovers from the Midlands herded cattle, sheep, and pigs to the capital for fattening and slaughtering, and some livestock arrived from as far away as the North Country, Wales, and Scotland. Goods left the city, too; city merchants and suburban workers and their masters depended on consumers in every county of the land. Year in and year out, villagers and townspeople were drawn to the metropolis for employment, entertainment, and a wide range of services that were harder to come by in their communities. Many a prosperous citizen's parents were living out their last years in the family's country homestead, left behind by a son seeking his fortune in the capital.

Overlapping public responsibilities had drawn together the city-based Samuel Pepys and a country gentleman, John Evelyn, despite differences in social background and temperament. The bon vivant Pepys relished everything the capital had to offer someone of middling income like himself. The accomplished gentleman gardener John Evelyn could not abide the unhealthy air and crowded housing of the capital. The two men met over their common interest in keeping the king's navy shipshape and its men healthy—Pepys as a procurer of naval supplies and Evelyn in charge of sailors sick or wounded in the line of duty. The bonds and the danger of their offices were soon to grow beyond the expectations of either man. Their experiences were recorded in their voluminous correspondence and their very different diaries. Evelyn's journal was an open accounting to his family of his public deeds and personal interests; Pepys' journal was a secret record of his thoughts, acts, and feelings, using his variation of a shorthand of the day.[2]

Pepys, a tailor's son, dreamed of being worth two thousand pounds and having his own coach and four horses. Having begun public life with cash balances approaching one hundred pounds, he had increased his wealth tenfold in five years, far above the average English household's annual income of about seven pounds. He was driven to gain more and more capital from his influential office, to make life comfortable for himself and his wife, Elizabeth, and to enjoy the services of his newly expanded household staff.[3]

How different life was for his new country-gentleman friend! John and Mary Evelyn did not have to think about money or status, thanks to his inherited wealth and station and her father's influential post as clerk of the king's Privy Council, which included a residence inside the Whitehall Palace complex. On occasion, John was persuaded to join royal commissions, including a special body to look into the urgent need to repair the crumbling medieval cathedral of Saint Paul's. When he participated in a public project, he did so with a sense of purpose and responsibility that could lead to danger. But his real passion was leisurely writing about exotic subjects, from tree planting to engraving, at his family estate of Sayes Court in the down-

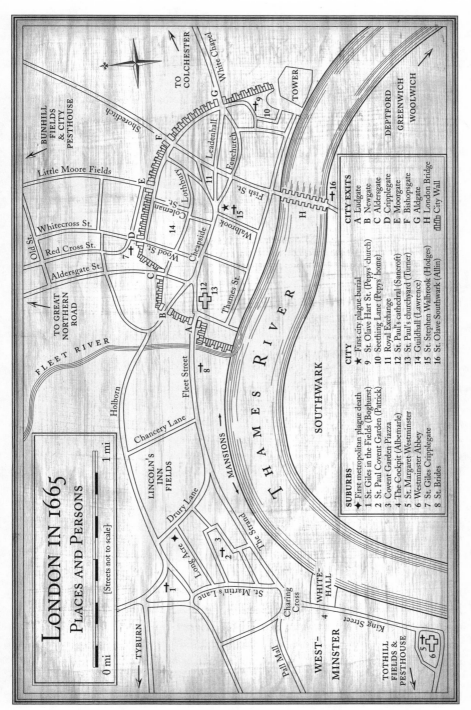

Map 1. London in 1665: Places and Persons

stream Thames River port of Deptford. The cultured life to which his city friend Pepys aspired was Evelyn's by birth and education.

Reverend Symon Patrick, too, had country associations. His father had been a country mercer, and Symon's first parish across the Thames River from Westminster had led to the closest of friendships with the Gaudens. Denis Gauden was the Navy Victualer and superior of Pepys, with a manor in the country and an apartment near the navy office in London. Symon Patrick and Denis Gauden shared a common interest in the welfare of the Anglican Church, the only recognized denomination at the time. With Denis's wife, Elizabeth, Symon's bond was more emotional and personal, though the two often debated serious points of theology and discussed the careers of clergy friends. When they were apart they corresponded regularly, once a week or more often when under stress.

A half-day's gallop to the northeast of London via the old Roman Road through the rich farmland of Essex lay the village of Earls Colne, where the local vicar and farmer, Reverend Ralph Josselin, could be seen ministering to the needs of his parish and tending his fields. Josselin's diary recorded his blessings and fears along with news of events in the capital and the local market town of Colchester.[4]

Farther away to the north of the capital, at the expansive manor of Donnington Park in the Midlands county of Leicestershire, resided a middle-aged, widowed noblewoman, Lucy Hastings, countess of Huntingdon. Lucy's closest relatives were currently at their London residences. Lucy had also sent a trusted agent, Gervase Jacques, to the capital to look into her legal affairs and make purchases for her and her children. The countess was relying on Jacques to relay any troublesome news about her city-dwelling relatives that they might not reveal in their letters to her.[5]

One other person in our story, John Allin, linked the country with the capital through a continuous correspondence via the public post. In 1662, Allin had been forced out of his pulpit at Rye on the English Channel when the newly restored monarchy ejected all clergy from the Puritan Era who would not subscribe to the Anglican Church's articles of faith. Widowed and with three young children, John relocated in a Southwark suburb across London Bridge from the walled city. Although he had the means to live and could add to his savings with clandestine preaching in private homes and by practicing medicine in his new neighborhood (quietly, and without a license), his was not an easy life. He had been compelled to leave his own children in the care of others in his old country parish; he depended on two close friends in Rye to keep an eye on them and on his wife's brother to help with their expenses.

Still, Allin enjoyed many skills and passionately followed his favorite pursuits of astrology, alchemy, and medical diagnostics. He would soon turn his talents to understanding plague, the disease everyone feared most.[6]

The people in these pages, along with thousands of their countrymen, experienced plague firsthand. It did not arrive as a totally unknown disease, however. The ancient Greeks had called any human scourge *plague,* from the word *plaga,* meaning a blow. The Romans added the Latin word, *pestis*— pestilence. Before long *plague* and *pestilence* became interchangeable. When a disease caused the calamity, the outbreak was called an *epidemic,* from the Greek *epi* (among) and *demos* (people). Hebrew scriptures narrated wide-ranging plagues inflicted on Pharaoh for keeping the Israelites in slavery and spoke of a three-day plague suffered by King David's subjects for his blasphemy of numbering God's chosen people in a census. The Greek historian Thucydides wrote dramatically about a hugely mortal "Plague of Athens" in 430–427 B.C., from which he personally suffered.

It is hard to tell what diseases caused epidemics like the one at Athens. Greek medical authorities, from Hippocrates (in the fifth century B.C.) to Galen (third century A.D.), defined individual maladies largely by symptoms and sorted them into chronic, endemic, and epidemic groups. This classical tradition continued to shape medical terminology well into the eighteenth century. But along with the continuing use of the words *plague* and *pestilence* to describe all epidemics, eyewitness observers began to apply the words to human morbidity and mortality associated with some bodily signs and symptoms that kept recurring.[7]

Modern histories of medicine distinguish three historical periods of repeated plague epidemics exhibiting these traits, calling them *pandemics* from the Greek *pan* (all) and *demos* (people).[8] The three plague pandemics were Justinian's Plague, which began under the late Roman Emperor Justinian in A.D. 541–544 and kept returning for two centuries; a second pandemic that started with the Black Death of 1347–52 and continued in Europe with fresh outbreaks well into the eighteenth century; and a third pandemic that affected five continents between the late nineteenth century and the mid–twentieth century. Since then, the disease has settled into an enzootic existence among wild rodents in scattered parts of the globe, with occasional transfers to individuals and sporadic epidemic outbursts among humans causing a few fatalities.

Apart from the physicians William Boghurst and Nathaniel Hodges, our protagonists of the Great Plague of London in 1665 knew little to nothing about the first pandemic, which had ravaged a wide area from the Mediterranean to China a millennium before their time. Even if they knew about Justinian's Plague, its sparse written records could have told them little about a disease over which modern epidemiologists continue to puzzle.[9] But literate men and women and many unlettered persons in 1665 certainly knew of the terrifying Black Death that entered Europe from the East in 1347. Plague tracts from the Black Death and its successor epidemics of the second plague pandemic had passed on a wealth of information about the symptoms and signs on victims' bodies, the terrifying climb in mortality that peaked in the hot summer months, and the erratic spread of the "infection" through a community. Most victims, it was said, bore the signature mark of a swelling on the neck, under the arm, or in the area of the groin and thighs, the infamous "buboes." People searched for words to describe the horror of this disease. Every new outbreak in England's capital was called "the Great Plague of London"—until the next one came along. English men and women called the disease a variety of names: *plague, pestilence, infection, distemper, contagion,* and *visitation*. But most of all it was known simply as *the sickness*, because it stood out from all other human ills.

Londoners in 1665 could not know that plague would never come back to their city after their epidemic. Nor could they imagine that within a few generations it would disappear from continental Europe. Western Europe suffered sporadic outbreaks well into the eighteenth century, most memorably at Marseilles, on the Mediterranean coast of France, in 1720–22 (inspiring Daniel Defoe's literary imagining of the Great Plague of London, *A Journal of the Plague Year*).[10] Thereafter, this second pandemic was confined to northern Africa and a wide area of Asia, from the Turkish Ottoman Empire to China, except for a few last sorties into eastern European lands, most spectacularly at Moscow in 1770.

In the distant future lay a third plague pandemic. It began in China in the 1890s, spread into Africa, and traveled by steamship to previously uninfected North and South America in the twentieth century. Classification and diagnostic techniques had changed dramatically between 1665 and 1894 because of the nineteenth-century microbial revolution, which traced the cause of infectious illnesses to pathogenic microorganisms. The bacterial agent of the third pandemic, *Yersinia pestis,* had probably also caused sickness and death in 1665, but definitive proof awaits future research. We will return to this subject after allowing our protagonists to recount their experiences with plague, as they understood it.

Whatever the "plague" disease of the second pandemic was, it remained the most dreaded malady known to early modern Europeans. Survivors of its first appearance in Padua in 1348 called it worse than Noah's flood. Later generations invented the term *Black Death* for this epidemic; perhaps, historians conjecture, they had in mind the dark blotches on the skin from hemorrhaging, or maybe a "black" death was the only way to picture so calamitous an event.[11]

Historians think the Black Death's most likely source was the steppes of Asia, from which it traveled westward along the Silk Road of merchant travel to the Black Sea and Constantinople, one of the greatest cities of the medieval world. From there it reached Sicily in 1347. In 1348 staggering fatalities were reported around the Christian and Muslim shoreline of the Mediterranean Sea, from Marseilles to Alexandria, as well as in the interior of Italy and France.

As the infection spread west, north, and east through the rest of Europe, it devastated capital cities and the remotest of villages. No place was safe. In Italy, Spain, France, Germany, the British Isles, the Low Countries, Scandinavia, and Eastern Europe, community after community braced itself for the onslaught, warned by graphic descriptions of the epidemic from elsewhere. Guarded, walled towns tried to keep the plague away but to no avail. Not even Venice, which responded more swiftly and thoroughly than most endangered centers, could cope with the huge numbers of sick, dying, and dead. This thriving Adriatic port may have lost 90,000 of an estimated population of 150,000 during its eighteen-month siege, an astounding 60 percent.[12] In Florence the dead were piled up in pits—"like cheese between layers of lasagna," an eyewitness said.[13] Historical demographers, who once thought contemporaries exaggerated the mortality, are now taking their figures seriously, saying that Europe may have lost close to half of its population to the Black Death.[14]

Today's readers may recall the nursery rhyme:

> Ring around a Rosie
> A pocket full of Posy
> Atchoo! Atchoo!
> We all fall down!

"Ring around the Rosie" characterized the red tokens of plague that appeared on the chest. The "pocket full of Posy" was a satchel of herbs worn as protection against infectious air. "Atchoo" was the sound of sneezing that spread the plague from person to person. "All fall down" was the sadness of sudden death, as people were known to collapse on the streets, sometimes with few symptoms of the sickness.

By 1352 the killing disease had come almost full circle to the Middle East, leaving Europe's survivors to ponder its meaning and take up their lives again. Then it returned, again and again. Some of the Black Death's characteristics—such as sneezing and coughing up blood—were missing from these later visitations, and the disease usually struck down fewer persons in cities and virtually none in remote country areas. But several continuities, including the painful, protruding buboes on victims, remained strong.[15] Common signs and symptoms were not always mentioned in contemporary accounts, but that did not mean they were absent. A historian of the Black Death, Rosemary Horrox, suggests that the brevity of some accounts may have stemmed from a belief that there was nothing new to say about plague and its effects.[16] Reports by some doctors of curing patients—which historian Samuel Cohn sees as a sign of the disease's decline in virulence—look suspiciously like a public relations gambit. Plague may have changed somewhat, but it remained an extremely deadly disease incapable of being cured.[17] Knowledge about plague acquired over time made its reappearances almost as frightening as its initial entry into Europe as a new disease.[18]

Until the sixteenth century, the plague's relentless return every six to twelve years kept the European population well below pre–Black Death levels. The demographic decline had begun before the Black Death from other causes, including famine, but plague accelerated the crisis. The population of Florence, which had been luckier than Venice in 1348, shrank by three-quarters from the cumulative effect of repeated plague attacks.[19]

After 1500 the intervals between outbreaks tended to be longer, up to fifteen or even twenty years. And Europe's population began to grow. But sooner or later London, Paris, Rome, Barcelona, and other early modern cities experienced another great plague. Although the loss of population usually remained under 20 percent, these visitations took more lives, for the post-1500 population explosion placed more persons in harm's way. At times the distemper continued into a second year with significant mortality, and in some areas it lingered still longer, with occasional further fatalities.[20]

Some of these epidemics took as large a proportion of the population as the Black Death had claimed. Venice, which kept excellent census records (a rarity at this time), reported 142,804 inhabitants in 1624, before the great epidemic of 1630–31; in 1633 only 98,244 residents were counted, a drop of one-third through death and emigration. Barcelona's last epidemic in 1651–53, chronicled in riveting detail by a local tanner, was its worst.[21] The great historical demographer of plague, Jean-Noël Biraben, places the mortality from this visitation at 45 percent (20,000 dead from a population estimated at 44,000), considerably greater than Barcelona's Black Death toll of 36 percent (15,000 of 42,000). Some of the fatalities were connected with the famine and war that accompanied this plague outbreak, but the impact of the disease was nevertheless enormous, compounded because the local garrison and neighboring peasants blocked all exits to prevent inhabitants of the city from fleeing. Then there is the shocking example of Digne, a river town in Provence, which suffered grievously from a killing epidemic in 1629. Assuming a population before plague of 10,000 and between 1,500 and 2,000 after plague, it has been estimated that Digne shrank by 80–85 percent. A *cordon sanitaire* of guards even more vigilant than at Barcelona two decades later had kept virtually the entire population inside. A century later, the town's numbers had climbed back to barely 5,000.[22]

The British Isles suffered along with the European mainland. Water was no barrier to the spread of the infection, thanks to the flourishing seaborne trade between London and other English ports and Amsterdam, Calais, Bordeaux, Lisbon, and Mediterranean ports of call. England's one stroke of luck was in avoiding the worst of the European wars that spread plague, dysentery, and typhus among helpless civilians to the drumbeat of marauding armies.

England's political upheavals, however, did not augur well for London's battle with the Great Plague of 1665. A takeover of London's civic government by political-religious radicals in 1640 helped plunge the nation into a civil war between 1642 and 1648. Oliver Cromwell and his Puritan-leaning army defeated forces loyal to King Charles I, executed the king, and abolished the Anglican state church and Parliament's House of Lords. An uneasy peace settled over the land under Cromwell's Puritan rule in the 1650s. On the left, radical religious sects, anticipating Jesus' Second Coming, pressed for more religious and social changes. On the right, Anglican royalists remained implacably opposed to the regicide of the nation's sacred ruler and the institutional destruction of the religious and social pillars of state. The Puritan Revolution unraveled after Cromwell's death in 1658, and in 1660 the king's older son was called back from his exile on the Continent to rule as Charles II.

The Restoration of the Stuart monarchy, Anglican church, House of Lords, and London's old civic governors managed to hold, but an undercurrent of unrest remained in England: Cromwell's surviving comrades resented their loss of power, and a ban on all worship except at Anglican services made all dissenters—from moderate Puritan Presbyterians to radical Quakers—potential threats to church and crown. No one knew how the capital and country would hold together against a destabilizing force like plague.

England had experienced sixteen plague visitations in the sixteenth and seventeenth centuries before this last one in 1665. The capital was especially susceptible, and popular almanacs included the "Great Plagues of London" in their chronology of memorable events since the Creation and Flood. A statistical study by the leading modern historian of plague in sixteenth- and seventeenth-century England, Paul Slack, offers comparisons (table 1).[23]

Of the seven "great" epidemics in London, the one in 1665 was by far the greatest in plague casualties and total fatalities, two times the comparable

Table 1. Major Plague Epidemics in London, 1563–1665

Year	Number of Burials		Index of Relative Mortality*	Estimated Population	Mortality (as % of Population)
	Total	Plague Burials			
City of London and its liberties					
1563	20,372	17,404	7.70	85,000	24.0
1578	7,830	3,568	2.29	101,000	7.8
1593	17,893	10,675	4.25	125,000	14.3
1603	31,861	23,045	6.74	141,000	22.6
1625	41,312	26,350	6.18	206,000	20.1
City of London and its liberties, plus some outparishes					
1636	23,359	10,400	2.25	313,000	7.5
1665†	80,696†	55,797†	5.41	459,000†	17.6†

SOURCE: Slack, *The Impact of Plague*, 151 (table 6.1).

*The index of relative mortality is an expression of mortality in a crisis year as compared to normal mortality. As Paul Slack cautions, these figures are very tentative because of the assumptions built into estimating "normal" rates of mortality and London's population.

†The figures in this table for 1665 are incomplete. Corrected totals were 97,306 (all burials) and 68,598 (plague burials). The rate of mortality, based on an adjusted population of 500,000, should be 19%.

figures for London's second most deadly epidemic, in 1625. The loss of nearly 100,000 persons from all causes in 1665 constituted a huge jump from the 15,000 to 20,000 fatalities recorded annually during the previous five years. The total death toll of nearly 100,000 was also considerable as a percentage of the metropolitan population: 20 percent of the 500,000 residents and visitors we estimate to have been in the capital at the beginning of 1665. And that figure of 20 percent masks a far deeper crisis because a huge number of Londoners had fled to the country to avoid the infection. If calculations from London's previous plague epidemics made by the contemporary demographer John Graunt held true for this great plague, 40 percent of the population (or 200,000) in the capital fled. That left 300,000 still in London, so the loss of 100,000 represented one-third of its actual population during the epidemic.[24] Another 100,000 succumbed in the countryside, where the Great Plague lasted into 1666. The Great Plague at Colchester, the longest lasting of all these local epidemics, was even more deadly. Its estimated toll of nearly 50 percent of the thriving provincial center's total population (and an even greater percentage of those who did not flee) allows us to see more clearly the profundity of this Great Plague.

How could any community cope physically or emotionally with this unwanted visitor?[25] Sex, age, privileged status, wealth—none provided a means of escape. Some epidemics seemed to strike the young most fiercely, others the old, still others those in the prime of life and in vigorous health. The increased danger for women during childbirth meant that large numbers of women died, even though many well-to-do women were sent with their children to safe havens while the master of the house stayed on. The one constant after the earliest epidemics was that far more poor persons died than any other group. There were more poor people than not, for one thing, but also their workplaces and homes were more likely to carry the infection and, of course, they lacked the resources to gamble on flight that took many wealthier persons out of danger.[26]

Still, communities did attempt to fight back. One of the most common resources was religious faith. Catholics and Protestants alike turned to prayer and repentance. The Virgin Mary was a favorite intercessor for Catholics, along with the fourteenth-century Saint Roch and the sixteenth-century Saint Charles Borromeo of Milan, whose fearless aid to plague victims— bodies and souls—became legendary. Anglican London joined Calvinist Amsterdam and Catholic Rome in celebrating the end of an epidemic with services of thanksgiving to God, following the traditional *Te Deum* of Christian ritual. In today's Vienna, Prague, Budapest, and Venice, commemorative monuments, votive altars, and even new churches stand as testimonies to the tragedy.

Artists recast saints who had lived long before the time of pestilence as heroic figures battling the unwanted invader. A favorite subject was the second-century Christian martyr Saint Sebastian. He had been executed after miraculously surviving the persecuting Romans' shower of arrows, which symbolized the pagan god Apollo's wrath. In early modern paintings, the arrows in this saint's flesh appeared as plague-poisoned weapons of a wrathful God's Destroying Angel, sent to punish humans for sinful acts. For Catholics, Saint Sebastian's survival offered hope that God would mercifully stay the angel's hand. In Protestant England and Holland, the menacing figure of the Destroying Angel, stripped of the association with intercessory saints, was deeply embedded in popular tracts and common speech. For Catholics and Protestants alike, the anguish of plague was chiseled in stone and painted on canvases by major and minor artists, including the great classicist Nicolas Poussin. Today, biomedical plague specialists and art historians turn to these visual representations as windows onto this world of unfathomable physical and emotional suffering.[27]

Material responses joined religious ones. Each community decided what public activities to allow (religious gatherings being favored, fairs prohibited), where to place the infected, how to bury the dead, and how to relieve the suffering. In some places religious hospitals for the poor were commandeered. Old leper houses, called *lazarettos* (after Lazarus, a beggar covered with sores in a parable by Jesus),[28] were also available thanks to the mysterious decline of leprosy—the most dreaded disease of pre–Black Death times. Gradually, major cities and some towns built lazarettos or pesthouse hospitals exclusively for plague patients, which in practice meant the sick poor. Wealthy households never sent a family member to one of these forbidding holding places, though some house servants passed through a pesthouse door.

Public and private agendas often conflicted, as magistrates placed restrictions on daily habits while residents improvised to survive. At Salisbury in 1627 and Colchester in 1631, angry women burned down the local pesthouse. Their motives were mixed, but much of their anger stemmed from the conditions in the pesthouses. Plague hospitals were widely perceived as places where poor people were sent to die and where their bodies were tossed in an adjacent plague pit.[29] In Florence, one of the most tightly controlled cities during epidemics, hundreds of women and men took to the streets in 1630 to demand that the large plague hospital be closed and all its patients returned to their homes for treatment. The authorities gave in temporarily, but when the soaring number of infected households made home care prohibitive, they resumed the policy of mass internment of the sick poor in the lazaretto.[30]

Most antisocial reactions to plague during its earliest visitations—vigilante-like attacks on Jews and other scapegoats accused of poisoning wells and other polluting acts—had virtually ceased by the sixteenth century, as had state violence against violators of plague regulations. Instead, persons who flagrantly violated plague regulations were imprisoned or placed in the stocks at a prominent square as an example; the gallows were sometimes on display but probably to scare people, since constables and judges had more pressing duties.[31]

The Italian city-states of Venice, Genoa, Florence, and Milan set the standard of care for the rest of Europe during plague epidemics. Venice's trailblazing "old hospital" for poor plague patients opened in 1424 on an island that had served as a hospice for pilgrims. A half-century later a "new hospital" was added for "suspects" who might carry the plague because of their contact with infected persons. The number of rooms or units in these two facilities was initially in the low hundreds; in later epidemics, as many as twelve hundred huts were set up on an island in the lagoon for the overflow of suspects. The need was obvious: in principle, all infected houses were closed up and the entire household was sent to some other facility until the home could be fumigated and clothing and other suspect possessions burned.

By the end of the fifteenth century, most other northern Italian cities had their own plague hospitals in place or under construction. The most ambitious of these, Saint Gregory Hospital in Milan, dwarfed the city's immense cathedral and Venice's pioneering plague facilities. Florence's lazaretto was more modest, but here and elsewhere a confraternity of Christian laypersons filled many needs the public authorities could not handle. In the sixteenth century the Florentine service group volunteered care for poor sick persons in their homes and provisioned hundreds of huts for persons who had been in contact with plague victims.[32] In one way or another, these Italian city-states handled a staggering number of plague cases in sickness and in death. During the epidemic of 1575–77, made famous by Saint Charles Borromeo's caregiving in Milan, Venice counted more than nineteen thousand persons who had expired in a hospital, plus some twenty-seven thousand who had succumbed in their homes or elsewhere.[33]

North of the Alps similar facilities came a century or more later. Amsterdam's large plague hospital was an impressive square structure with drinking water for the inmates coursing through the courtyard in the middle. Paris's

Hôpital Saint Louis was part of an evolving grand scheme of specialized hospitals called the General Hospital. At Poitiers and probably some other provincial cities, civic officials added to the usual pesthouse a recovery center for those who had survived the illness.[34] But many places in northern Europe chose the least expensive expedient, erecting a small, makeshift facility at the start of an epidemic and letting it fall into disrepair after the plague ended. Such a primitive hospital could not have housed many persons nor been of much comfort to its overcrowded inmates. Even the most expensively maintained lazarettos in Italy often failed their patients. The hospital at Venice was likened in 1576 to the Inferno in Dante's *Divine Comedy,* with its patients running through the wards amid the stench and groans, shrieking with the voices of the Damned.[35]

English cities lagged behind both northern and southern Europe in providing facilities for the infected poor. English pesthouses, where they existed, were often a small cluster of huts capable of handling no more than a few dozen inmates. The vast majority of the infected poor were shut up in their own homes along with healthy relatives, servants, and nurses until forty days had elapsed since the household's last plague fatality. England was also much slower than continental states in creating a national health body and municipal boards to oversee plague control. The Italian city-states established permanent public health bodies within a century of the Black Death. The rest of continental Europe moved gradually in the same direction, with physicians and surgeons working under the direction of lay officers and boards. The English state and its cities started from scratch each time plague broke out.

In other respects the English nation had gone just about as far as other countries in fighting plague. England had a set of Plague Orders for the capital and another for the rest of the kingdom. The quarantine of ships coming from infected foreign ports and their cargo and passengers was the nation's first line of defense, and placing guards at a city's gates a second, more desperate gesture. Sanitation measures were haphazard, as were many on the Continent, and none seemed to stem the pestilential flow.[36] England did not take a census, as did some places on the Continent, but London began tracking plague deaths in printed weekly Bills of Mortality in the early sixteenth century, almost immediately after Milan and Venice. This told officials and householders where the infection had been spreading. Although English cities and towns did not have the extensive control over the surrounding countryside that Florence exercised during epidemics,[37] they made far better use of the institution that was closest to the people—the neighborhood parish. In Italian cities, civic hospitals and private confraternities carried the burden of plague relief.[38] The parish was to be the prime source of assistance in London during the Great Plague of 1665.

The story that we tell in this book is really two stories intertwined, a tale of two Londons. One was the city of the working poor who lived in alleys and cellars and tenements throughout this bustling metropolis. Their story has never been told because they were unlettered, and there was no one like the tanner of Barcelona to record their actions and feelings.[39] Something of their struggle emerges from parish records and the personal observations of people in the other London, however. That other London was the city of the rich and titled as well as the middling merchant and professional people, whose struggles are revealed in the accounts written by our protagonists. Many of them lived cheek to jowl with the poor, on the main streets and courts of the old merchant guild center inside London's wall and the fast-growing suburbs that radiated into the countryside. How the struggles of these two Londons made them interdependent—if unconscious of the bond between them—will become apparent as the plague story unfolds.

Some of our readers may anticipate the darkest of tales, recalling the great Renaissance storyteller, Giovanni Boccaccio, describing popular reactions to Florence's Black Death in *The Decameron*: "All tended to a very barbarous conclusion, namely, to shun and flee from the sick and all that pertained to them, and thus doing, each thought to secure immunity for himself . . . Brother forsook brother, uncle nephew and sister brother and oftentimes wife husband; nay (what is yet more extraordinary and well nigh incredible) fathers and mothers refused to visit or tend their very children, as they had not been theirs."[40]

This view of plague epidemics as catastrophic events has long prevailed in literary and historical writing because it rings true.[41] Some have gone so far as to see plague as an inversion of the normal order, with criminal elements among the poor threatening the powerful and others among the lower orders fatalistically laughing at death. "Like carnival, plague inverted the normal world," suggests Brian Pullan, a distinguished historian of the rich and poor in early modern Venice.[42] But without exploring how individuals reacted to them, can we truly call these events disasters that undermined political, social, and economic order? Historical demographers come at the issue from an opposite vantage point, contending that early modern plagues were not disasters at all because the population shot up within a few years after every epidemic. These exponents of viewing the "long run" in history have a point, but perhaps this view goes too far in concluding that "the dramatic nature of the occurrence of plague attracts attention which is out of proportion to its importance."[43] What of the fight for survival that people waged at the time? Wasn't that important?

Louis Landa, who spent some time studying the Great Plague of London for his edition of Defoe's *Journal of the Plague Year*, pointed the way to our own study when he wrote: "Although large numbers fled and certain activities ceased, we know from Pepys, Evelyn, and others that many of the customary routines of life continued."[44] But how were these "routines" maintained? The historian Charles Mullett hinted at what personal testimonies might reveal: "Devotion matched desertion; conscience stood beside crime; and on occasion comedy relieved tragedy."[45]

Having lived for some time with the writings and evidence of our real, flesh-and-blood characters and their unraveling world, we believe we can provide some insight into how they coped. We hope our readers will appreciate the various roles played by medicine, religion, commerce, the Crown, court, and guildhall as our protagonists grappled with what Reverend Josselin up the Roman road in rural Essex called "the greatest plague in England since that in Edward the Third's time [the Black Death]."[46] Reflect on the haunting last words of Defoe's *Journal:*

> A dreadful plague in London was
> In the year sixty-five,
> Which swept an hundred thousand souls
> Away—and yet I alive!

PART I

Beginnings

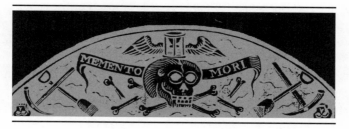

Winter, 1664–1665

This is the terrible enemy of mankind, that sends its arrows abroad by day, and walks all stained with slaughter by night; that turns the vital into noxious air, that poisons the blood and kills us by our breath . . . Before it are beautiful gardens, crowded habitations and populous cities; behind it, unfruitful emptiness and howling desolation.

—*The City Remembrancer, Being Historical Narratives of the Great Plague*

In a remote, squalid section of Saint Giles in the Fields, outside London's wall, on Christmas Eve in 1664, the parish's "searchers"—old women paid to determine the cause of death—pronounced that Goodwoman Phillips had died of the plague. The searchers were paid two pence for their efforts, the house was locked up, and "Lord Have Mercy on Us" was written on the door in red paint. The parish quickly saw to the needs of the bereaved family; on December 30 the sum of five shillings was paid to "Goodman Phillips and his children being shutt upp and visited."[1] With a shilling worth twelve pence (12d.), or one-twentieth of a pound (£), this poor family of three or four persons had been given enough money to get them through a week, perhaps more, assuming that the guard at their door was paid by the parish and the food he passed through a window was cheap. Three pennies would buy them a penny loaf of wheat bread, a pound of cheap cheese, and three herrings. For a few more pennies, they could strengthen their bodies and spirits with some sausage or a chicken plus some beer.[2] The parish had undoubtedly paid for a cheap wooden coffin for the children's mother; if anyone else came down sick, a poor neighbor woman might be paid to live in as a nurse until the last survivor recovered or died.

Frightened whispers in a few other run-down parts of the suburbs spread the word of a neighbor suddenly turning ill with suspicious symptoms. A month before, two other persons had been struck down and carried off by the pestilence. Such reports could not be brushed aside as idle gossip. During the Christmas season, Dr. Nathaniel Hodges attended a feverish young man and prescribed "a course of Alexiterial medicines," a common antidote to contagious infections. After two days "two risings about the bigness of a Nutmeg broke out, one on each thigh; upon examination of which I soon discovered the malignanty, both from their black hue and the circle around them, and pronounced it to be plague, in which opinion I was afterwards confirmed by subsequent symptoms although by Gods blessing the Patient recovered."[3]

No personal letter or published newssheet of the time mentioned the solitary plague fatality in Saint Giles. It appeared only in the week's printed Bill of Mortality—a single-sheet tabulation of metropolitan fatalities and their causes distributed at minimal cost every Thursday by the head office of the London parish clerks from reports by the clerks of the 130 parishes throughout Greater London.[4] The official report raised no general alarm. Every year the odd case of plague carried away a poor person like Goodwoman Phillips in some dense alley of a suburban parish. Certainly, the illness was a concern for her poor neighbors, but it would not worry the better-off residents of Greater London. Plague had not swept through their quarters of the suburbs and city for decades. Moreover, plague epidemics in England flared up during the hot summer months, not in the dead of winter. Everyone knew that.

Something else gave Londoners second thoughts about the deadly pestilence, however. That same Christmas Eve, a comet streaked across the dark winter sky. From London to Devon people stared in wonder at the sight; reports came in from as far away as Holland, Spain, Germany, and Austria. The brightly colored, fiery orb first appeared in the southeast sky on November 18, 1664, about 3:00 or 4:00 A.M. and again on the first of December. John Gadbury, a distinguished astrologer and member of the newly formed Royal Society for the advancement of science, commented darkly on the event. "This comet," he wrote in *De Cometis: or a Discourse of the Natures and Effects of Comets*, "portends pestiferous and horrible windes and tempests."[5]

The ambitious Royal Navy official and man about town, Samuel Pepys, heard about the comet while gossiping at one of London's coffee houses. King Charles II and his queen, Catherine of Braganza, sat up late on the seventeenth of December to see the comet for themselves.[6] The most fanciful report described "a Blew and Purple cloud, full of leprous spots and a Great Black Coffin in the sky over Hamburg and Flanders."[7]

Astrology was a respectable practice despite the skepticism of some literate people, and medical astrologers read the seasons and stars for advice on public health as well as public affairs. A conjunction of Saturn and Jupiter in 1663 had been followed by the approach of Saturn to Mars on November 12, 1664, surely an ominous sequence. Almanacs for 1665 prophesied war between the two great maritime powers, England and Holland, plus fire, famine, earthquakes—and "pestilence." William Andrews's almanac, *News from the Stars*, predicted "a MORTALITY, which will bring MANY to their Graves."[8]

At his comfortable home in Covent Garden, the wealthiest parish in Greater London, Thomas Rugge remarked on the "great discourse" about the comet all around town as he entered a friend's doggerel verse "Upon the Blazing Starr" in his gossipy diary. The friend mused about the comet as a possible portent:

> To treat of Comets or the Starres
> That doe portend as some say Warrs
> If anyone wish Pestilence or other change
> That unto many, may seem strange
> Bee it what it will if God decree
> So pleaseth him, it pleaseth me.[9]

Many Londoners, especially religious dissenters, took the comet's appearance more seriously. Upset by the Restoration's crushing of the religious liberty they had enjoyed under Cromwell, they consoled themselves that this comet foretold God's punishment of their oppressor ruler and his profligate court.[10] Dissenters in the countryside echoed these sentiments. In Leicestershire, the youthful Theophilus Hastings, earl of Huntingdon, received word from a friend at court that the "gallants" of London would soon pay for making light of the "astereal portents of great calamities."[11]

Prophesying continued into March, when a second comet appeared in the skies of southern England.[12] In Southwark, just south of London Bridge, an alchemist and astrologer named John Allin observed the blazing star, night after night, "riseing about northeast at one or 2 of ye clocke in ye morning, and continuing till day light hides it." Allin did not know what to make of it. He was apt to see any unnatural change in the heavens or on earth as a sign of God's judgment. In January, he had heard that Secretary of State Morice's cistern of water had turned to blood overnight. An "ominous matter," he declared.[13] But the remaining months of 1665, despite all the untoward signs, frightened people less than did 1666. Astrologers warned that this next year was really the one to look out for, because 666 was the number of the Beast of the Apocalypse in the Book of Revelation.

The winter of 1664–65 passed quietly enough. Europe was in the throes of a little ice age, and sharp frosts and bitter cold had descended on London before Christmas. A heavy snowfall blanketed the city early in January, and the Thames River froze over for the second winter in a row. The weather turned worse in February. On Shrove Tuesday, Samuel Pepys managed to enjoy a plate of fritters with his wife, Elizabeth, before embarking on the forty days of Lent, when he would have to give up some of the indulgences he periodically vowed to forego. (In January he had made a private oath to "leave the ladies alone" for a while but failed to keep it.) His mind dwelled on the weather outside: "One of the coldest days, all say, they ever felt in England," he wrote in his diary. Pepys fretted about coming down with an ague, brought on, he feared, by wearing a coat that had lain unaired too long.[14] London's poorer residents faced a much grimmer prospect: the price of sea-coals (the coal shipped into London from Newcastle and other northern mining centers) had soared beyond their means, leaving their dank living quarters without heat.

The adverse weather offered one pleasure to substantial citizens like Pepys. A frost fair, a tempered Protestant English version of Catholic Europe's pre-Lenten carnival festivities, was in progress right on the solid ice of the Thames.[15] Wrapped in long coats of wool or fur, skaters whirled around on blades of bone or wood. Up at the Musique House near Saint Paul's cathedral, a grand assortment of rarities could be viewed. A popular newssheet of the time heralded the thigh bone of a "gyant," a twenty-foot serpent, a dragon, a rare Egyptian mummy with hieroglyphics, "the antbeare of Brasel," a remora, a moonfish, numerous salamanders, and a twenty-eight-inch "Camelion," among other wonders. Sporting games such as bear baiting, always popular on the south bank of the Thames, added to the capital's carnival spirit.[16]

The Lure of London

O London is a dainty place
A great and gallant city!
For all the Streets are pav'd with gold
And all the folks are witty.

Well-to-do Londoners had much to be thankful for as they tallied their gains and losses on the first of January 1665.[17] The political scene seemed harmonious by comparison with the turmoil of the previous two decades.

Merchants in the commercial center of the capital inside its ancient walls were enjoying a brisk trade with the usual winter throng of country visitors. If they stopped to think beyond their profits, merchants could count their blessing of living in the healthiest part of the metropolis. Although the plagues of Henry VIII's and Elizabeth's days had struck hardest at the city center, the last epidemics had concentrated in the crowded, run-down suburbs, with only a few parishes inside the wall being heavily infected—in 1603 in the wharf area by the Thames River and in 1625 on either side of the city gates.

Elizabeth and Samuel Pepys celebrated New Year's Day at their apartment in the Navy Board building near the Tower of London. They indulged in a venison pasty and a turkey and were "very merry." After dinner, Samuel slipped out to his adjoining office to go over his last year's income and expenses. A hard frost covered the ground the next day, but his growing profits gave him a confident gait as he walked through the old walled city toward Whitehall Palace in suburban Westminster, buying New Year's "boxes" as gifts for his business associates and hiring a coach to the impressive new Piazza of Covent Garden for a noble French dinner with aristocratic friends. Speeding homeward through the wall at Newgate, he stopped off at the shops in Saint Paul's yard and came upon Robert Hooke's new book on the microscope, "so pretty," he wrote, "that I presently bespoke it." Samuel was a month shy of his thirty-second birthday. Elizabeth was twenty-four. This rising star in the navy's civilian administration had the ear of cabinet officers of the Crown and did business with brokers in town who arranged supplies for the Royal Navy's ships and men.

Born and raised above his father's tailoring shop in the shadow of suburban Saint Bride's church and nearby Bridewell prison, where pestilence had struck hard during the Great Plague of 1625, Samuel Pepys had come a long way in a short time. After graduating from Cambridge in 1654, he started out as a servant in charge of the personal affairs of a distant relative, Lord Sandwich, who had lodgings at Whitehall. Soon Pepys was at work in the government's financial office, the Exchequer. In 1660 he joined the four-member Navy Board as Clerk of the Acts in charge of recording its meetings and preparing its correspondence. He greatly expanded his duties until he was now indispensable to the board, the navy, and the king. Among the benefits of office was the Pepys' handsome apartment at the Navy Building on Seething Lane in the well-off parish of Saint Olave Hart Street. Their spacious new quarters were quite a contrast to the cramped turret room at Whitehall that Samuel and Elizabeth had called home as newlyweds and to the portion of a nearby house they had rented later in a dark cul-de-sac.

Most Londoners would have been content with attaining Samuel Pepys' comfortable place within the middling ranks of contemporary English society.[18] Pepys was different. He lived life on the edge, engaging in risky business arrangements, indulging in a wide range of erotic adventures, and at times engaging in death-defying acts that set him apart from others in his class. Consider his activities the day after New Year's. At his barber's he had little chance to talk to "his Jane" alone but gave her something; at the Piazza he regaled friends with a new "ballet"—a musical ballad "made by the seamen at sea to their ladies in town." He had "good sport" with a kinswoman of the proprietor of the Swan, "without hurt." And he was lucky in love at Mrs. Martin's lodgings, where he did "ce que je voudrais avec her most freely" (a typical lingua franca allusion in his secret journal to a sexual encounter).[19] This dalliance cost him two shillings in wine and cake, plus bearing with the woman's "impudence," but he could afford it. The only disturbance of the government entrepreneur's happy-go-lucky world occurred at the end of the day. His wife was waiting up with a passage for him to read by the Elizabethan poet Sir Philip Sydney on marital jealousy, which, he said, "stuck in my stomach."[20]

Samuel and Elizabeth Pepys lived in the oldest part of Greater London, a barely one-square-mile area known as "the city." A remarkable conglomeration of short, narrow streets, clattering with heavy foot and carriage traffic, the city contained no fewer than ninety-seven churches, twelve great merchant and craft guilds with sumptuous halls for their wealthy members, and row after row of multistoried shops and houses. Bounded by an ancient Roman wall on the east, north, and west and the Thames to the south, the city and its liberties (a series of enclaves just outside the wall that came partly under its jurisdiction) were governed by the lord mayor, a legislative council, and the executive-judicial court of aldermen who held forth at the twelfth-century Guildhall.

Beyond the walled city, London's suburbs spread out along ribbonlike roads leading to the open country. These suburban outparishes had once been villages or fertile farmland. Now they housed four-fifths of the households in the metropolis, including the vast majority of its laboring families. While most of the ninety-seven parishes within the wall took in only a few blocks,[21] the thirty-three suburban units each covered many acres. Saint Giles Cripplegate reached northward from the wall for a mile and a half and stretched half a mile from east to west. It was home to 130 trades and a hundred times the population of the largest city parishes. Coal-fueled industries had sprung up everywhere, providing employment in sugar and soap boiling, brick and metal work, tanning and brewing and glass making. Youths worked side by side with their uncles and cousins as weavers or dyers for wealthy employers. Many hoped to make their mark as apprentices to specialized tradesmen, such as Henry Foe the saddle maker, east of the wall, or John Moore, who dealt in lead in the city. In the city and suburbs, three thousand shoemakers were employed.[22]

This configuration of a prosperous "city" surrounded by much poorer "suburbs" was typical of early modern Europe's metropolitan areas. In Paris, Madrid, Florence, and a score of other cities on the Continent, the population explosion that followed recovery from the Black Death had brought prosperity to the merchant-dominated city center while drawing huge numbers of working-class men and women to cheap housing in the adjacent suburbs.[23] These European city centers were something to behold, with half-timbered residences of three, four, and five stories and adjacent large shops with enticing mercantile displays. The squalor of poorly built housing predominated in working-class suburbs, but the city centers had their own pockets of poverty hidden away in narrow alleys, where unsanitary conditions and overhanging roofs choked out sunlight and air and were thought to breed disease.

London differed from the European urban pattern in one major respect. Other capitals had their royal court and palace in the heart of the old city; London's palace and the surrounding courtier district were situated a mile southwest of the city wall amid the teeming working-class suburbs. Royal Whitehall, a major residence of English monarchs since Henry VIII, boasted two thousand rooms to accommodate high officers of state and many of the courtiers who congregated around royalty. So Greater London really had two centers: one for metropolitan and national commerce, and the other for the nation's court and government. Although they were separated by the city wall and had different political jurisdictions, London's two centers developed a thriving symbiotic relationship. The royal court and government in suburban Westminster needed the city for its goods and services and its wealth, which could be tapped for taxes; the courtiers did their share of fueling the city's economy with their extravagant tastes.[24]

Nothing, it seemed, could hold London back. Its trade with the rest of England was enormous. Its huge merchant fleet and mile-long wharf area beckoned the riches of the entire world, rivaling the success of the greatest international traders of the day, the Dutch. And, unlike most European capitals, which produced few goods of their own, London's manufacturing strength equaled its trading prowess. The city and suburbs made or finished an enormous variety of products, concentrating in the clothing, building, metal, and leather trades, with an ever-expanding victualing trade.[25]

Trade and manufacturing went hand in hand with the surge in population. In 1550, London's population had been about 70,000. A half-century later it approached 200,000. By 1650 it had more than doubled again. London in 1665 was home to at least 450,000 persons, with visitors and transients raising the total population to around 500,000. These are, of course, rough, working approximations; no one at the time knew the true population count.[26]

By the time of the Great Plague of 1665, London had exceeded in population all the capitals and major cities of Europe except Paris and had drawn almost even with that great metropolis. Metropolitan London had outstripped Paris in the ratio of the capital to the rest of the country: London had close to 10 percent of the total English population of five million; Paris held less than 3 percent of France's reputed twenty million.[27] This explosive growth came largely from the overpopulated English countryside, whose youth and adults were drawn to the capital by the lure of a job with better wages.[28] From the fourteenth century, when, after the Black Death, Dick Whittington had walked barefoot to London from Gloucestershire, urged on (the legend says) by church bells pealing a message that he would be "thrice Lord Mayor," London had attracted outsiders. The pace quickened in the sixteenth century and accelerated again in the early seventeenth century, causing the first Stuart monarch, James I, to exclaim, "Soon London will be all England." He scarcely exaggerated. Under James, his son Charles I, and Oliver Cromwell's revolutionary Puritan regime, London welcomed, on average, six thousand immigrants each year.[29] So great was the lure of the capital that, when Charles II took back his father's throne in 1660, one-sixth of his subjects who survived to adulthood would live at some time in the metropolitan area.[30] Immigrants from the Continent, especially the Low Countries, added to the burgeoning population.

The number of mouths to feed was a concern, for famine occasionally stalked the land. But production by country farmers had kept pace with the gargantuan appetite of the capital.[31] A greater danger to life came from within; more Londoners died than were born each year. This dark side of London's growth was masked by the inflow of immigrants, which more than made up the difference. As calculated by the London haberdasher-turned-demographer John Graunt from the metropolitan Bills of Mortality, the city and suburbs filled up quickly with a surge of new births and immigration even after the Great Plague of 1625. London was not a healthy place, but it had become an extraordinarily prosperous and attractive venue.[32]

In the 1630s, the energetic young Charles I and his advisors had tried to limit new building within the walls and clear the suburbs of vagrants, cutpurses, and precarious housing—lean-tos, shacks, and sheds—but royal regulations failed dismally. After Charles I's execution, expansion resumed under Oliver Cromwell's republican rule in the 1650s. The monarchy was restored in 1660 under the late king's oldest son, and the pace of building quickened. Plague or no plague, it was hard to argue with Graunt's statistics, which predicted a bright future for the city and suburbs of the nation's capital.

A City of Guilds

Write to Mr. Reurgot to send the cloths as soon as might be. If the waters frozen then by land, and if he can with ye first parcel of the Spanish fashion.
—SIR WILLIAM TURNER to his Paris partners, March 3, 1665

A wealthy importer of European silks and other fine fabrics shared Pepys' and Graunt's upbeat feelings about the magical square mile of the old city. Sir William Turner had the ideal spot for his shop, the Golden Fleece, on the south side of the large churchyard that surrounded Saint Paul's cathedral. The gigantic "yard" and nearby Paternoster Row, with all their bookstalls and shops, symbolized the inner city's prosperity. Here in January 1665 Pepys bought his copy of Robert Hook's *Microscopy* and had it handsomely bound. Saint Paul's yard was a meeting place for gossip, a designated spot to pick up odd jobs, and a paradise for "gull-catchers," the con artists of the day. Idlers could expect to see poets and painters, and the wares of makers of pins and looking glasses were a short walk away.[33] Best of all for Sir William, the Golden Fleece was accessible to wealthy wholesale buyers in the neighborhood and fashion-conscious courtiers a carriage ride away in Westminster. The nearby docks and Custom House on the Thames held cloths he imported by ship from Flanders, France, and the Italian city-states. He probably thought as little as possible about the shabby alley dwellings behind the cathedral, rented out by the dean of Saint Paul's, William Sancroft.

The square-mile city within London's wall thrived on the close connection between private enterprise and civic governance. The councilmen, aldermen, and mayor (chosen annually from the aldermanic ranks) came almost exclusively from the city's merchant guilds. The guildsmen were among the richest persons in England, eclipsed only by the great landed magnates, who divided their time between the court and the country.[34] There were scriveners (notaries) and goldsmiths (the bankers of the era), grocers and vintners, fishmongers and ironmongers, and haberdashers and merchant tailors like Sir William Turner.

Turner embodied a characteristic overlap of economic power and civic leadership. He was both a past master of the prestigious Merchant Taylor's Guild and a lifetime member of the executive city court of aldermen. The city government at the Guildhall gave legal protection to his guild and the many other "worshipful companies" of trade and crafts in the city, as they were fancifully called, against competition from unincorporated businesses in the suburbs. The guilds, in turn, funded a large measure of civic undertakings. They also supplemented the philanthropic actions of the city's parishes, the main source of help for the poor. The guilds maintained regular supplies of grain for the bread and beer consumed by the poor and of coal for heating their modest homes, as well as providing almshouses and educational endowments for their own pensioners and members' widows and orphans. In good times and bad, members of guilds often contributed individually or collectively to exceptional hardship cases—enough to keep the "deserving poor" from starving.

A confirmed bachelor without Pepys' carefree ways, Sir William had amassed a small fortune while participating actively in civic affairs. He was not yet fifty and stood out among his peers. At the Guildhall he kept his eye on public health and the moral behavior of the poor. At the Golden Fleece, his success in trade was evident in his working motto, "Keep to your shop and it will keep you," and his meticulous ledgers, headed by a joyous paean to business and religion: *"Laus Deo"*—Praise to God.[35]

In January, Sir William imported rare silks and other colored cloths from Florence, Milan, Genoa, and Lucca worth thousands of pounds. One shipment alone cost him £1,515 plus £16 in customs dues at Dover and London. But what a shipment it was! Taffetas in rose, scarlet, pearl, green, yellow, gray, and silver poured forth from cartons filled to the brim. His usual wholesale buyers, Smith and Company and Howard and Company, purchased part of one shipment within a fortnight. They expected another shipment to arrive around the same time, with others to follow right through the winter and into the spring. On February 23, Mr. Taylor the milliner bought a small consignment. On March 23, the king came through with an order for 3 ¾ yards of rich brocade at £8 a yard, to be made up into royal robes. As usual, the price was marked up for His Majesty, who could afford it and did not mind. (Besides, Sir William had loaned the king £1,600 in 1664 when the royal treasury was in dire straits.) Noble ladies stood in line for his rare silks, as did Roger L'Estrange, who made a comfortable living publishing the *Intelligencer* every Monday and the *News* on Thursdays, with upbeat columns on town and court doings.

Of course, Turner gambled by engaging in a luxury trade, with high operating costs as well as high profit margins. Goods might be impounded by customs, or war with Holland or France could impede the flow of goods through the English Channel. Profits were split with partners Pocquelin père et fils in Paris (probably relatives of the popular French playwright Jean Baptiste Poquelin, better known by his pen name, Molière) and with brokers and buyers on the Continent, whom he paid through bills of exchange. The inventory of unsold cloth sat on the shelves of his shop in the heart of the city, a considerable debt tied up at any time. In July 1664, his account books listed the value of this cloth as three thousand pounds.[36]

Still, Sir William sincerely felt that his financial world could not come crashing down. His business was as sure as that of the goldsmiths on Lombard Street and Cheapside. The Backwells and Vyners, for example, made a tidy sum serving as early modern bankers, offering 6 percent on deposits. They were happy to advance cash to the king for 10 percent (his credit being a bit shaky). The arrangement benefited everyone: the king got an advance on hearth tax collections; the goldsmiths got their 6 percent; and opportunists like Pepys, who advanced their own cash to the bankers for this purpose, pocketed the extra 4 percent.[37] The thriving commercial city inside the walls seemed to have something for almost everyone.

Approaching Turner's city was a heady experience for a newcomer. From far away one had a commanding view of "old Saint Paul's" and its six acres of leaden roofs. The medieval cathedral soared above the jumble of half-timbered, red-roofed merchant houses grouped in courts, the scene punctuated by church towers looking down to wharfs on the Thames.[38]

Entering from the rich farmland of Essex to the east, visitors passed through an old, narrow opening in the wall called Aldgate, leading to Leadenhall's meat and produce markets, the goldsmiths of Lombard Street, and the dazzling Royal Exchange. Built in 1547–50 on the plan of Antwerp's bourse, the Royal Exchange stood between Cornhill and Threadneedle Streets near the commercial center of the walled city in Cheapside.[39] The four-story Renaissance building, featuring a central courtyard and bell tower, was one of northern Europe's leading centers for the trading of commodities and *the* place in London to catch up on the rise and fall of private fortunes, the latest public news, and tantalizing rumors and gossip. Inside its marble-arched arcades topped by imposing statues of England's kings and queens,

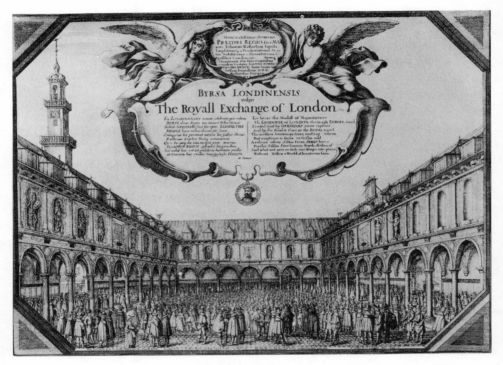

Fig. 1. The Royal Exchange of London. This major center of London commerce, finance, and gossip, crowded with well-dressed men and women in Wenceslaus Hollar's mid-seventeenth-century print, would become virtually deserted as the plague spread through the city in 1665. The caption boasts of the array of luxury items in its many shops, from Arabian perfumes and Chinese silks to precious jewels and cloth of gold. Notice the statues of the rulers of England above the arcades. Guildhall Library, Corporation of London

fashion-conscious shoppers found women's apparel, fine fabrics, apothecary powders, and dozens of incidental items. Bargain hunters went straight to the many pawnshops. Here the needy left linen (*pawn* is from the Latin *pannus,* meaning linen) as credit if they couldn't pay for their purchases. The exchange was also the hub for London's financial market. Merchants and shipowners conversed here. Samuel Pepys visited frequently to transact navy business, pick up the latest political news, and buy whatever caught his fancy.

The big attraction from the south was London Bridge—the only crossing over the Thames River for the entire metropolitan area.[40] Navigating the long, narrow span was a feat in itself; nineteen stone arches supported a passage 910 feet long and 20 feet wide, crowded with structures on both sides. Visitors gaped at 20-foot houses reaching to three or four stories. There was also a chapel, a square for festive events, a drawbridge to allow river traffic through, and a curiosity like none other, appropriately called Nonesuch House—a veritable palace on the river put together without nails. At peak hours it was anyone's guess how all the carts and carriages got through the narrow space into the city or back to suburban Southwark and the countryside of the southern counties: Kent, Sussex, and Surrey. The Thames could also be crossed by boat, of course. Hundreds of watermen living in cheap housing at the water's edge ferried persons and their goods for moderate fares. Those traveling in the best style could hire a flat-bottom wherry to take a coach and horses across the river.

Several roads from the north served as a vital lifeline for Londoners' appetites, conveying produce and livestock each week to the city's markets and slaughterhouses. The farm-country carters and their wagons competed for space with carriages bringing in people from the Midlands and North Country. Samuel Pepys' father and mother shuttled back and forth between the city and the family's ancestral home in Cambridgeshire. Samuel frequently took to the northern roads, passing through Aldersgate and Bishopsgate. Two other openings in the northern wall at Cripplegate and Moorgate eased the congestion. Still, on a busy day traffic could be bottled up for hours at these narrow gates. Conveniently, taverns clustered around the gates, beckoning weary travelers.

For Londoners with interests at court, two additional gates led to Westminster and on through the southwestern countryside to Salisbury, Portsmouth, Southampton, and Bristol. Ludgate connected Whitehall with Saint Paul's busy churchyard. North of Ludgate, Newgate linked the nerve center of London commerce at Cheapside via poor suburbs to open land where some of the most powerful persons in the realm were building new mansions. Pepys frequently took that route on business with high officers of the crown, stopping on the way at the inn of his cousin Kate and her husband in a less desirable neighborhood.

Ceap is an Anglo-Saxon word for *barter* or *trade,* and Cheapside lived up to its name, emerging from Newgate's thriving livestock "slaughters" and food markets and proceeding eastward to the Royal Exchange and the poultry markets, where it branched into Threadneedle and Cornhill Streets and the more southerly Lombard Street. The jousting bouts and small structures of Cheapside's olden days had given way to row upon row of shops three, four, or five stories high, featuring the wares of goldsmiths and mercers. But

Cheapside, like other parts of the walled city, blended merchants, artisans, and laborers; travelers, lodgers, and tenement families lived among some of the most illustrious members of Restoration society.[41]

The city boasted a dozen markets inside the walls, all of them just a short walk away for householders. "Herb markets" featured vegetables and fruit, and "white markets" offered poultry; there were "flesh markets" for meat and fish markets. Housewives had the pick of the market from six to eight in the morning. After that, street traders bought perishables to carry in baskets on their heads as they hawked their wares. The city contained numerous bakers' shops and taverns and inns, for bread and beer were staples for everyone.

Full-fledged markets were scarcer in the suburbs, and the best of these were in the aristocratic neighborhoods of royal Westminster. Suburban markets had followed a population shift within the metropolis that made eminent sense to the courtier class but could not have pleased Turner's civic pride and business interests. He and Pepys tolerated the coal smoke constantly blowing into the city from industries and housing in the western suburbs. But those same conditions had been too much for the last great noble residents inside the walls and others with independent incomes. For some time upper-class Londoners had been leaving the city's congested streets and polluted air for new luxury housing outside the western wall. They still bought fine cloth from Turner and played a role in Pepys' business affairs, but their lives were centered in royal Westminster, a cultural and political world apart from the city of guilds.

Royal Westminster

Up and abroad to Paul's churchyard, to see the last of my books new-bound—among others *The Rise and Fall of the Family of Stewarts*. Thence in Mr. Grey's Coach to Westminster, where I hear the King met the Houses [of Lords and Commons] to pass the great bill for £2,500,000. After doing a little business, I home.

—PEPYS, *Diary*, February 10, 1665

Economically, the city and suburbs depended on each other, but they had no common political structure to bind them together. Only the weekly Bill of Mortality provided the illusion of shared public space, with its tabulation of the total numbers of christenings, marriages, and burials that had occurred during the previous seven days throughout the metropolis. Even these vital statistics could not hide London's political dysfunction, for the front side of the weekly sheet counted the burials in each of the 130 parishes within four groupings. Most of the page was taken up with the week's burials in the city, parish by parish, followed by the caption: "Buried in the 97 Parishes within the Walls." Below this came parish-by-parish tabulations within the other three categories: "Buried in the 16 Parishes without the Walls, and at the Pesthouse," "Buried in the 12 out Parishes in Middlesex and Surrey," and "Buried in the 5 Parishes in the City and Liberties of Westminster." The reference to the "city" of Westminster was especially misleading. All urban areas in England with a cathedral were called *cities*, so royal Westminster with its ancient abbey held that honor—but no self-governing body like London's Guildhall.

Routine maintenance of public order was left to justices of the peace in their separate jurisdictions at Old Bailey inside the walls, royal Westminster, and the counties of Middlesex and Surrey. The Guildhall's political jurisdiction stopped just beyond the seven gates and single bridge. The king and his councilors, while calling Westminster their home and London the nation's capital, did not meddle in most metropolitan affairs. They kept an eye on taxes from the city and suburbs, reckoned by the number of hearths in each building (always a large part of the royal budget), and maintained a military force at the Tower of London and around Whitehall to intimidate restive dissenters. However, it was unthinkable that the carefree Charles II would focus his attention on the capital unless a major crisis erupted there—like the foiled plot of diehard Puritan soldiers immediately after the Restoration in 1660 or something on the order of another Great Plague. The king's passions were his personal pleasure and the Royal Navy. The possibility of war with England's greatest rival on the seas loomed large in his thoughts.

English and Dutch fleets were already engaged in piratelike skirmishes on the high seas and in the channel, capturing each other's merchant ships and removing the bounty to their respective ports. A Major Holmes had been clapped into the Tower by King Charles—not for seizing a Hollander off the coast of Guinea but for stashing away as private booty its three chests of gold worth £100,000. The king wanted his share![42] Windfalls like this would, it was hoped, tide the king over until the "Royal Aid" voted by Parliament to fight the Dutch was gathered.

Fortunately for the king, the merchant guildsmen who ran the Guildhall government in London desired his good will as much as he eyed their money. They wanted peace and order in their city, and supporting Charles II's Dutch war would help them gain his support when the city faced its next crisis. They also expected to benefit commercially by wounding Dutch shipping—the archrival of London's maritime trade. Finally, they knew any money they spent on the king's war would help remove the last vestiges of mutual distrust left from the revolutionary era, when radicals had taken control of the Guildhall and financed much of the civil war that had toppled Charles II's father from the throne and taken his life.

The Guildhall's rapprochement with Whitehall had begun with Charles II's return to the throne of his Stuart forebears in 1660 and his subsequent marriage to the Portuguese princess Catherine of Braganza. The drab garments of the Puritan Interregnum were shed for the finery and flash of the restored court. The city fathers joined in the fun by opening wide the city coffers, which they usually guarded jealously, for the royal coronation. The city chamberlain spent almost £5,000 just for "His Majesties entertainment at ye guildhall." Another £1,000 went to Charles and Catherine as a freewill gift. The "show upon the river Thames" when the king and queen came to Whitehall cost more than £500, and entertaining the royal couple at Cheapside came to £112. By the time the chamberlain counted up his expenses for the royal couple, the sum reached a whopping £8,044 and one penny. This far exceeded the city's entire yearly budget.[43]

On coronation day, city dwellers turned out to watch the royal procession, swelling with pride at such a sight. "It is impossible to relate the glory of this day, expressed in the clothes of them that rode," Pepys wrote. "The king, in a most rich embroidered suit and cloak, looked most noble. The streets all graveled, and the houses hung with carpets [from balconies and windows] . . . and the ladies out of the windows. So glorious was the show, with gold and silver, that we were not able to look at it, our eyes at last being so much overcome."[44] The parade of twenty thousand persons on horse and foot began at the Tower at the eastern end of the old walled city and arrived seven hours later at Whitehall Palace.

Charles and Catherine settled into the immense spread of Whitehall, a maze of buildings on both sides of Westminster's King Street that included galleries, apartments, a chapel, a tennis court, and Inigo Jones's Banqueting House, the architect's masterwork.[45] Southwest of Whitehall, the buildings in the palace yard served the high justices and Parliament in Saint Margaret parish, which was also home to Westminster Abbey. To the west of Whitehall, in a gigantic private park enclosed by an immense wall, Charles II's brother and presumptive heir, James, duke of York, and his duchess, Anne Hyde, daughter of the lord chancellor, resided at Saint James Palace, awaiting the birth of their child.

The nation's nobility flocked in for the coronation and stayed on with their families and servants, attending the House of Lord's sessions at Parliament and occupying grand estates bordering the Strand thoroughfare that connected Whitehall with Fleet Street and the city. These Strand estates, boasting dwellings with twenty, thirty, even fifty hearths, combined elegant living with isolation from clutter and crime outside their gates. The immense grounds of Bedford House, designed by royalty's architect, Inigo Jones, stretched from the north side of the Strand all the way to Covent Garden's Piazza. Its neighbor, Exeter House, featured a turreted, Tudor-style façade and a chapel where Samuel Pepys and a throng of Londoners had secretly worshiped according to the illegal Anglican rite near the end of the Puritan era. Set back behind protective high walls from the south side of the Strand lay a series of miniature palaces also called "Houses," named after their distinguished founders, York, Worcester, Somerset, Arundel, and Essex. Most of these palatial complexes had a great hall, a chapel, stables, extensive gardens, a commanding view of the Thames, and private stairs leading down to the water. The duke and duchess of York were married in Worcester House at the beginning of the Restoration, and the queen mother, Henrietta Maria, moved into Somerset House at the same time.[46]

Country gentry and squires who aped these social betters added to the swelling throng. As historian Roy Porter has written, "Squires weary of the idiocy of rural life rode up to town for business and pleasure—to dabble in politics, beg favors from the great, sell acres, borrow gold, arrange marriages for daughters, purchase fine fabrics, see the sights, and sup with boon companions in the dozens of hostelries, inns and . . . coffee houses."[47] Many of these squires stayed for only a fortnight; others rented lodgings for a season or for years on end. The presence of all these socially conscious folk and their bulging purses attracted many other groups to Westminster. Scriveners and barristers stood poised to write legal documents and plead cases. Doctors, apothecaries, and surgeons prescribed regimens and cures for the health-conscious. Shops and inns proliferated. Household servants and coachmen abounded.

Of the five parishes in royal Westminster, Covent Garden was the jewel. Its tax base showed it off as the wealthiest parish in the entire metropolitan area. Its array of peers and high royal officials in residence made it *the* society parish of Greater London. And it was beautiful. The earls of Bedford were real estate developers par excellence. Acquiring a sparsely populated forty-acre area where Westminster Abbey had a convent garden, they transformed it into a showpiece of the suburbs. The present earl's father had struck a bar-

gain with the king's father. Bedford could employ the royal architect Inigo
Jones to create breathtaking Covent Garden Piazza, with its redbrick row
houses in imitation of London's Royal Exchange and the Rialto in Venice. In
return, Bedford was to maintain a major east-west route, Long Acre, a little
to the north. Bedford kept only one part of the bargain; Long Acre, which he
had agreed to "pave and keep . . . as well as any street in London," began to
deteriorate. By the 1660s it had attracted brothels and coachmakers, and
newly constructed ramshackle dwellings lay just out of sight in alleys.[48]

A new market on the south side of the Piazza was one of the rare suburban supply points for food. At the western end stood another landmark,
the Inigo Jones–designed church of Saint Paul Covent Garden. The classical
façade was not especially appealing, but inside one heard the most edifying
sermons in London. The new minister, Symon Patrick, enjoyed powerful patrons led by the Bedfords, an ability to stir the consciences of his wealthiest
parishioners, and a rare knack for understanding the plight of the parish
poor. Patrick was a thirty-eight-year-old bachelor, seemingly at the peak of
his career. Some of his parishioners with influence at court were grooming
him for even greater things.

As Greater London entered the sixth year of the Restoration monarchy, it
continued the tumultuous growth that had thrust it into the top rank of European cities. To economic dynamism and geographic expansion was added a
remarkable flourishing of the arts and sciences. John Dryden's first rhymed
heroic play, *The Indian Emperour*, with Montezuma battling Cortez, was set
for a spring opening. Attendance at plays in Westminster had never been
better. Charles II's future mistress, Nell Gwyn, titillated courtiers and people
of Samuel Pepys' rank with a new kind of farce, pitting a rakish hero against
an independent-thinking heroine. On January 4, Pepys attended *The Comical Revenge, or Love in a Tub*, which wittily probed Restoration manners. On
the fourteenth Pepys saw Ben Jonson's comedy of 1606, *Volpone, or the Fox*,
and declared it "a most excellent play—the best I think I ever saw, and well
acted."[49]

The great Puritan thinker of the late revolution, John Milton, was finishing *Paradise Lost* in the poor suburban parish of Saint Giles Cripplegate. On
the cusp of the scientific revolution, Robert Hooke and other members of
the new Royal Society in the heart of the old city were engaged in ground-
breaking scientific experiments. Some were fanciful, others daring. In a
memorable treatise William Harvey, not long before, had described the circulation of blood. William Sydenham and other physicians were distinguishing different fevers, from the simple kind to spotted fever and the dreaded

plague, and prescribing quinine for malarial fever, which was proving beneficial. The microscope was revealing a new world—a new frontier.

London's access to the sea placed it on another frontier, as goods came from around the world—spices from the East Indies, sugar from Barbados, silks from the Levant, tobacco from Virginia, and that new delight, tea, from the Far East. A less inviting import, however, loomed across nearer waters. The homegrown variety of plague might continue to be contained in a few remote corners of London's suburban parishes densely populated with poor workers, but the foreign variety had made a new march across the Continent, from port to port and country to country. A decade before, it had infested the Italian and Iberian peninsulas and then moved northward until it reached the North Sea shores of Holland and Germany. Amsterdam had suffered one of its worst epidemics in 1663, and the infection had continued there through 1664.

Samuel Pepys had ended his diary for 1664 with reflections of how good God had been to him and how fortunate he was in estate, office, and health. But with an Anglo-Dutch war about to become official on both sides of the North Sea and English Channel, it was anyone's guess whether the physical health of Londoners could be sustained as their city's economic vigor had been. Pepys' new associate in naval matters, John Evelyn, had just been appointed one of the king's commissioners to care for the throngs of sick and wounded royal sailors and Dutch prisoners who were expected to come on shore as the warmer weather of spring followed the bitter frosts of winter. If the city-dwelling Pepys did not think about what darkness might lie ahead, the country gentleman Evelyn certainly did: he began his search in London's hospitals for vacant space that could be used for stricken sailors. Unfortunately, the city and suburbs had only two hospitals with any significant capacity, Saint Bartholomew's just beyond the western wall (with room for 200 to 300 beds) and Saint Thomas across the river in Southwark (with about 250 beds).[50] For the worst disease of the age, only two small pesthouses served the half-million persons in the capital. Though conveniently distant from the city and court, they were woefully inadequate if plague should be carried in by Dutch prisoners from Amsterdam and other infected Dutch ports.

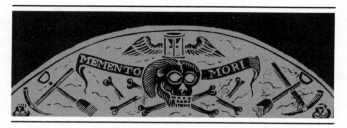

The Other London

It was a Received Notion amongst the Common People that the Plague visited England once in Twenty Years, as if after a certain Interval, by some Necessity it must return again . . . It greatly contributed both to propagate and inflame the contagion, by the strong Impression it made upon their Minds.

—Dr. Nathaniel Hodges, *Loimologia: Or, An Historical Account of the Plague in London in 1665*

Life had been kind to Reverend Symon Patrick. As rector of metropolitan London's wealthiest congregation, he had the ear of prosperous merchants and the personal backing of powerful patrons at the royal court and in government, who had made possible his meteoric rise on the ecclesiastical ladder. Within the enormous range of possible incomes and degrees of social status, Reverend Patrick stood far above the "common people"—the vast majority of Londoners.

If Patrick had been asked to explain his good fortune, he likely would have attributed it to divine providence, for the idea that God shaped human ends was common during his lifetime, and both of his parents believed in it strongly. He was born into a family that lived comfortably and appreciated both sacred and secular learning. His mother was a minister's daughter, his father the sixth son of a country gentleman. As a younger son, Symon's father had to work for a living; he did well as a mercer, and Symon, as his father's first son, could have continued the trade. Instead, he turned to the world of learning. After surviving a nearly fatal childhood fever, Symon completed grammar school and graduated from Cambridge University in 1648 as Cromwell's Roundheads were defeating the royalist Cavaliers. A promising scholarly career was cut short when his college passed him over for a permanent post. Symon altered his career path and was secretly ordained as an Anglican priest in the mid-1650s, when the Puritans still had a monopoly over religion. He immediately became the household chaplain of Sir Walter St. John, son-in-law of the chief justice. Through St. John's patronage he was appointed vicar of the church of Battersea, in rural Surrey across the Thames from Westminster, in 1658.

Patrick had been flattered by the invitation from the earl of Bedford, whose father had developed the Piazza area of Covent Garden, to move to Saint Paul Covent Garden as its minister in 1662. His delicate health was holding up well despite his concern at leaving the fresh country air of Battersea, and the new courtier congregation was almost as friendly as his old parishioners, easing his fears that they might not take to him. To be sure, he missed dropping in at his younger brother's Battersea home. And no one could replace his closest friends at the old church, Denis and Elizabeth Gauden, and their beautiful manor house in nearby Clapham. Patrick went back to Clapham to see Denis and Elizabeth now and then, but his new congregation was taking virtually all his time and energy these days.[1]

As he stepped out of his church on the Piazza and headed for Maiden Lane and Ward Alley for the day's pastoral calls, Patrick knew what to expect. Here at the crossroads of privilege and poverty, two Londons met. The London most familiar to Samuel Pepys and Sir William Turner was found in places like the Piazza, where Pepys' pleasure-loving associate on the Navy Board, Lord Brouncker, and the good-hearted Lady Abergavenny owned splendid townhouses. Uncomfortably close by was the "other London" in shabby spots like Maiden Lane and Ward Alley. Here Patrick encountered the one-hearth homes of Goody Cocke and Goodman Hall, whose first names were likely known to a few neighbors but were omitted by the parish's churchwardens from their accounts of payments to the neighborhood poor. In good times the Goody Cockes and Goodman Halls of this other London made up a quarter of the metropolitan population; in times of great want, sickness, or economic downturn, their numbers approached one-half of the population. The proportion could grow quickly because many unskilled laborers and workers in specialized crafts lived on extremely low wages or in seasonal jobs that left them perpetually on the edge of subsistence.

The easiest gauge of poverty in the capital was the royal hearth tax, an ingenious, basic direct levy on Charles II's subjects at the rate of two shillings a year for every fireplace in a dwelling. The rationale was simple: the number of hearths gave a rough idea of the size of the dwelling and, by inference, the financial status of the occupying renter or owner. The lowest rate of two shil-

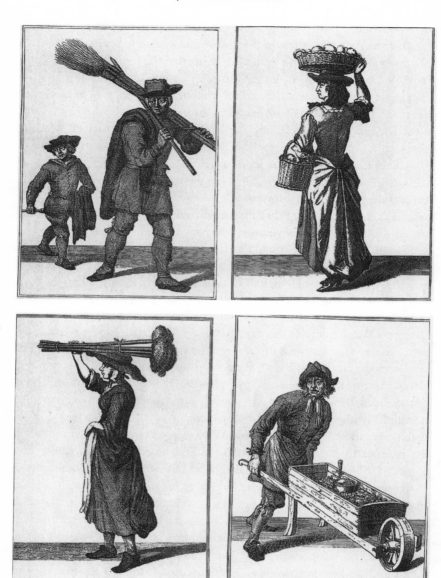

Fig. 2. Street peddlers in seventeenth-century London. These contemporary prints of the working poor are as close as we can come to visualizing the clothes and deportment of the "other London." Clockwise from upper left: a chimney sweep, fruit seller, oyster man, and mop peddler.

lings, however, was what it cost the most frugal poor person to subsist for a week on bread and cheese and without any purchase of clothes or shoes. The king's tax assessors, therefore, looked more closely at the assets of a single-hearth or two-hearth family, usually granting them an exemption on the basis of poverty. Not too far away a mansion boasting seven hearths or more housed the family of a very wealthy tradesman or peer, taxed at the high end of the hearth tax assessments. At the center of the walled city, 1.5 percent of the population was poor by these hearth tax calculations. Down at the city's waterfront, poverty averaged 5.2 percent. Beyond the old wall, the percentages rose dramatically: the poor were 25.7 percent of the western parishes (including affluent Whitehall), 49.1 percent in the north, and 51.9 percent in the east. Across the river, poverty in Southwark's parishes reached 43.7 percent.[2] The percentage of poor Londoners who were struggling to survive on their own or subsisting with the help of parish relief was greater than these figures indicate, however. Modern investigations show that tax officials and other official records missed up to one-third of the capital's households. Most of these undocumented families and individuals were surely poor people doubling up in the same quarters, hidden in cellars or shacks, or boarding at someone else's dwelling.[3]

Parish Priorities

Church expenses: To Mr. Symon Patrick, rector, in full for the year, £150.
    To the bricklayer for mending churchyard walls and bellfrey, £9.
    For rosemary, bayes, holley, and ivy for the church, 5s 6d.
Poor-tax payments: To a woman having 2 children sick of ye small pox, 2s.
    To the nurse for keeping a child till sent back to St. Martin's, 2s 6d.
    For a coffin for a child that dyed in Holborne, 1s 6d.
—From the account book of Saint Paul Covent Garden, Easter 1664–Easter 1665

To the problem of poverty in medieval England, voluntary Christian charity was the response. The surging population and migration of the sixteenth century, however, greatly increased poverty, unemployment, and homelessness. The crisis was greatest in the capital, whose economy even in the best of years could not fully integrate the thousands of immigrants from the countryside and abroad. Queen Elizabeth and her parliaments responded with a compulsory Poor Law system.[4] Able-bodied beggars and drifters were whipped and put in a "house of correction" or Bridewell, while the "deserving poor" were taken care of in the parish of their residence by a special poor tax on householders who could afford to be Good Samaritans but often were not.

This rigid division of the poor into deserving and undeserving groups was logical to middling and upper-class families, who believed that every able-bodied person should work and who abhorred "masterless men" who lacked the skills to set up their own trade and were too stubborn to become someone else's servant. Some adults clearly needed help to survive: they were sick, infirm, or indigent because of widowhood (often associated with old age) or widower status (often with a large number of dependent children). Foundlings had to be put out to nurse at considerable cost. Orphans must be housed and apprenticed until they could fend for themselves, another considerable expense. But able-bodied poor adults who had no job deserved no handout, it was thought.

The flood of immigrants to London made the distinction between the meritorious and incorrigible poor difficult to uphold. Although a proclamation by Charles II in 1662 still referred to "rogues, vagabonds, beggars and other idle persons" flocking to London to live "by begging, stealing and other lewd practices," a parliamentary amendment to Elizabeth's Poor Law that same year admitted that many immigrants and residents could not find work through no fault of their own other than lack of the proper skills. "Defects in the law of relief and employment," the new law declared, "doth enforce many to turn [into] incorrigible rogues and others to perish for want." Up to this time, immigrants had had to wait three years before going on parish relief; now they could claim residency after forty days and get immediate assistance.

With a stroke of the royal pen endorsing the new law, Charles II greatly expanded the legal burden on his London parishes. What were they to do, especially in the densely populated suburbs, where most of the unskilled laborers lived? In principle, every parish was supposed to have a supply of raw materials for unemployed persons to work on, preferably in a prisonlike enclosure. But there would be virtually no such workhouse arrangements in London until the eighteenth century.[5]

Still, the machinery existed to implement the amended Poor Law. Mixing the secular with the sacred, every royal government since Queen Elizabeth had folded a political calendar of poor relief seamlessly into the familiar ecclesiastical one. Every Easter the thirty to forty leading members of each parish gathered at their church to elect its main lay officers, substantial householders who served without pay (or paid a fine of about ten pounds to avoid the onerous duties). The new churchwardens and overseers of the poor revised the previous year's budget for poor relief, assessing all taxable households according to their means. Collectors for the poor would gather the money periodically, and the churchwardens would disburse it to those in need. The two churchwardens (senior and junior) and two to four overseers of the poor kept close watch on their pounds, shillings, and pence, recording every sum and its use.

The heavy-bound ledgers listing the shillings and pence doled out weekly to widows, orphans, and indigent old men offer rare glimpses of the hard-luck lives of this other London. The chronically indigent were kept alive, and the churchwardens, though burdened with their own business and volunteer activities, prioritized unexpected cases of need. A chance fire (a common occurrence) destroyed the lifetime possessions of a family; an accident at work maimed a healthy man for life; one of the illnesses that were endemic in working quarters struck down the breadwinner in the family. Even when the winter was kind, springtime employment plentiful, and the summer harvest bountiful, unexpected expenses sometimes put the churchwardens' account in the red; they were to make up the difference with their own money until the next assessment. The Elizabethan Poor Law, now three generations old, was not a perfect instrument of caregiving, even in Symon Patrick's affluent parish.[6]

Covent Garden, with a median of 7.7 hearths per household (the highest in Greater London), was the victim of its own privilege.[7] Pregnant girls, down on their luck, came trudging in to give birth at the parish's expense. Vagrants were found lying dead on the streets at dawn; no relative offered to pay for their burial. Unwashed beggars stumbled upon the Piazza and paused at the doorstep of one of its illustrious householders. Perhaps that generous noblewoman, Lady Abergavenny, or Lord Brouncker, who had designed King Charles's yacht, would take pity on their plight. But maybe not; most well-to-do residents were content to pay their poor tax and let the churchwardens decide who merited poor relief.

From Easter 1664 to Easter 1665, the parish's 485 ratepayers had funded relief for 50 pensioners, orphans, and homeless children, along with an equal number of emergency cases. An outsider, including a woman about to give birth, was quickly hustled back to her home parish (if it could be determined), which was expected to bear the burden of support as the law required. It was odd to see an elegant coach taking a poor person along the Strand to the countryside, but the churchwardens of Covent Garden felt they had to limit poor-relief expenditures to the needy of the parish.

The harsh winter had placed an exceptional burden on the year's poor-tax income of £160. Symon's patrons, the Bedfords, dutifully paid their £4 16s., and Lady Abergavenny and Lord Brouncker their £2. But other ratepayers were delinquent and were about to shirk their duty again when the new assessment came around. Privileged Covent Garden parish was running a poor-relief program with arrears averaging 15 percent of the budgeted amount. The parish's church-related priorities also cost money from the pockets of the same people. The collection plate at Sunday and midweek "Fast Day" observances and incidental income from such things as burial plots and nuptials had to take care of everything from the minister's salary to the gravediggers and crude wooden coffin that the parish poor could not afford when their loved ones departed this life. Reverend Patrick's salary of £150 just about equaled the poor-tax assessment. His hard-working clerk, whose duties ranged from assisting at every funeral to recording the parish baptisms, marriages, and burials in his register, was paid an annual salary of fifteen pounds and twelve shillings (twenty shillings to a pound).[8]

The budgetary problems at Saint Paul Covent Garden paled by comparison with those at the largest suburban parishes. Nearby Saint Margaret Westminster, for example, had six times the documented households of Covent Garden and a large number of unlisted poor persons. There were probably fifteen thousand persons in this one parish, more than in virtually every English city outside the capital. When icy winds swept in from the river in November 1664 and again in February as the Thames became a sheet of ice, Saint Margaret's overseers of the poor scoured the courtier quarters in search of a Lady Bountiful or Lord Charitable to meet the exceptional needs of the season. "The court of Whitehall is mostly in St. Margaret parish," they pleaded with Charles II. His father had given the parish one hundred pounds every year, they said, and his brother's wife, the duchess of York, was giving generously, as she always did to this and other suburban parishes in need. These pleas failed to move the king, even when the overseers pointed to the extra medical costs Saint Margaret's absorbed in treating sick or injured royal troops who were quartered in the parish.[9]

Throughout the metropolis the unusually cold winter of 1664–65 strained to the limit the health and income of the poor. Coal for heating and cooking was in such demand and its price so high that cooks began to use wood. That other great sustainer of life in winter, when vegetables and fruit were scarce—one's daily bread—was jeopardized by a shortage of grain. The Guildhall and Whitehall responded as best they could. Following an old practice, the Guildhall set the weight of a penny loaf of wheaten bread or three halfpenny white loaves every week. As temperatures plunged in January and February and the supply of flour in city bakeries dwindled, Alderman Turner and his colleagues decreased the weight from its normal 11 ½ ounces to 10 ½ ounces and in March to 9 ½ ounces. The weight was listed in each week's metropolitan Bill of Mortality, so bakers in the suburbs as well as the city observed it. For coal, the control was over the price. The king's privy council became concerned at the end of the winter when seacoals became too expensive for poor families. The king's councilor for such matters, the earl of Craven, ordered the price of a bushel of coal down to twenty-eight shillings.[10]

These stopgap measures could do only so much in the face of an ever restricting vicious cycle. The wretched weather had increased sickness and unemployment, pushing ratepayers below the poverty line and triggering new shortfalls in poor-tax collections when the need was greatest. By March, a desperate lord mayor turned to the merchant guilds to lay in new stores of grain for the bakers in the city. The next day, Mayor Lawrence dipped into the well of inducements for additional charity. Playing on the "hard season and dearness of coles, and ye smallness of the [poor tax] collection" in city parishes, he asked the masters and wardens of the guilds to make a "liberall and charitable contribution for the number and necessitys of the poore in every parish . . . in a time of so great extremity."[11]

Easter Sunday, March 26, was fast approaching, when the vestry of each parish must elect its officials and make a new poor-tax assessment. No one looked forward to that task when collections for the past year were badly lagging. The prospects were bleak. The Royal Navy ship the *London*, which the city had paid for, accidentally blew up on its way out to sea to fight the Dutch. Eighty brass cannon and three hundred men went down with the city's man-of-war. The king needed every available warship to fight the Dutch. Its replacement, the *Loyal London*, would cost city merchants an astronomical sum.[12]

The mayor and aldermen soldiered on. Turner and his colleagues solicited subscriptions for the new ship from their guilds and exhorted the better-off city parishes to make liberal poor-tax assessments so that some of the money could be transferred to needier parishes inside the walls and in the liberties. The deadline for the new budget lists was May 8.[13]

When that date arrived, something more foreboding than escalating poverty and poor-tax shortfalls was on the minds of the city fathers. Plague had turned up in the metropolis and was spreading. Those who had experienced the last major epidemic in 1625 recalled that it had concentrated in filth-ridden "pestered places" in the suburbs, whereas the epidemics of Henry VIII's and Elizabeth's times had centered inside the wall.[14] But once the infection started to spread, could it be kept out of the courtier quarters in Whitehall and Covent Garden or halted at the city gates?

Pestered Places

Increases of buildings in and about the city.

Inmates by whom the houses are so pestered [overcrowded] they become unwholesome.

Carrying up of funnels to the tops of houses from privies.

Neglect of cleansing common sewers and town ditches.

Slaughter-houses in the city; butchers killing unsound cattle; tainted fish. Baking unwholesome corn and selling musty corn in public markets.

Churches overlaid with burials.

—London College of Physicians' list of "annoyances" leading to plague in 1630

The plague death in suburban Saint Giles in the Fields on Christmas Eve 1664 had been followed by uneventful weekly Bills of Mortality in January.[15] In the week of February 7, another plague death was recorded out in Saint Giles. The rest of February passed without incident, as did March and early April. Then came the bill for April 18–25, listing two more plague deaths in the same parish near the winter fatalities. Elizabeth Pepys' parents, Dorothea and Alexandre St. Michel, were right in the path of the infection.[16]

Alexandre le Marchant de St. Michel was an adventuresome French gentleman who had come to England in the entourage of Charles II's mother, Henrietta Maria, and been cast adrift after a religious quarrel with a staff member. He had had the good fortune to marry Dorothea, the widowed daughter of an Anglo-Irish landowner, and hoped to strike it rich on both sides of the English Channel with various inventions (a perpetual motion machine, devices for curing smoky chimneys, a scheme for making ponds fit for horses to drink). None of his ideas caught on. He was a hapless noble, dependent on a pension from the fashionable French émigré church that held Anglican services in Westminster and on offers of odd jobs from his son-in-law Samuel Pepys at the navy office.

In 1664, Dorothea and Alexandre settled into the Saint Giles neighborhood on Long Acre north of Covent Garden. Long Acre was just the right place for the couple. The street had a mixture of upscale and inexpensive housing, with Irish, French, and Dutch neighbors for easy conversation. The King's Company staged plays nearby on Bridges Street, and its rising actress, Nell Gwyn, lived around the corner from Long Acre in Drury Lane—a favorite haunt of theater people. Perhaps the new neighborhood would bring a turn in Alexandre's luck, for the king's influential aide, the earl of Craven, was just up the street from the St. Michels.

However, there were problems with the new setting right from the start. Alexandre's son-in-law spoke dismissively of the St. Michels' "ill-looked" lodgings "among all the bawdy-houses."[17] In fact, Samuel Pepys had as little contact as possible with his father-in-law. He had married the man's daughter for love, not money, and wouldn't darken his door (sending a few pounds by a servant if Elizabeth nagged him). There had been a considerable amount of construction around Long Acre and Drury Lane in recent times, most of it illegal. One developer, John Ward, had created blind alleys off Long Acre no wider than sixteen feet, each crammed with a dozen or so cottages having two rooms each on the ground and first floors.[18] The plague death on Christmas Eve 1664 was (historical legend would later hold) right on the St. Michels' street. Now, in April, plague returned to the neighborhood. Two houses had been shut up in the Drury Lane area.

Rumors flew thick and fast, outpacing the posting of the weekly Bills of Mortality. "Great fears of the Sickeness here in the City," Pepys wrote in his secret journal on April 30. "It [is] said two or three houses are already shut up. God preserve us all." He tried to keep his wits about him, knowing that people called the pestilence "the poores plague." Samuel turned to his month-end accounting, a reassuring ritual. "Herein I with great joy find myself to have gained this month above £100 clear," he wrote. His assets totaled more than £1,400, "the greatest sum I ever was worth."[19]

Across the river in Southwark, word of the infection reached John Allin a day before the bill announcing the return of plague. "I heard yesterday there are 2 houses shutt up about Drury lane for the sicknes," he informed Philip Fryth at his old country parish near the English Channel. "I comitt you to God, Your loveing friend, John Allin."[20] Allin said that he had no time "to enlarge." What brooding thoughts and dark fears was this unlicensed physician and devoted alchemist-astrologer withholding from his old friend? Saint Olave Southwark was a notoriously unhealthy waterfront parish, with hundreds of immigrant families and watermen crowded into cheap housing along the Thames and thousands more in nearby alleys.

Rich and middle-income Londoners believed that the "sluttishness" of the poor and their overcrowded housing, called "pestered places," bred disease, especially the "feavers." Westminster's justices, reflecting the royal court's nervousness, took dead aim at Saint Margaret's "close and insalubrious lanes, courts and alleys." A few paces from the fancy inns on King Street where Samuel Pepys consulted with high royal officials, the locals found relief from their daily burdens in back-room alehouses. Every fourth building had one of these dens of iniquity, if one believed the authorities. They harbored "Lewde and bade people [whose] squalid misery and poverty struggle with filth and wretchedness," warned the justices. All of this created an "atmosphere in which the worst diseases are generated and diffused."[21]

There was something to be said for linking the living conditions of the poor with disease, for day laborers and skilled workers were sicklier and died younger than those higher up on the economic ladder. But environmental stress was not just the product of an unholy trinity of poverty, uncleanliness, and immorality. Many "nuisances" and "annoyances" in the Greater London area were not connected in any way with uncleanly living conditions. Most Londoners breathed miasmatic air emanating from effluvia in the soil, traversed streams fouled by slaughterhouses and tanneries on the banks, and contributed to the rubbish that piled up on the streets. Pollution was a common hazard, and public health was everyone's concern.

The country gentleman whom Charles II had put in charge of the king's sick and wounded sailors had a blueprint for attacking this sickly condition of the nation's capital as well. John Evelyn had already served on a royal commission for the "improvement" of the streets and sewers of London and Westminster and on an advisory board drawing up badly needed repairs for Saint Paul's cathedral. These patchwork projects and the lack of clean air and public health facilities in the nation's capital frustrated this bold dreamer, who had traveled the Continent and declared Milan's great plague hospital fit for a king.[22]

Evelyn penned a study bristling with ideas and aimed it directly at the king. "One day as I was walking in Your Majesties Palace at Whitehall," he boldly began, "a presumptuous smoak" created such a haze that courtiers could scarcely make each other out. This page opener led the king to Evelyn's solution: The capital's "atomical effluvia" and "epidemicall aer" would be cleansed by the removal of industrial coalfires, animal slaughterhouses, and human burial grounds to the outskirts of Greater London. In their place Evelyn would plant trees and shrubs to sweeten the air with their perfumes.[23]

Despite Evelyn's urgings and the justices' diatribes against pestered places, the environment of London remained little changed. There was not even a decent facility for sick people, like the Hôpital Saint Louis for plague victims and other units of the General Hospital in Paris that Charles I's French physician had wanted to replicate in London. The Guildhall and regional justices concentrated on keeping the streets and streams and slaughtering places as clean as possible.

If citizens swept the passageways in front of their homes and shops, the justices said, London's infamous effluvia and miasmas would be reduced. Property owners could be fined for allowing "nuisances" around their buildings, though they seldom were. The parish raker periodically carried dung-pots away. When neighbors complained of "noisome smells" emanating from the parish churchyard, its graves were covered with additional soil or quicklime. Tanners, brewers, butchers, and others whose livelihood resulted in polluted public space were largely left alone.

Water was of great concern. Since the Middle Ages, London had developed an impressive conduit system, with miles of pipes carrying water from country brooks and the Thames River to collection spots largely within the wall. A lucky few in the city had water piped right into their homes or delivered by servants or water carriers, but the great mass of people inside the wall fetched water from the neighborhood conduit. This water could be trusted, by and large, but the poorer suburbs ringing the wall fell back on neighborhood wells or, worse, polluted streams that drained into the Thames.

Since early times, small boats traveling up from the Thames to as far as where Saint Pancras station stands today had used the Fleet stream. Over the years, numerous tenements and shanties had been built on either side of the once beautiful stream that wended its way southward from the countryside. The results can well be imagined. A historian of the Great Plague, Walter George Bell, describes the stream in the 1660s as no better than an open sewer. Its appalling condition affected three adjacent parishes in the city's western liberties: Saint Bride, Saint Sepulchre, and Saint Andrew Holborn. All three parishes had been hard hit in years of pestilence.[24]

Water-filled ditches ringed the northern wall, remnants of marshlands that once had stretched from Mooreditch in Saint Giles Cripplegate all the way to the parish of Saint Leonard Shoreditch. Choked with rubbish and filth, the neighborhood ditch slipped from desirable to derelict. Persons assigned to the task by their parish periodically hauled away refuse from the ditch.

Wells were no longer the pristine sources of water that old-timers remembered. A few stood next to land that had been appropriated by parishes for burying the dead. Outside the north wall lay Crowders Well alley in Cripplegate parish. Folk memory held its well water to be "very good for sore eyes to wash them with," a preservative against "distempers," and containing "fumes" to sober up drunkards. There now stands a Crowders Well Pub on the Cripplegate well site, dispensing drinks that are undoubtedly more salubrious to the well-being of today's patrons. Land leading up to the well had been appropriated for burials in 1662.[25]

Horses for riding and drawing coaches and all sorts of wagons and carts were kept in stables throughout the area, and cattle, swine, and goats were herded through the streets to the city slaughtering yards. People in the suburbs kept their own domestic animals. When neighbors complained of hogs roaming the streets or the smell of the slaughtering areas near Newgate, the government fined the offending owner and had the parish scavenger remove the animals or carcasses. Otherwise, people shrugged their shoulders; these sorts of "nuisances" were part of city life.[26] Unless plague came, as was happening now.

Apprehension

These [orders] are in His Majesty's name to be given to all inhabitants within your ward that from henceforth every morning they cause the streets and channels before their doores to be watered, swept and cleansed of all manner of dirt, filth and rubbish.

—Order of the Lord Mayor of London to the city aldermen, May 11, 1665

The new infestation was tracing a path eerily similar to that of the Black Death three centuries before. From its seat in Asia, the pestilence had traveled westward in epidemic form. At Naples 300,000 were said to have died in five months in 1658, and at Genoa 60,000 for the year. During the next four years, the disease raged in Spain, France, and Germany. By 1663 it had traveled via the European interior and Atlantic coast all the way to major ports dotting the North and Baltic Seas—vital sources of timber and cloth for England's war fleet. That fall, word reached the Great Coffee House on Cornhill that the king would forbid any Dutch ships to sail up the Thames, Holland being England's nearest trading partner and rival—and heavily infested with plague.

England's first line of defense against the threat of plague from abroad was an external quarantine, and Pepys and his navy friends knew it better than did the rumormongers sipping coffee on Cornhill. By the end of 1663, the king's council ordered all ships from Amsterdam to be detained at the mouth of the Thames for a thirty-day "triantine." Early in 1664 Rotterdam was added to the list. The civic officials of Rotterdam and London lobbied the privy council to let a perishable cargo of barreled cod and peas pass through to London for the coming Lenten season. However, a line was drawn: "NO PASSENGERS TO STIRR until triantine done." Then ships from Holland stopped briefly in the neighboring province of Zeeland to hide their infected place of origin. The royal council responded by including Zeeland stopovers in the embargo. In May 1664, the nervous councilors of Charles II extended the triantine in British ports to forty days, or "quarantine."[27]

The holes in the dike were opening faster than the privy councilors' fingers could plug them. In August 1664 a Dutch ship captain broke quarantine. He was sent back to his ship, and the houses of Dutch immigrant friends he had visited were shut up for forty days. How many foreign sea captains were trying the same thing? English royalty itself bent the rules when its special interests were at stake. Sixteen horses were brought ashore for the duke of Albemarle, Master of the Horse. Cordage was unloaded for the duke of York, Lord High Admiral. Glazed tiles reached the king's palace at Greenwich. The brewing war with Holland prompted other exceptions by Denis Gauden as Surveyor General of the king's maritime victuals. The Dutch ship *King David of Rotterdam* promptly unloaded a cargo "useful for the king's fleet." This was business as usual: the two states were unofficially at war, and selling and buying naval supplies took precedence over pestilence.

As 1664 neared its end, a navy informer reported that the infection had come into the East Anglia port of Yarmouth, but he remained optimistic. Only one person had died from this sickness, he assured Whitehall. A few days later, he was all confused, writing that reports of new deaths were not to be believed because the searchers were the usual ignorant old women chosen by parishes to view corpses and determine the cause of death, and they were debauched and drunken as well. Yet he had to admit that a pesthouse was taking in sick persons, and the contagion had spread to a house in the interior. The external quarantine of England's shores had failed.[28]

In February 1665 the monarchy officially declared war on the Dutch republic and pressed commercial sailors into naval service. Between engagements at sea, sailors slipped into London to explore the sights and while away the time. Danger lurked in the clusters of immigrants in the city and suburbs, who had personal and business contacts with Holland, Flanders, and France. Many were engaged in importing and finishing cloth, one of the suspected carriers of pestilential seeds. Still, Pepys' diary made no mention of plague until that first entry at the end of April, when the deadly disease entered suburbs far from the docks of the city.

The plague death counts in the Bills of Mortality for the next three weeks did not seem to have any pattern. The first two announced fatalities were followed by a week of no deaths. Then there was a sharp increase and almost as sharp a dip (table 2). It was somewhat reassuring to see only fourteen deaths and a relief that they were concentrated in the pestered suburbs of Saint Andrew Holborn, Saint Clement Danes, and Saint Giles in the Fields some distance from Whitehall. However, the Bills of Mortality missed at least one fatality—in the choicest part of Westminster. On the twelfth of April, the clerk of Saint Paul Covent Garden had made a secretive entry in his parish register: "Margarit Daughter of Dr. John Ponteus Buried Church, plague."[29] This little girl's death had occurred at least a week before the two plague fatalities in Saint Giles in the Fields. More frighteningly, a society physician's household just off the Piazza was infected! The family and friends gathered in the church for the funeral and interment of the leaded casket beneath the church floor, as if nothing unusual had occurred. Afterward the clerk took his tallies to the clerks' hall in the city, listing NO PLAGUE BURIALS. The doctor's family did not want their house and all its inhabitants shut up as the Plague Orders of past epidemics had required. Reverend Patrick also kept quiet.

Friends of the king who lived around the Piazza of Covent Garden may have passed word of this plague death to him. If so, that is as far as the news traveled, for denial came fast on the heels of fear. Lord Brouncker and the ever inquisitive diarist and overseer of the parish's poor, Thomas Rugge, did not want nearby tradesmen and professionals to flee, nor did they welcome draconian plague controls in their neighborhood.

Courtiers may have assured the thirty-five-year-old Charles II that children and old persons were more vulnerable to the infection than was someone in the prime of life—especially one so virile as their sacred ruler. But this "merry monarch" always struck a carefree pose. He did so now; we do not know whether he knew of the plague death at Covent Garden and was feigning nonchalance or whether he was simply happy in love and war.

The naval conflict with the Dutch was going well despite misgivings by Pepys and others in the know about the navy's preparedness and supplies. On April 3 His Majesty had enjoyed the play *Mustapha* with his mistress Lady Castlemaine, soon to give birth to their fifth child. On the fifteenth the king's schedule drew him to the College of Physicians for an anatomy lecture. The *Intelligencer* reported him "enquiring into the seat and causes of infectious diseases and . . . the most rational Means and Methods of preserving and advancing the health of his subjects." The ruler's curiosity ranged from

Table 2. Parishes Infected and Number Buried of Plague,
April 18–May 16, 1665

Week	No. of Infected Parishes	No. Buried of Plague
April 18–25	1	2
April 25–May 2	0	0
May 2–9	4	9
May 9–16	2	3

NOTE: The weekly Bill of Mortality in London and elsewhere, including Colchester, was listed as being from Tuesday to Tuesday, but it covered the seven days from Tuesday to Monday, with the second Tuesday being a day of tallying the counts for the previous seven days.

the Royal Society's experiments to the meaning of planetary movements. He consulted astrologers about dealing with his parliaments. He asked them the odds on his Dutch war and inquired about the prospects for his health. He undoubtedly had been talking with his favorite astrologer about the latest comet in the heavens.[30]

The weekly Bills of Mortality reached the king and lord mayor a day before they were made public. On the morning of April 27, as Londoners awoke to the first public word of the fatalities out in squalid Saint Giles in the Fields, Charles II's council chamber was poised to act. The stakes were high, the mood tense. The king and his closest advisors knew that more than one parish was infected; Whitehall itself was in danger. The council register revealed the panicky truth: "Plague has broken out and Vehemently suspected to be in some houses within the parish of Saint Giles in the Fields and other out parishes."[31]

Action came swiftly. The chief justice of the Court of King's Bench ordered all suspected houses in the nearby suburbs inspected. If infected, a residence was to be shut up, and everyone inside, whether well or sick, sealed off from the outside world. For forty days, counting from the time of the last plague death inside, a "watcher" would guard the house and a live-in nurse would care for the family's needs, with medical supplies and food passed through a window by a courier. If the inmates could afford it, they would bear the costs; if not, the parish would pay from its poor-tax fund.

The king was following the Plague Orders of his father and grandfather to the letter. There was no time to rethink the logic of protecting the general public by shutting up entire households when one person inside caught the plague—a practice that ensured the death of many more persons. Nor was there any mention of the unwritten custom of quarantining only the poor in this sacrificial act. Isolating the infected poor apart from their healthy family and neighbors was a pipe dream; only small pesthouse sheds, at the far end of Saint Margaret Westminster, and the other makeshift facility, north of the city wall up in Saint Giles Cripplegate, remained from the last Great Plague.[32]

Reaction in Saint Giles in the Fields to the forced incarceration was swift and ugly. A "ryett" broke out at the shut-up Ship Tavern. The red cross on the door was ripped off by friends in the street, "the door opened in a vicious manner and the people of the house permitted to go abroad into the streets promiscuously with others." The king countered with an order to the Westminster justices "to inflict upon the offenders in the said ryett (for such of them as they shall find) the severest punishment."[33]

Charles II was acting like the legendary King Canute ordering the waves back into the sea. Watchmen from Saint Giles were posted on the major roads to prevent persons suspected of carrying the plague from leaving the parish. The neighboring parishes mounted their own watch as self-protection. These futile gestures at a *cordon sanitaire* were soon given up. The disease had no trouble crossing parish boundaries.

Across town another drama unfolded. Two weeks after the riot in Saint Giles in the Fields, the plague entered old London's merchant center. The bill for May 2–9 told the story: a house in tiny Saint Mary Woolchurch parish had suffered a plague fatality. The family lived on Bearbinder Lane just off Lombard Street. To the east were the Royal Exchange and the Great Coffee House. To the west was the Stocks market, with its butchers' and fishmongers' stalls. The stricken household was not identified in the official record by class, religion, or national origin, but the neighbors were Anglicans and dissenters, native English families and French and Dutch immigrants. A few doors from the infected house, Quaker dissenters knew all about the fatality and passed the word through the network of communications established by these religious Friends in the metropolis.[34]

Knowledgeable doctors and apothecaries had their own ideas about what was happening. Out in pestered Saint Giles in the Fields, the neighborhood apothecary William Boghurst surmised that the endemic plague in his parish had spread eastward with the end of cold weather. Dr. Thomas Cocke, who tended rich and poor patients in the city, traced the beginnings to "a parcel of skins brought out of Holland into St. Giles." Dr. Nathaniel Hodges weighed in with the fullest explanation. The disease was definitely contagious, he argued, and not just carried through the air by miasmas. It had doubtless come in on "packs of merchandice" from Holland; the original source was likely to have been Turkish "bailes of cotton or silk which is a strange preserver of the Pestilential Steams." On plague's arrival in Westminster, he continued, the local authorities had failed to shut up the first infected house. Some "timorous neighbors, under apprehension of the contagion, removed into the city of London, who unfortunately carried along with them the pestilential taint." The Bearbinder Lane fatality was the inevitable result.[35]

Over time this story became embellished. We next pick it up during the plague epidemic at Marseilles in 1722. As Londoners braced themselves against the prospect of another Great Plague, Daniel Defoe wove the Bearbinder Lane episode into his *Journal of the Plague Year.* The journal begins with the riveting fictional account of two "French-men" living at the juncture of Drury Lane and Long Acre in Saint Giles in the Fields who die of plague in December 1664. In the spring, a Frenchman living "near the infected houses" in Long Acre, where the plague had claimed its initial French immigrants, flees across town to Bearbinder Lane. There he dies, "to the great affliction of the city."[36] Defoe's whodunit omitted only one tantalizing detail: the strong link between immigrant status and religious dissent. Perhaps the Frenchman who carried the plague across town was a Quaker, like the neighbors of the person he unwittingly infected.

Other storytellers copied Defoe's version more or less verbatim during the rest of the eighteenth century. The old reference to Frenchmen opening infected goods from Holland gradually took on the mythic truth of legend.[37] It remains so to this day.[38] The truth will probably never be known.

The king and mayor were informed of the Bearbinder Lane fatality a week before it came out in the Bill of Mortality for May 2–9. On May 4, Whitehall quietly ordered the city's justices of the peace to shut up all infected houses. The Guildhall was empowered to take all action to stay the progress of the plague. A week later, when the plague death became public knowledge, the mayor ordered all householders and shopkeepers in the city and liberties to clean the street in front of their places every day. Like the king, the mayor of London was following old Plague Orders to the letter. There was no time to review past policies and try something new. Sir John Lawrence had to hope that daily street sweeping and scouring would be more successful against the worst disease of the age than occasional cleansing had been against lesser maladies. To convince the aldermen and general public (and possibly himself) that he was on the right track, he added that health and safety were their responsibility, and they would neglect it "at their peril."[39]

To the consternation of Mayor Lawrence, Londoners were slow in complying. Tradespeople with a shop and residence on a main street may have considered daily watering in front of their building a meddlesome chore, but they had ready access to water and little excuse for evading their duty. A poorer artisan or laborer had better reason to resist the mayor's command. Living in a miserable alley that was neglected by the authorities and working elsewhere in the city from dawn to dark six days out of seven, they had neither the time nor the money to fetch water from the nearest cheap source.

An angry Sir John issued a second mayoral command on May 26, accusing citizens of "obstinacy and heedlessness to obey." All householders must sweep and water their streets and lanes "to prevent those unsavory and noisome smelles and stenches thence ariseing (which hath a pestiferous influence on man's body)." Lawrence hinted that the aldermen themselves had not borne down hard enough on the parish scavengers and beadles to convince people to do their civic duty. Each alderman was to hand in to the mayor "a weekly certificate of every person failing therein." Those who did not obey would face legal prosecution.[40]

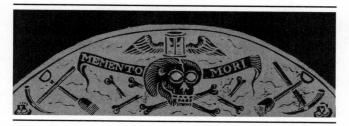

Signs and Sources

A mantle wrought with purple spots she wore
Embossed with many a Blane and many a Sore
She had a raving voice, a frantic look,
A noisome Breath, and in her hands she shooke
A venom'd Spear which where it toucheth fills
The veins with poison, and distracts and kills.

—GEORGE WITHER, *Britains Remembrancer*

The spring came in with blue skies, warm breezes, and picturesque white clouds, as if by mockery. April and May were always a reviving time, but this year the thawing ground and warm air were not happy harbingers. If plague was about to run rampant through the capital, the moist soil was a likely major source of its pestilential poison. In times of plague, common wisdom said, the bowels of the earth released their "feces" as venomous exhalations from refuse and other corrupt effluvia in the soil and water. The warm rays of the midday sun turned the putrefied matter into miasmas, which the gentle spring breezes carried off to unknown destinations.[1]

Now was the season for spring cleaning, when a household's mistress and maids worked at airing rooms and ridding them of moths and fleas and all the other household pests. With spring also came the strongest urge to go out of doors and greet friends, linger at the local herb market to inspect the fresh vegetables that had replaced winter's leftovers, and visit a neighborhood tavern or alehouse for drink and conversation. But this springtime the master and mistress and their servants were all at risk on the street and even in their own homes. When the miasmas of plague swooped down on a neighborhood and sickened a family, it was subsequently thought to spread contagiously by an infected person's breathing or maybe just by a frightening gaze at a stranger passing by. It was not even safe to open the windows and let in the fresh air. People hesitated to allow their pet dogs and cats out for fear they might become carriers of the infection, as had happened in past epidemics. Stray animals were most suspect, so when the master went out on business or a servant was sent on an errand, they had to stay clear, if they could, of wild cats and dogs. No place was completely safe, for these wild creatures roamed the streets even in Cheapside and on the Strand.

From peer to pauper, foreboding thoughts like these conjured up a familiar image of God's Destroying Angel punishing a sinful people with her poisoned spear and noisome breath. How easy it was for writers like George Wither, who was both a religious person and a keen observer of past plagues, to personify this unpredictable curse of human society as an inscrutable agent of the Lord.[2] With all the elusiveness of a femme fatale, pestilence made a sudden arrival without a prior appointment and remained mysterious about its itinerary. "Where oh where will ye take your flight? God's arrows fly by day, as well as night," warned a gloomy rhymer, before he himself was struck down in the prime of life.[3]

With a street map and Bills of Mortality in hand, one can trace the plague's early advance. In the six short weeks after the acknowledged fatalities at the end of April 1665, death marched eastward from Saint Giles in the Fields along the Holborn road to Saint Andrew Holborn and on to Saint Sepulchre by the polluted Fleet River, perilously close to the inn kept by Samuel Pepys' cousin and her husband. From Holborn the pestilence veered south along Chancery Lane, where panicky law teachers and their students at the Inns of Court recessed their classes and vacated the premises. Turning into the Strand, the infection settled into the parish of Saint Clement Danes near Drury Lane. From there the malignancy made its progress along Fleet Street, bringing death to the middle-income parish of Saint Dunstan in the West and to the poor, densely populated parts of Saint Bride's, where Samuel Pepys had grown up (see maps 1 and 3).

By mid-June the rampaging contagion had gone completely around the wall. It was close to Ludgate and Newgate on the west, Cripplegate and Bishopsgate on the north, and Aldgate on the east. From outside Aldgate it had leapt across the Thames to John Allin's parish of Saint Olave Southwark. If it were to branch westward along the southern bank near the palatial headquarters of the Church of England at Lambeth and leap back over the Thames to Saint Margaret Westminster, the king and queen at Whitehall would be hemmed in on all sides by the contagion.

At the Guildhall, the mayor and aldermen had been on alert since the single plague fatality in Saint Mary Woolchurch. Four weeks passed without any parish clerk inside the wall acknowledging another plague death. But during the second week of June, four city residents succumbed. Two died in a cluster of shacks near London Bridge, a third near Cripplegate exit at the northern wall, and the fourth in a fashionable parish near the navy offices just inside the eastern wall. This last fatality and the spread of the disease to the nearby house of a physician, infecting one of his servants, struck fear among the professional people of the quarter. The doctor was Alexander Burnet, a member of the prestigious College of Physicians, whose patients included Samuel and Elizabeth Pepys. Dr. Burnet had sent his sick servant to the city pesthouse north of the wall, a customary medical practice. But he had defied middle-class custom by inviting the authorities to shut up the rest of his household, including himself, for the statutory forty-day quarantine of infected buildings. How many professional persons, including his fellow physicians, would have protected their neighbors this way at the risk of their own lives and livelihood? Samuel Pepys stared at the cross on the door and wondered how the sickness had entered such a substantial household. The Burnet residence was one of the finest in the city, boasting nine hearths.[4]

The city physician Dr. Hodges warned that the pestilential disease could strike anyone, regardless of age, sex, or social condition. The suburban apothecary Boghurst estimated that half of those who caught the infection would succumb. Some physicians put the figure much higher. A few doctors said it could strike like apoplexy, as had happened during the Black Death. But even Boghurst's more measured observations could not have calmed his patients' families and neighbors. The venom spread through the vital organs rapidly, he acknowledged, but "I saw none dye under twenty to twenty four hours."[5] The rising toll from the plague's first appearance inside the wall to its return five weeks later told a tale of approaching disaster (table 3).[6]

Signs and Symptoms

Of the Tokens . . . I have ranked them in the forefront of the evil Signs, making them the fore-horses of Death's Chariot, because among all the evill signes there are none so common or conspicuous, soe dispatching, certain and infallible signes of death as this.

—WILLIAM BOGHURST, *Loimographia . . . a personal account of the Great Plague from November 1664 to May 1666*

In rare moments of reflection, when he wasn't with patients, tending his herb garden, or relaxing with the lute he played expertly, William Boghurst might be found atop the church tower of Saint Giles in the Fields, gazing at the city below. In the distance stood the cathedral and throngs of people passing by the shops of Cheapside. Beyond lay the River Thames, dotted with wherries navigating around the supports under London Bridge. From the perspective of his poor suburban parish, which perpetually had more chronic illness than most places inside the walls, the prosperous city must have looked inviting to this overburdened caregiver. Pulmonary troubles and gastrointestinal ailments were extremely common in his neighborhood. The high incidence of childbed and infant mortality was disturbing to a man dedicated to saving lives. Smallpox frequently reached epidemic proportions, killing some and disfiguring others for life.

Boghurst took special note of a clustering of ills that were all identified by their common symptom, a high fever. He knew the common fever well and was an expert on the dangerous spotted fever (sometimes called *jail fever* because it flared up in prisons and other crowded quarters).[7] He knew less about malarial fever than did physicians with patients near the ditches north of the city. However, he had firsthand knowledge of the worst kind of fever, plague.

Pestilential fever had continued to rage in the capital for a decade after London's last Great Plague in 1636, but with fatalities steadily decreasing

Table 3. Greater London Bills of Mortality: Plague Burials,
May 2–June 13, 1665

	Number of Plague Burials			
Week	St. Giles in the Fields	Parishes inside the Walls	All Parishes	Number of Infected Parishes
May 2–9	3	1	9	4
May 9–16	1	0	3	2
May 16–23	7	0	14	3
May 23–30	9	0	17	5
May 30–June 6	31	0	42	7
June 6–13	68	4	112	12

from 12,000 that year to 4,000 in 1647. During the next three years, the number of plague deaths dropped sharply, to 693, 71, and 15. After that, plague lurked in a few of the suburbs year after year, with an average of 9 fatalities in each of the three years before 1665.[8] Boghurst knew the specific localities: the disease, he declared, was "endemicall" in his Middlesex outparish of Saint Giles in the Fields and in three adjacent parishes in Westminster: Saint Clement Danes, Saint Martin in the Fields, and Saint Paul Covent Garden (see map 4).

The isolated deaths in Westminster's pestered alleys drew little attention at Whitehall Palace or inside the protective walls of noble estates on the Strand. But plague was an ever-present concern for medical professionals who practiced in the four endemic plague areas and a worry to practitioners in places now free of the pestilence but prime candidates for its return (because of their dangerous combination of poverty, overcrowded dwellings, and high incidence of other disease). In the extreme north of the suburbs, in the densely pestered parish of Saint James Clerkenwell, the French doctor Theophilus Garencières kept his eyes open for plague on his patients, having known its terrible toll in northern France in the 1630s while training to be a physician at Caen.[9] And because the infection kept entering a few poor dwellings in Saint Giles in the Fields, the native English apothecary William Boghurst kept abreast of medical understanding of the disease by reading everything that was available in English and European sources.

Boghurst could quote Thucydides on the Plague of Athens and speak with authority on Justinian's Plague. A treasured copy of Dr. Thomas Willis's pathbreaking work on the range of fevers, published in 1659, shared space in his library with weighty Latin tomes and shorter English tracts on plague. Some of these works dated to the Black Death; others had appeared during recent plague visitations. Laypersons and even some professional caregivers could not easily tell what was new and what was recycled information.[10] But Boghurst's experience with plague patients helped him pick out anything that broke new ground. The best research was done by medical specialists in Europe: the German Jesuit polymath Kircher, who had trained his low-powered microscope on human blood; the Flemish nobleman van Helmont, a leader among the avant-garde "chymical physitians" who were challenging the methods of the Galenist old guard of medicine; and the influential Dutchman Diemerbroeck, whose *Tractatus de Peste* was now being translated into English. Boghurst had all their books at hand.[11]

When the pestilential distemper reappeared in Saint Giles in the Fields in April and fanned out in May, Boghurst knew the disease had advanced from an endemic to epidemic state.[12] He needed to look closely at the "signs" on all his patients' bodies and listen to their professed "symptoms."[13] Although plague acted like no other bodily ill, many medical authorities believed it could develop from lesser maladies. Even ordinary fever had to be watched because, it was thought, it could lead to spotted fever, and that disease might develop, in turn, into true plague.[14]

Plague could be suspected whenever a family member or servant developed a high fever or shuddering cold along with frequent vomiting, headaches, and dizziness. Between three and ten days after these initial symptoms, if plague was really at work, the visible marks or signs started to appear. Boghurst listed "carbuncles, buboes, blains, blisters, [and] spots riseing on the body." Not long after that, terminal signals began. There could be a "griping" (or cramping) in the guts, faltering speech, faintness or an unusual pain in one area, sudden looseness of the bowels, and shortness of breath. Frenzy, hysterical laughing, swooning, or staggering also sometimes occurred. Many patients experienced cold sweats and an irregular pulse. Any two or three or four of these indicators coming together, Boghurst wrote confidently, "were infallible signs of death now at hand and they seldom came single."[15]

The most recognizable proof that someone had become infected was a bubo, a swelling of the lymph nodes in the groin or neck or under the arms. With chilling detail Boghurst later described the chief varieties of buboes in his own account of the plague of 1665–66, *Loimographia: Or an Experimentall Relation of the Plague.* The wedge-shaped, red swellings rose slowly and receded gradually. More dangerous were the white ones, appearing suddenly, soft and puffy. "Few live that have them," he claimed.[16]

Everyone knew that buboes characterized plague. When Dr. Burnet, having survived quarantine, showed Pepys the pesthouse master's postmortem report on his servant, Samuel noted in his diary the mention of "a Bubo on his right groine, and two Spots on his right thigh, which is the plague." The buboes did not always appear, however. Boghurst had a ready explanation: the infection moved so quickly through the body that a victim succumbed before the swelling started. Attention was paid to another trademark sign, which everybody called "tokens" because they betokened almost sure death: "Spotts riseing on the body," as Boghurst called them. These spots came out early on the victim's chest—small, round, hard, and red, "like flea bites," Dr. Garencières wrote.[17] It was a helpful description; almanacs featured fleas in their checklist of vermin to be cleared out during spring cleaning, and everyone knew what fleabites looked like.

The sight of the tokens on their bodies stunned people. "God's Marks," the religious murmured. A divine sign upon the heathen, the judgmental proclaimed darkly. Sometimes no tokens appeared on a victim until after death, if at all. Contemporaries who knew this looked for additional "infalli- ble signs." An obvious candidate was an extremely high fever. Despite the range of diseases with fevers, the learned society physician, Dr. Thomas Wil- lis, had asserted in his work *On Fevers* that the acute plague fever could be distinguished from lesser fevers by its intensity. Dr. Thomas Sydenham ex- pressed the same opinion in a paper published in 1676, drawing on plague cases he saw at his Westminster office in 1665 before removing with his family to the countryside. Sydenham had the advantage over Willis of seeing both peers and paupers, charging high fees to the wealthy to subsidize his care of the poor. Finally, there was Dr. Gideon Harvey, an accomplished city physician who combined practice with theory and a fair measure of common sense. In *A Discourse on the Plague,* published while the plague was raging in 1665, Harvey described the range of signs and symptoms, from an initial weak pulse to an irregular heartbeat, including raging headaches and frenzy. These, in conjunction with a high fever, he said, were a strong indication that the illness was plague. Still, he cautioned that one could not be absolutely certain the disease was plague "unless the said Feaver prove Infectious, as two or three dying in one house, or several in a Neighborhood, of one and the same kind of fever."[18]

Boghurst objected that Harvey and several other physicians who claimed to write from personal experience had been too afraid of plague to come close enough to their patients to verify their theories. The suburban apothecary was undoubtedly frustrated that he had no time to write up his own experiences at present. Perhaps there was also a twinge of jealousy; Harvey's university train- ing and doctor's license gave him a professional status superior to that of an apothecary, though this made no difference to their medical methods.[19]

Death Counts and Denial

In this year the weekly bill was filling with the death of new borne children and women in childbed.

—Thomas Rugge, *Diurnal* (1665)

Talk of plague made the rounds in London's cafes and inns. Everyone knew that *the sickness, distemper, infection,* and *contagion* were code words for plague and plague alone. From the Royal Exchange to Covent Garden Piazza, citizens spoke of buboes and tokens and the terrifying frenzy or stupor of a victim's last hours. But could one be sure it was plague? What about all the other possible diseases?

Since the previous autumn physicians had noticed an unusual amount of sickness for any number of ailments, from the ever dangerous smallpox to a respiratory ailment called *tissick*. Dr. Hodges had a heavier-than-ever workload of city patients. Out in Westminster Dr. Sydenham was finding the same thing. The pattern held in the northwestern suburbs. "Small pox was soe rife in our parish," Boghurst reported, that about forty families were infected by it within 120 paces of the church.

By all reports the increase in these sicknesses persisted through the winter and was continuing into the spring season, along with the onset of plague. But were all these other maladies killing people or just making them sick? In short, were Londoners heading pell-mell into another great plague, or had a Pandora's box of many killing diseases sprung open?

Take smallpox, for example. It was a very serious contagious disease, and a moderate epidemic of it was clearly under way. However, smallpox was not known to be as lethal as would be indicated by the numbers reported in the Bills of Mortality this April and May. In the winter, the city barrister Bulstrode Whitelocke had kept his children at the family's country home because of the threat from smallpox. Four of them came down with it despite precautions, one after the other in a matter of days. By mid-February, all were fully recovered, "through God's goodness." Smallpox epidemics could occur in any season, and mortality could reach as high as 20 percent—high enough to send waves of terror through any infected household but far lower than the 50–80 percent routinely observed for plague.[20]

Smallpox told only part of the story of increased mortality. In April and again in May, an unusual variety of diseases claimed high numbers of victims, according to the reports of the parish clerks for the metropolitan Bills of Mortality. The trend for these eight weeks broke sharply with that shown during the same weeks in the previous decade (see appendix A). The causes for the unusually high incidence of fatalities reported during this April and May ranged from enteric ailments and dropsy (a swelling of the limbs) to consumption (tuberculosis) and several nonplague contagious diseases, including fever, spotted fever, measles, malaria, and smallpox.[21]

Metropolitan London's system for reporting its deaths started with a parish searcher (sometimes accompanied by a physician) viewing the body and reporting the cause of death to the parish clerk (and possibly the parish priest). The parish clerk tallied the burials for the week and their causes and took his figures to the head office of the parish clerks in central London.

The searchers were widely considered the weak link in the chain, garnering an unsavory reputation as unreliable old women, usually on the parish dole and occasionally befogged by drink. Why bother to depend on such untrustworthy sources? Because someone had to undertake this disagreeable task, and the parish authorities were able to dragoon these poor women into service with the threat of withholding their pensions, food, and clothing. In times of plague, the searchers were segregated from the public out of fear of contamination and were forced to share lean-tos with gravediggers in the neighborhood's burial ground.

But were these parish pariahs so untrustworthy at fulfilling their sworn duties? The head clerk of the company of parish clerks said the bills were "of great use and necessity," and these "ancient women" were chosen by "some of the eminentest men of the parish."[22] If that sounded like a defensive tactic to save the reputation of the bills, one could not say the same about the balanced opinion of John Graunt, whose work on the bills had won him a seat at the prestigious Royal Society.

Graunt gave the searchers a mixed grade. He judged them competent enough to determine most causes of death, from old age and the falling sickness to gout and palsy. One could easily forgive them their quaint way of describing these diseases. What difference did it make if they described a corpse as "very lean and worn away" rather than saying that the person died of consumption? They erred badly on plague, however, Graunt said, underreporting it by 25 percent during the Great Plague of 1625. They had obviously put down other causes of death in many cases when they should have listed plague. They were doing the same now, judging by the jump in nonplague mortality in April and May over the figures for the years just past. Graunt left the matter there, not wanting to probe human motivations. He was a demographer, not a mind reader. The only thing he would suggest as an explanation was that these old women were "perhaps ignorant and careless."[23]

But if they were less than candid about plague, so were most Londoners. Denial took second place only to fright. Samuel Pepys kept his mind off the emerging epidemic by steadfast devotion to his pleasures and obsessive attention to his profits. Yet he could recognize a bubo as well as anyone.

Denial easily found support in good intentions. The Reverend Symon Patrick and his parish clerk had colluded in covering up the plague death of Dr. Ponteus's daughter, which the parish searcher had dutifully reported. They

were about to do the same with a second fatality, though this time the interment would be in private, in the churchyard, not in the sanctuary surrounded
by family and friends of the departed.

Given that buboes occasionally didn't come out until after death, it was
hard to blame a searcher for not reporting plague after viewing a corpse
without that sign. Word was spreading that the nurses whom parishes hired
to care for shut-up families were covering the warm bodies of newly deceased persons with a blanket to keep the tokens from coming out. This
saved the nurses from being shut up in the infected house with the rest of the
household for the obligatory forty-day quarantine.[24]

The searchers were pressured from all directions. Who except for courageous public-minded persons like Dr. Burnet would rush to have their house
shut up or admit there was plague on their street? A poor searcher entering a
dark alley and approaching a grief-stricken household could anticipate pleas,
sometimes accompanied with money, not to report the fatality as plague.
Neighbors naturally wished to avoid having the neighborhood labeled as
plague ridden, with the accompanying associations of immoral, sluttish behavior that people said bred the disease. The leading newsletter publisher in
the city, Roger L'Estrange, catered to this sort of denial by continuing to report the usual court and city news and gossip and asserting that plague did
not come to the better neighborhoods.

Dissembling and inaccurate reporting did not fool the doctors. Spotted
fever and other ailments suddenly became a very popular cause of death. But
spotted fever did not carry off the high number of victims that plague did. "I
had many patients of [spotted fever]," Boghurst later recalled, "but few
died." Likewise, fatalities from tissick and consumption had occurred last
winter, as normal for the season. But this year they were reported in increasing numbers as the weather warmed up, which did not make sense to medical authorities. Convulsions and dropsy were not prone to the epidemic gy-
rations and greatly increased mortality being reported for them. And death
from disorders of the stomach and intestines usually formed a gently rising
curve to plateau in the summer, yet the Bills of Mortality recorded a much
earlier increase this year in deaths from "griping in the guts," "stopping of the
stomach," and "surfeit" (overeating).[25]

There was one group of related causes of death in the Bills of Mortality
whose soaring figures could not be attributed to false or inattentive reporting. Pregnant women and the fetuses they were carrying were always at great
risk. In a plague epidemic, pregnant women were probably more vulnerable
than any other group.[26] A poor pregnant woman increased her exposure to

the infection when she visited the marketplace to purchase food, herbs for medicines, and other "necessaries." If she caught the distemper, her chances of surviving were decreased by the weakened physical condition associated with her pregnancy. Not surprisingly, in April and May of 1665 fatalities connected with childbirth, listed as "abortive," "childbed," "stillborn," and "infant," were 4.7 times greater than in previous years. In addition, "teeth" (or teething) of early childhood and the closely related "worms" claimed 1.4 times more lives than in the recent past. (See appendix A.)

The shadow of plague was distorting normal patterns of mortality. Plague was either the direct cause or a contributing factor for much of the increase in deaths related to motherhood. And this was just the beginning of the epidemic. What might happen to expectant mothers and motherless infants who remained in the city when death, unemployment, scarcity, and deserted streets became the order of the day?

There was yet another concern about people's health as plague entered the nation's capital. Out in Essex, whose farms fed Londoners, Ralph Josselin prayed that "God good in outward mercies" would grant "a gallant seed time. Lord remember us with rain." In the fields surrounding the capital, there was only a "little sprinkling shower or two," Boghurst said, presaging "a pitiful crop of hay." With dearth might come death as city people's ability to fight off vagrant diseases wore thin. Famine, Dr. Hodges believed, greatly increased mortality during pestilential contagions.[27]

Even without the looming prospect of starvation, people were dying in alarming numbers. There was only one explanation: a single disease, the most horrifying, deadly, and mysterious of all illnesses known to this age, lay behind most fatalities, and Londoners were learning to identify it. The harder question was how to protect oneself from the infection. A wise person would want to learn everything that was known about the propagation and spread of the pestilential poison. This was not easy; the invisible poison left no calling cards until it entered human bodies and the tokens, buboes, and high fever appeared.

On the Nature of Causes

Diehard Puritans and a scattering of Anglicans, Catholics, and Quakers thought God alone brought the plague as a judgment on a sinning people. If a plague struck a community, these fervent believers called for repentance and hoped that God would remove the Destroying Angel's hand. For others, this austere view was mixed with a varying degree of attention to natural causes: God was the first or prime cause of plague, but He allowed it to come about through the forces of nature—the second causes that He himself had created.[28]

Reverend Patrick, groping to make sense of the plague's invasion of his wealthy parish, reached for his Bible. He turned to a favorite among David's spiritual guides, Psalm 91. We are special creatures of God, the psalmist says, and should not fear "the arrows [of war] that flee by day, nor the pestilence which worketh in darkness." Plague comes from God and cannot be escaped any more than any other human tragedy. "If we are not saved from the Destroying Angel," the pastor told his congregation, "there is a good reason for our dying." To be sure, Patrick believed that plague was a physical malady, and he relied on his physicians as well as God's will. Still, he reserved first place for the divine.[29]

Dr. Hodges began at the other end of this spiritual-natural discussion. He methodically traced the epidemic to "pestilential steams" carried on bales of cotton or silk from the seat of the infection in Turkey to Holland and then on Dutch merchandise to England. Soon backtracking, however, he asked his friends in the religious establishment not to think him an atheist simply for not first proclaiming what he never doubted, that the first cause was always that of the Almighty.[30]

Medical astrologers also subscribed to the idea of first and second causes for disease and other human calamities. John Gadbury, while asserting astrology to be "the only science that can give the cause and effect of plagues," acknowledged God as "the chief and supreme cause." Gadbury knew how to cover all possibilities. Before the plague appeared he'd forecast a quiet year for the capital: "London now / Some petit discontents begin to know!" As the plague unfolded, he made an artful dodge: "I called them petit because I wished them so."[31]

Across London Bridge, that interesting combination of alchemist, astrologer, ejected minister, and unlicensed physician, John Allin, believed in divine judgment with a fervor that few could match. The Destroying Angel was hard at work, he said. The only human recourse was repentance; all was in God's hands. Yet there seemed to be a contradiction in this man's thinking: he also leaned toward natural explanations, at least for the spread of plague. "The infection," he informed a country friend, "may be taken by the scent of smelling, and . . . grosse savour of a foggy infected aire, or the corruption of an infected person or place."[32]

Then there was Robert Boyle, a bright star in the Royal Society's galaxy of scientific experimenters. Robert and his sister Katherine, Lady Ranelagh, could not help being concerned as the epidemic approached her comfortable

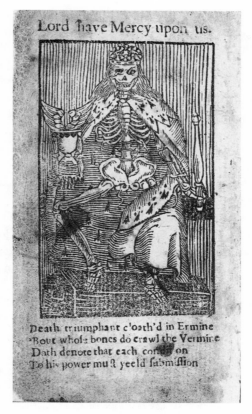

Fig. 3. Frontispiece of *The Christians Refuge: or Heavenly Antidotes against the Plague in this time of Generall Contagion* (1665). The figure of death as a monarch with scepter and crown reveals beneath his ermine cloak a worm-eaten skeleton holding an hourglass. The four lines "Death triumphant cloth'd in Ermine / 'Bout whose bones do crawl the Vermine / Doth denote that each condition / To his power must yield submission" suggest that plague comes from God and cannot be escaped even by royalty. The Wellcome Library, London

Pall Mall residence in Westminster. For Lady Ranelagh, God was a powerful first cause and life force guiding her every move. Soon she would hold vigils at the bedside of infected friends, praying continually through the night for their recovery. Meanwhile her brother believed the Almighty gave humans a "divine spark" of wisdom to probe the natural, "second causes" of disease. Yet he was also a strong believer in God as the "first cause" of everything, including plague.[33]

Accepting God's right and power to strike down anyone, good or bad, young or old, rich or poor, several writers proceeded to discuss the possible natural causes through which He was inflicting this misery. Richard Kephale put down a dizzying list of "sources," from surfeit and rotten mutton in London's pestered suburbs to a pack of carpets from Turkey and a dog from Amsterdam.[34] William Boghurst listed the movement of comets through the sky, changes in the weather, and children "aping at funerals." These random approaches suggest that their authors were cribbing creatively from earlier plague tracts, with a few personal observations thrown in for good measure.

"Swarms of ants covered the highways," Boghurst remembered; there was a "multitude of croaking frogs" and flies lining the sides of houses "like a rope of onions." Boghurst's reading took him back to a biblical plague unleashed on Pharaoh's Egypt: it had been preceded by a strange alteration of the water supply, unusual hail, murrain in cattle, and an attack of locusts. He then noted the eerie absence of swallows in London in 1664, which continued into the present year. And there were strong winds blowing from the heart of the city to the western suburbs as the plague came in. The suburban apothecary's mental meandering coincided remarkably with Reverend Patrick's reaction on hearing that many birds died just before the epidemic. He scanned his reference books and found the explanation: "These airey creatures feele the alteration in [the air] sooner than wee."[35]

There was one common element in all this probing—miasmatic air. It was both a prime conveyer of the infection and the product of such things as contaminated soil, the motion of the planets, or even earthquakes. The ancient medical authority Galen had defined plague to be "nothing else but changing aire into a putrefying pestilent quality," Boghurst recalled. "Miasmas" were suspected of spreading the plague in the air, though the seeds or atoms were invisible. "Contagion," the other prime suspect, was a much more elusive idea, for how could one come in contact with the infection? Still, it made sense that the poison, however it was produced, could be passed from person to person by touching or by breath, even from someone who had not yet shown signs of the plague. Or the poison might be carried by dogs and cats, or material, especially light-colored cloth (which was often found near a stricken family).

Most often the miasmist and contagionist views were combined. Boghurst nimbly wove these views together. He began with the winds blowing in miasmatic poison. Especially susceptible to the miasmas were people who had engaged in disorderly living, overeating, and excessive physical exertion (including sex). Then the plague exploded, and Boghurst saw contagion as the main vehicle for spreading the infection. Like many others, he knew to protect himself against miasmatic air and equally to avoid persons carrying the infection, especially vagrants and beggars. In addition to closing windows and fumigating rooms, the shutting up of infected houses would be primary strategies against London's raging epidemic.[36]

The most ingenious blending of miasmist and contagionist ideas emerged from Europe's battle, during the previous century, with the new disease of syphilis. What could explain this fast-spreading disease new to Europeans? A brilliant Italian medical observer thought he had an answer. Girolamo Fracastoro saw promise in an idea, propounded by some ancient authorities, that the world was composed of invisible atoms. He suggested that individual diseases had atomlike seedlets, or *seminaria,* as he called them. Syphilis fit the theory perfectly; Fracastoro could imagine its seedlets flying through the air like miasmas and then becoming dormant for a long period before re-emerging or vanishing. While these seminaria remained in the atmosphere, they would pass contagiously from person to person until they gradually died out in people's bodies.[37]

A decade after Fracastoro proposed his grand theory, a great plague epidemic broke out in Venice, and doctors familiar with his theory started talking of plague-specific seminaria. The idea entered London's medical vocabulary, pushing the frontier of medicine to its outermost edge as the Great Plague unfolded. "The seeds of the pestilence," Boghurst wrote, "are so hidden and removed from [our] senses that we can [only] perceive their effects."[38]

These plague seminaria were more plausible and far more frightening to imagine than were conventional miasmas and contagion. They flew great distances through the air. They spread from person to person. They could even pass indirectly from contaminated objects. They might be produced by celestial or atmospheric alterations. Ultimately, they were traceable to God, the creator of everything from seminaria to their human prey.[39]

Was there no avoiding them? Symon Patrick's wealthy parishioners on the Piazza and others with itchy feet and a large purse suspected that all expert wisdom on the sources and signs of this grotesque killer added up to one conclusion. The adage from past plague epidemics put it most succinctly and convincingly: "Go early; stay far away; return late." But what were persons to do who had the resources to leave, yet hesitated out of moral and practical concerns? And what of those lower on the economic ladder, who faced the dilemma of staying and facing possible death or fleeing to unfamiliar places without friends to receive them or the wherewithal to enter an inn? Could they leave and should they leave?

PART II

Confusion

4

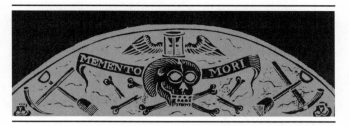

Fleeing or Staying?

Loveing brother: I hope these lines will finde you and yours and all our friends in the country well, as (blessed be God) I am and all my family so long as God pleases. For we have a crasie sickly time att London.

Now knowing young persons are most apt to take infection, thought good to give you an accompt of it to have your advice about Cosen John, to know your mind whether you do not desire him home again.

—JOHN MOORE, London, to Charles Moore at Little Appleby,
Leicestershire, June 18, 1665

A Country Servant

In the crowds milling around the city, Gervase Jacques might be seen looking over girls' and women's gowns in the shops of the Royal Exchange or stopping at a haberdasher's or tailor's shop to inquire about making up boys' clothes. To a casual observer, these activities might have looked like routine errands for a middle-income London household. But Gervase Jacques was no ordinary house servant.

As a highly skilled employee of Lucy Hastings, the countess of Huntingdon of Donnington Park manor in Leicestershire, Jacques earned an annual income far above that of the 20 percent of London's population who worked as servants or apprentices. The best-paid waiting woman or chief male servant might earn ten pounds a year in the capital. A scullery maid or footboy, clinging to their yearly two pounds plus clothes, lodging, and meals, could scarcely imagine the security and prestige of someone like Jacques.

Jacques had a confident air as he shopped around Cheapside and the other main streets, which were monopolized by London's wealthiest merchants.

His rounds took him through the narrower but respectable lanes lined with shops rented by wood and metal master craftsmen. The city's dark alleys just off the lanes and streets were another matter, best avoided by someone like Jacques. The mapmakers of the day didn't include these miserable dwellings in their bird's-eye views of the city's buildings. Workers in the many stages of cloth and leather making lived there, attracted by some of the lowest housing rentals in the city. The thriving dock area was more attractive to Jacques, despite the warehouse squatters. He could be seen making his way among the import dealers and victualers to consult with a relative, Francis Jacques, a silk buyer.[1]

Gervase's employment also took him to fine city residences like the house of Sir Gervas and Lady Alice Clifton. Lady Alice was a sister-in-law of Jacques' Midlands employer, Lucy Hastings, countess of Huntingdon. He knew all about the Cliftons' preparations for the society marriage of their daughter, Jane, which was about to take place in their London townhouse. And he was equally at home in the best parts of Westminster, where Henry Hastings, Lord Loughborough, a brother of Lady Clifton and brother-in-law of the countess, had a residence.

The countess of Huntingdon depended on Jacques' trustworthiness, good judgment, and knowledge of a wide range of her business, legal, and other concerns. She had sent him down to London from her Leicestershire manor during the Lenten season in 1665 to negotiate the settlement of her past and current accounts with London merchants, to order Easter clothes and household furnishings, and to check on "her great affaire" (possibly a lawsuit or a petition to the House of Lords, with which she was associated as the widow of a peer).

The forty days of Lent were long since past, and Easter had been happily celebrated at the Donnington Park manor house. Many items remained on Lady Lucy's list for the late spring rite of Whitsuntide commemorating the descent of the Holy Spirit to Christ's followers after his Resurrection and Ascension. Time was running short; Gervase Jacques would be hard-pressed to send everything up to Leicestershire before the holiday.

Jacques knew Lucy Hastings, countess of Huntingdon, to be a strong yet caring head of her household. Her privileged childhood had given her a command of several foreign languages and Latin and Greek. From her father, Sir John Davies, who had been King's Attorney in Ireland and then a practicing lawyer in London, she had learned to pay attention to the changing fortunes of public life, which had thwarted his ambitions for high office. But she also had acquired emotional security from a belief in divine providence, which came from her mother, Lady Eleanor Davies. Fortunately, Lucy never followed her mother's penchant for inflammatory millenarian prophesies in voice and print, which landed Lady Eleanor briefly in Bedlam, the London hospital for the insane. (Lady Eleanor had prophesied that the plague and the Civil War were signs of the imminent end of the world.)[2]

Married when she was only ten years old to the sixth earl of Huntingdon, Ferdinando Hastings, Lucy had coped as a child bride with an imperious mother-in-law and as a middle-aged woman with the death of her husband in 1656. Amid the tension and loss, she had raised her four children well (carefully choosing their tutors and her household servants), married her eldest daughter to a country gentleman of fine character, and turned her attention to her only son, Earl Theophilus, as he approached manhood.

Tragedy struck again in 1664 with the death of her married daughter after a long illness. Lucy bore the loss well but wondered how her grief-stricken son-in-law, Sir James Langham, would manage on his own. He had taken his children down to London while he saw to his business affairs. The distance bothered her, but on the other hand Sir James and the children were near Lucy's brother-in-law, Lord Loughborough, and her sister-in-law, Lady Clifton. She could also count on Gervase Jacques to check on her London relations and tell her how they were faring.[3]

Jacques' latest letter to the countess was not a happy one, despite his efforts to set her mind at ease.[4] The traffic on the Great Northern Road was all heading toward the capital as April came to a close, and the city and court were crowded with visitors. Among them was a dear friend of Lucy's, Anne Stavely, who had left her oldest child at Donnington manor and gone south with her younger girls. Nothing untoward had happened to the Stavelys or the Langhams, but Jacques' other news was truly dreadful. Lord Loughborough's son and heir, Henry Hastings Jr., had gotten into an argument over a gaming and drinking bill at a tavern in Covent Garden. Noble honor called for settling the matter with a duel, and Lucy's nephew had been struck fatally in the head by his opponent's sword. The solemn funeral cortege and torchlight burial in Saint Martin in the Fields parish had drawn a huge throng, led by the grieving peer and his many relatives and friends at court.

The nuptial story involving Sir Gervas and Lady Clifton's daughter was just as dramatic. The groom, Mr. Packe, and his party had arrived on the wedding day only to learn that the bride was sick in bed. Jane Clifton tried to dress and come down but was overcome with dizziness. "After some little tyme," Jacques related, "the small pox appeared."

Jacques was keenly aware of Lucy Hastings's uncommon skill in diagnosing illnesses and prescribing treatments for neighbors and friends of the gentry, who could easily have afforded a doctor of "physick." "My mother doth believe Your Honors study and practice in physicke is above our doctors," a worried friend of Lucy's pleaded. The local physician was "good and proficiente," she admitted, but none of his pharmaceutical pastes, powders, and pills had done anything for the suspected palsy. No one but the countess could put the sick woman and her worried daughter at ease.[5]

Jacques chose his words about Jane Clifton's condition carefully: "She is very full," he said of the rash, "but great hopes she may recover." This was encouraging, considering the risks of disfigurement and death from this malady. But the next lines were not so calming. "Sir Gervas and his family are removed into Holborn," he said, adding "this [smallpox] and the [common] feavour are much in towne." Jacques was admitting that not one, but two diseases had become epidemic in London.

This mention of the common fever's running rampant in the capital surely caught the countess's attention. Fevers, she knew, could progress into spotted fever and plague. If the pestilence had suddenly returned to London after several years' absence, that would explain the precipitous flight of Sir Gervas's family far better than smallpox, which Jane Clifton had clearly contracted but recovered from quickly with no sign of infecting the rest of the family. And if it was plague they were running from, High Holborn (just west of Newgate and home to members of the legal profession and other substantial citizens) offered a temporary safe haven while Jane regained her strength and her family prepared to move farther out of harm's way.

Jacques wrote his letter on April 25, a Tuesday. For the past fortnight the searchers in the metropolitan area had been reporting a surge in fatalities from the simple fever and spotted fever. When the printed Bill of Mortality came out that Thursday, it listed the two plague fatalities in Saint Giles in the Fields. Across London Bridge John Allin heard the news before it was official. Perhaps Gervase Jacques knew in advance from his city contacts or Lord Loughborough at the royal court.

Two weeks passed before Jacques picked up his pen again.[6] Whitsuntide was just five days off, and he was full of entertaining news for Lady Lucy and gossip for Earl Theophilus as titular head of the family. Foreign ambassadors were filing into Whitehall with their credentials and falling all over themselves to impress the king, Jacques chortled. The best court news, however, was a splendid funeral at the Abbey for the chief justice, Sir Robert Hyde, who had died suddenly of apoplexy. Jacques described the hundred carriages bearing bishops, high justices, and peers that had followed red-coated heralds and mounted escorts in full mourning dress as the coffin wended its way from Westminster toward Salisbury for burial with the judge's ancestors.

The tone of the letter grew more serious as Jacques got down to the personal affairs of his masters. He admitted having a hard time prying commitments from the countess's and earl's favorite tailors in time for the holiday. Full payment of past and current accounts had to be promised to secure the making of the suit and hat the young earl desired and of dresses for his sisters. Surely, they knew the countess would pay up eventually. Yet they were pressing Jacques and their regular customers for cash.

Finally, Jacques came around to the likely reason behind the merchants' urgency. "Here is still greate feares of the plague, and I wish it bee but only our feares," he admitted. "I am credibly informed that two houses are shut up in Axe Yard nere St. Clements church in the Strand." No sooner had the master of the pesthouse shut up the infected residences than the householders broke open their doors and escaped.

Jacques' graphic account conjured up images of people with plague sores breathing out the infection on the Strand, the best street of Westminster. And while he did not say so directly, he certainly implied that merchants inside the wall were preparing to flee to the countryside. Lacking the resources of great families like the Hastings, they had been gathering in as much cash as they could from their customers to tide them over in a country inn or boarding house until the plague abated. No doubt the countess of Huntingdon, on reading Jacques' lines in the safety of her Midlands manor (a four-day carriage ride from the capital), hoped her relatives in the city and at court were thinking of speeding northward toward Leicestershire. Nothing in London could keep them back. If their country houses were not ready for immediate habitation, the countess's hospitality at Donnington Park would be extended to them, as it had been in the past, for as long a stay as necessary. Furthermore, they were reasonably secure in leaving their London residences behind. Like royalty who took some of their belongings from residence to residence, peers and gentry could take some valuables to their country manors and leave the rest under guard by house servants they chose not to take with them. By contrast, many city tradesmen lacked the staff to guard their premises; if they left, their livelihood was in jeopardy, since their personal property consisted of tools and goods in their ground-floor shop, plus furnishings in the family's living quarters above.

The metropolitan Bill of Mortality for May 2–9 was being readied as Jacques wrote. When it appeared on the eleventh, the news was worse than he had suggested. Among the nine reported plague fatalities was the first one inside the wall. The infected house in Saint Mary Woolchurch parish was not far from his relative's cul-de-sac abode off Thames Street. Gervase surely wanted to get back to the safety of the countryside, but he knew his duty as a servant; he still had to check on the countess's "great affair," settle the last of her accounts, and pick up the Hastings' last orders. The Loughboroughs and Cliftons and Langhams, we know from their later correspondence, were all heading for the Midlands at this very time. So were the countess's friend Ann Stavely and her children; there was no point in keeping these young ones in the path of the pestilence, as the great mass of poor London mothers surely were obliged to do with their children, hoping that their offspring would be among the survivors when the plague had run its course.

On May 26 John Allin broke the news of the early departures from Westminster to his friends down in Sussex. The weekly bill from London had listed three plague deaths a week before, he said, and fourteen this week, "but its rather believed to be treble the number," he confided. "At ye upper end of the towne [Westminster], persons high and low are very fearful of it, & many removed." The flow of traffic in and out of London had suddenly changed. Only four weeks before Jacques had remarked on the crowds of people flocking in from the country. Now there was a surge of outward-bound coaches, accompanied by wagons piled high with clothes and other personal belongings. Fifty miles away in the far reaches of Essex (a long half-day for the fastest male rider and an arduous two days by coach), Rev. Ralph Josselin looked at the bill for the first week of June, listing forty-three plague deaths, and exclaimed: "The plague certainly in London. Lord helpe us . . . to turn away thy wrath." He was relieved that an ailing parishioner was back home after having a stone cut from his bladder by a London surgeon. Reverend Josselin's eldest son had been planning to go down to the capital on business; that trip had to be postponed.[7]

Among the escapees from the western suburbs was the rector of Covent Garden parish, Rev. Symon Patrick. On May 13, his clerk had recorded a second plague burial in the parish register. Again Mr. Ramsbury and Reverend Patrick hid the true cause of death from the metropolitan bill. Shortly after the body of Mistress Bowler had been lowered into a freshly dug churchyard gravesite, the minister started northward toward Northamptonshire. He wanted to see his parents because of their age and his father's faltering health, and a Midland spa at Astrop near their house would be good for his own health. After moving from rural Surrey, Patrick had survived his first years in the bad London air better than he had expected, but he felt in need of rejuvenation.[8]

The timing of this society pastor's removal from his rented Westminster lodgings and his church and congregation suggested another reason for this action. Patrick's renowned physician friend, Dr. Thomas Willis, had discovered the spa at Astrop the year before and was there at this very time. Perhaps part of the draw was this medical wunderkind's knowledge of plague, which he had discussed in his recent book on fevers.

Or perhaps the Reverend Patrick may have been avoiding the thought of an approaching epidemic, as were many Londoners this May. The metropolitan bills sustained this denial by false reporting to spare people the ignominy of plague in their family or neighborhood. During the last week of May, there had supposedly been 23 burials for spotted fever—an astonishing figure. Surfeit had claimed 13 lives, and "teeth" or teething 19 persons of a tender age. Rickets was right up there, too, with 14 fatalities. The first week of June saw the figures for these and other diseases shoot up even higher. The terrifying figure of 43 plague deaths alongside 20 for smallpox and 16 for spotted fever made the accuracy of the latter two attributions suspect. And how to account for 31 deaths from convulsions, 27 of dropsy, 27 caused by griping in the guts, and an astounding 63 attributed to consumption? Some of these counts were 40 percent higher than those reported for the same malady during the same time in prior years (see appendix A).

The unofficial spinner of good news about the king and capital tried to nourish this social amnesia. On June 4, Roger L'Estrange's *Intelligencer* decried the rumors of "multitudes that dye of the Plague in this Towne . . . I shall very briefly deliver the truth of the matter," L'Estrange editorialized: "There have dyed 2, 9, 3, 14 and 17 in these five last weeks (45 in all, and none of these within the walls and but 5 parishes infected of 130)." This bland reassurance was plainly at odds with the increasing number of advertisements in the *Intelligencer* hawking all manner of plague preventives and remedies.

Any merchant inside the wall could see through L'Estrange's claim that only a few of the suburban poor were dying of the sickness. At the city pesthouse, two burials had already been reported by the end of May—perhaps servants of an unlucky merchant or professional household in the central business district. Pepys' physician's servant would be among the later casualties.

The toll in the western suburbs was more alarming and not just in numbers. By the first week of June, plague burials had occurred in ten parishes, ranging from the very poor to the extremely wealthy. At the high end stood Symon Patrick's Covent Garden, with its 7.7 mean number of hearths—the top figure for London's 130 parishes. At the other end was

Saint Sepulchre—where Samuel Pepys' cousin, Kate Joyce, and her husband had their busy inn—with a median of only 1.7 hearths.[9]

Gervase Jacques was caught between the down-and-out poor of Saint Sepulchre, who were trapped by their meager resources in a neighborhood that buried in an average year 750 persons out of 1,015 documented households, and the titled and wealthy of Covent Garden's Piazza, who could leave their servants as guards and flee to their spacious country homes. The return of the plague to the city, with four deaths one week and ten the next, made Jacques restive. He took up his pen once more, unsure exactly what to say but knowing he must alert Lady Lucy and Earl Theophilus to his plight.[10]

Jacques apologized for yielding too much to the "pressing importunityes" of the Hastings's creditors. Alas, he had paid some of them "more than was intended," and still they were not satisfied! This was uncomfortable to relate, but it prepared him for an even more difficult admission. The ravages of time have obliterated parts of the ending, but enough remains to show the gist of it. "I humbly entreat your perusal and speedy pleasure concerning [past and present bills] that my stay now intended may bee short," he began. After suggesting that his prolonged stay was costing her a great deal of money, he finally threw himself at the mercy of the countess: "For besides the great charge [my stay] gives your Honour, my own health and safety doth a little concerne mee if I may not bee otherwise serviceable to you [back] in the country." The complimentary closing fragment pleads his mistress's attention to "my preservation in this sickly Cittye, Madame y'r Honours most dutifull most obedient servant G. Jacu."

Jacques' surviving correspondence does not resume for two more years. Presumably, after his letter reached Donnington Park and the countess sent her approval by "express" courier (a turnaround of four days by a fast rider changing horses frequently), he followed the Langhams, Loughboroughs, Cliftons, and Stavelys on the Great Northern Road. But what were the great mass of London servants, apprentices, artisans, and small shopkeepers to do? Their livelihood depended on their masters or their trade. If they left everything behind but their meager savings, they would soon run out of money; transportation and lodging alone would cost them half a pound over the three-month duration of a minor plague epidemic.[11] And what of professional persons like Dr. Hodges and merchants like Alderman Turner and high royal officials like Samuel Pepys, on whom poorer Londoners depended directly or indirectly for employment and charity?

Dilemmas

Question: Is it lawful to depart from our own place and habitations in time of
plague?

Answer: Provided a man be not tyed by the relation of a Husband to a Wife, a
Father to his Children, a Master to his Family, a Governor and Overseer of
good Order in the place he lives in, and bee otherwise free, hee may Fly.

—RICHARD KEPHALE, *Medela Pestilentiae* (London, 1665)

Seeking to recapture that frantic moment of his early childhood, Daniel Defoe opens his *Journal of the Plague Year* with two brothers arguing about
whether to flee or stay. "H.F." is a city-dwelling saddler with an eerie likeness
to Daniel's late uncle Henry Foe, whose saddler shop in 1665 lay on the road
out of Aldgate to the Essex countryside. H.F.'s argumentative brother is an
international merchant who has returned from Portugal with a healthy respect for the hazards to life in the Mediterranean world. The fictional dia-
logue between the siblings remains the most believable recreation of how
middle-class tradespeople actually thought, felt, and acted in the panicky
days of June 1665.[12]

The merchant's travels make him suspicious of anything that resembles
the fatalism about plague he has witnessed in the Muslim world.[13] He has
only one word of advice to the saddler: "Save Thyself!" This merchant's wife
and children are already safe in the country, and he is winding up his affairs
to join them. H.F. has his shop and his faith, however. He will stay with his
trade and his goods—"all I had in the world." He misses one chance after
another to arrange for a person with fewer resources to guard his shop in his
absence and, finally, as he wavers, opens his Bible randomly at Psalm 91.
"Thou shall not be afraid of the terror by night, nor the arrow that flieth by
day," he reads. "There shall no evil befall thee, neither shall any plague come
nigh to thy dwelling." He decides to await his destiny. In real life one can imagine many Bible-reading Londoners putting on the same providentialist ar-
mor against the pestilential steams of that early summertime.

H.F.'s brother thought his reasoning utter nonsense; he was surely tempting God to let him die by risking plague so directly. In real life that was the
way many persons saw things. An Anglican bishop put fleeing Londoners'
consciences at ease with a simple question: "You say [plague] is God's Visitation? What evil is not? Because death will overtake us, shall we run and
meet him?"[14]

One would have had to be blind and deaf not to be pulled in contrary directions as the debate over flight raged in print and voice.[15] Single-sheet broadsides appeared like magic that June, with the sad title, "Lord Have Mercy Upon Us," repeating the words placed on the door of every shut-up household to signal it was infected with the plague. The borders of these tracts were peppered with hourglasses, pick and shovel, and skull and cross-bones. To drive home the point that no one could escape God's judgment, even through flight, there was almost always an Avenging Angel holding a poisoned arrow. Crammed into the corners were hackneyed verses pillorying hard-hearted citizens for not giving generously to plague relief. The most arresting feature of these sheets was their lists of burial totals from previous great plagues in London, capped by a column of figures for 1665, week by week, down to the time of printing. Surviving broadsheets often have subsequent weeks' totals penned in by the people who bought them.[16]

Beyond these scary images lay moral concerns. "If we go away," one tract asks with disarming rhetoric, "what's that to you?" The response is swift and unyielding:

> What sottish question is't this Carter asks?
> When Doctors leave their patients, Priests their tasks,
> Is't nothing to the Sheep [that] their shepherds leave them?
> Is't nothing to the sick, if Doctors deceive them?[17]

Practical issues compounded these ethical dilemmas. *The Run-Awayes Return* made people think twice of taking to their heels:

> What fury dogs and hunts you up and down,
> First from the City and then the Country Town?
> But when you'r there, you are afraid to stay,
> And a nimble pace do Run away . . .
> For suppos'd Safety, yet you are much worse,
> Having both Plague of Body and of Purse.

A well-known woodcut from earlier plague traumas portrayed the tension between city anguish and country inhospitality with stunning images: country officials attach ropes to the feet of deceased Londoners and drag the bodies to an open pit; in contrast, a city funeral cortege moves in quiet grief to a neatly tended churchyard where a single marked grave awaits. Up in Oxford, an avid collector of news, Anthony Wood, paused over a newly printed London tract with the eye-catching title, *Iter Boreale, the Country Clown,* which excoriated rural "barbarity" toward fleers. At nighttime, Wood saw the torches of mounted guards at the four bridges of Oxford, keeping watch against the entry of unwelcome Londoners.[18] Who could blame this self-protective behavior? Fear and suspicion of Londoners gripped townspeople in the heart of the interior. Along the coastline, ports from Bristol to Newcastle turned away ships from the capital.

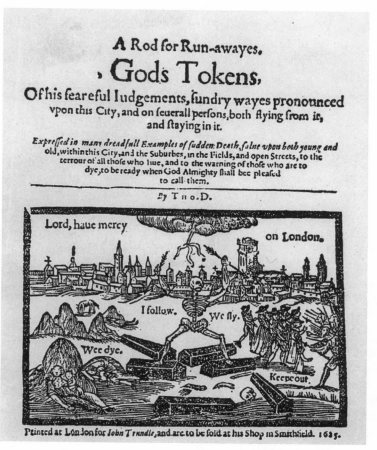

Fig. 4. Frontispiece of *A Rod for Run-awayes, Gods Tokens of his fearful Judgements*. This woodcut from the Great Plague of 1625 features God's Destroying Angel as an arrow-wielding skeleton pursuing fleers from London who fall exhausted and die in the fields on the left and are held back by armed country people on the right. The caption warns of death to "both young and old, within this City, and the Suburbs, in the Fields, and open Streets" and tells Londoners fated to die "to be ready when God Almighty shall be pleased to call them." The Wellcome Library, London

At Samuel and Elizabeth Pepys' dinner table, the conversation turned to flight. The questions did not come easily, but come they did. How long could he wait before pressing his mother to go back to the family home in Cambridgeshire, which she had left for London out of boredom? And where could he and his wife go if the plague got worse? Cambridgeshire was too far from the downstream ports where much of his navy business took him. There were also Elizabeth's maids to think of—Mary and Alice and the little girl Su. With her husband's rise in the world, Elizabeth Pepys had been able to take on all this household help, and she couldn't think of doing without them. But if they came along, who would guard the family's possessions in Seething Lane?

Pepys also worried about his assistant, Will Hewer. Will had become indispensable, first as his manservant and then as his clerk at the navy office. But Will was spending a considerable amount of time looking after his own parents in Saint Sepulchre parish, one of the centers of the raging plague. Pepys feared that Will might catch the infection from his folks' neighborhood. He couldn't afford to lose Will. And if truth be known, Pepys was wary of his assistant carrying the infection into Seething Lane.[19]

Dark thoughts of encroaching death were interrupted by a great naval victory over the Dutch near Lowestoft on the North Sea coast. "The Lord good in our wonderful success," Josselin wrote.[20] Londoners heard the cannon shots and hoped the Dutch would sue for peace. Bonfires and bells and dancing in the streets rivaled the celebrations held after the Spanish Armada's defeat and the foiled Gunpowder Plot to blow up the king and Parliament.

The celebrations were premature. The Dutch escaped total disaster when a bungling English officer called off pursuit of the battered and retreating fleet. Hundreds of wounded royal sailors and thousands of captured Dutch seamen streamed ashore. Evelyn's prison and hospital costs soared to one thousand pounds, and he began to despair of a war he called "bloody" and "miserable."[21] The Anglo-Dutch conflict would go on for three years, with astronomical costs for maintaining the navy with ships, men, and supplies—a nightmare for the navy high command, though an opportunity for Pepys to increase his profits.

By a cruel fate, war and pestilence became connected by ritual and reality as well as by the forecasts of popular almanacs. Pepys went down to the naval port at Woolwich and engaged rooms for Elizabeth and her maids "for a month or two." The king had set aside a national day of celebration *and* sorrow. On June 20 the English people were to gather at their churches to thank

God for the "signal victory" at sea and give generously to households suffering from the "sad disease of plague or pestilence." "The town grows very sickly," Pepys wrote.[22]

Pepys kept up his spirits with an energy that knew no bounds. At the Royal Exchange he purchased stockings at a shop frequented by a class of people thought unlikely to catch the infection. He placed orders at Sir William Turner's Golden Fleece in Saint Paul's churchyard and stopped by his goldsmith-bankers, Vyner and Colvill, on Lombard Street to negotiate loans for navy supplies. The pestilence had done nothing to rein in his libido; as his hand reached into his purse to claim a dozen silver salts costing almost seven pounds, a roving eye caught sight of Colvill's pretty wife.

Three days before the national day of thanksgiving and mourning, Pepys' spirits were at a peak as the king's brother and other high naval officers returned from sea to Whitehall, "all fat and lusty and ruddy at being in the sun." Pepys hired a coach and proceeded along the Holborn Road, which a few short weeks before had been a safe haven from the Cliftons' smallpox episode. He was not so lucky; at the end of the road, he found the home of the high royal official he was to see boarded up "because of the sickness." The entire family had fled out of town; Pepys' meeting on finances was cancelled.

On his way home Pepys had one of the great frights of his life. The hackney coach driver, whom he had hailed from the direction of Saint Giles in the Fields, picked up speed and then went slower and slower until he came to a stop, telling Pepys that he was "suddenly stroke very sick and almost blind." Pepys found another coach to take him home, but the terror of the moment lingered "with a sad heart for the poor man and trouble for myself, lest he should have been stroke with the plague—being at [the infected] end of the town that I took him up. But God have mercy upon us all."[23]

It was time for bold measures. While Samuel attended to navy business, Elizabeth shopped with his mother, Margaret, in preparation for sending her off to Cambridgeshire. Then Elizabeth checked on her own mother, Dorothea St. Michel, who was staying put with her husband. They had no money to tide them over in the country, and their son-in-law was not offering help. He simply told his wife to avoid the streets and lanes most likely to be infected around her parents' neighborhood.

On the twenty-first of June, Pepys took a break from his business rounds at the Cross Keys tavern by the Cripplegate exit from the city. He was in a somber mood after the special service of victory and humiliation at his church the day before, still muttering over the miserable sermon by the pastor, whom he thought a shallow man. "I find all the town almost going," he exclaimed as he looked out the tavern windows, "the coaches and wagons being all full of people going into the country." Pepys lingered with the tapster's wife, spent time at his office, and went home for dinner and sleep.

But sleep he could not. His mother was balking at going back to the boring country. On the twenty-second he finally persuaded her to go, pointing out that the sickness was worsening, Elizabeth was about to leave, and there would be no female company left for Margaret. It was left to Elizabeth to see that her mother-in-law did not change her mind again. But Margaret Pepys put off her departure until the carriage was full of passengers and she had to ride in a wagon hitched to the back of the coach.

Seven or eight houses were now infected near the Guildhall. It was rumored that several aldermen had fled to the country. Ever the optimist, Pepys stopped at Saint Paul's churchyard to order some new books. Out in Westminster he came across shut-up residences, some on King Street and one "great house" right on the Piazza. At Whitehall he found the court "full of wagons and people ready to go out of town." He sought to quiet his nerves but found his favorite west-end mistress, the newly married linen draper Mrs. Betty Martin, gone from Westminster Hall to the country with her husband. Pepys had to settle for idle chat with Mary at the Harp and Ball by Charing Cross.[24]

The city and suburbs suffered another demoralizing loss on July 6, the day after Elizabeth Pepys departed to Woolwich. King Charles sent last-minute instructions to the mayor and aldermen to stay at their posts and then took a boat upstream to Hampton Court with Queen Catherine and the duke and duchess of York. The privy councilors followed, except for the duke of Albemarle, captain general and admiral of the kingdom, and his assistant, the earl of Craven. They were entrusted with keeping an eye on the mansions of royal Westminster and preventing disorder in the poorer suburbs. The lord mayor, Sir John Lawrence, assumed full control of security for the merchant community and sustenance for the poor throughout the city and its liberties beyond the wall.

Twenty-three Londoners dead of the plague were buried in the city's churchyards during the king's last week in his capital. Another 438 plague corpses entered suburban churchyards. Five others died at the city pesthouse, and four at the facility in Westminster. These were the official figures in the bill for June 27–July 4.

Refugees and Rescuers

Question: How are men to fly into the country?
Answer: No one should depart his house except to an house of such distance as
   that he may conveniently travel thither without lying by the way.
   —KEPHALE, *Medela Pestilentiae*

"All Doors and Passages are thronged for escape," Dr. Hodges exclaimed.[25] Three thousand watermen turned London into a Venice of the North, as venturesome persons took up residence on boats anchored in the Thames River and pressed every available boatman into service for their ongoing needs. The noise and dust from horses' hooves on the city's narrow, crooked streets evoked memories of Civil War battles, as Londoners fled by the tens of thousands during the last week of June and the first week in July.

Horse-drawn coaches jockeyed for room with wagons piled high with baggage. Squeezing in between were laborers on foot, taking their chance of bedding down by a country hedge. As traffic converged at the city gates, the severity of the bottlenecks was beyond anything in memory. London Bridge was a madhouse. Out in Westminster, carters transported mattresses, furniture, and clothes to the country and turned around to do it again. Peers and gentry accustomed to smooth rides in their elegant carriages found the broad suburban passages clogged beyond belief. The exodus would continue right through summer, reaching 200,000 if Graunt's estimates from past plagues (repeated in two new editions of his *Observations on the Bills of Mortality*) held for this epidemic.[26]

This mass migration, the largest London had ever experienced, affected every class, trade, and occupation in the city and suburbs. After his own flight from Westminster, Dr. Sydenham claimed that "at least two-thirds of the inhabitants had retired to the country to avoid infection." The wealthy area around Whitehall, which sustained a population of twenty-five thousand or more through employment and service associated with the royal court,[27] was emptied out. Almost all of its noble and gentry families fled, followed by most of the professional lawyers, notaries, merchants, and other middling residents who catered to their needs. Covent Garden parish was "very empty," Reverend Patrick recalled later on, "all the gentry and better sort of tradesmen being gone."[28] The other center of metropolitan wealth, within the walls, experienced a considerable exodus of the merchant and professional classes that sustained its economy. More of them stayed on than in Westminster, however, hoping the plague would not reach their streets.

John Allin had commented on people "high" and "low" joining the early exodus, but the lower a person stood on the economic ladder, the less likelihood there was of leaving. Common laborers could not have saved much for a long stay in the country; the median daily wage of the working population in England was seven pence, and one-sixth of these workers earned only two pennies a day, according to Sir William Petty.[29]

Transportation costs put travel to safety beyond the reach of most Londoners. Only the peers and gentry could set out in a coach seating six persons for a distant county at thirty to thirty-five miles of travel a day. A daughter of Lady Lucy Hastings had recently taken the four-day trip between the Midlands and London by coach at a cost of ten pounds, one-third more than most persons earned in a year.[30] Even the five shillings Petty said it would cost for the cheapest transportation to the immediate countryside was far beyond the means of London's skilled craftspersons.[31] Beyond this initial expense, fleeing artisans risked starving under a hedge, shunned by the local inhabitants because of their poor dress and appearance—which would be associated with carrying the plague.

And so they stayed en masse: the skilled artisans, unskilled laborers, porters and coachmen, and maids and servants left behind by their masters. Even in Covent Garden, deserted as it was by almost everyone else, the "ordinary sort of people continued," Patrick said. They were to be admired, Sydenham said with genuine awe, for carrying on "heart and soul . . . with danger all around [and] the thousand shapes of death before their eyes."[32]

Pepys and his naval colleagues settled their families in the royal ports downstream, Elizabeth taking her maids to Woolwich and Navy Treasurer Carteret and Vice Admiral Sandwich moving to staff quarters and family housing at Deptford. Navy Commissioner Lord Brouncker forsook the Piazza for his county estate outside Greenwich. Dr. Busby, the headmaster of King's School in Westminster, ferried his pupils upstream to the school's country place at Chiswick. Dr. Busby calculated that the water route was safer than facing down pitchfork-wielding vigilantes on the road.[33]

The first few miles could be the most dangerous. West of Westminster, at Hayes, the locals attacked Londoners with clubs. On the northern road, at Whetstone, they were turned back with muskets. A caravan that crossed London Bridge and headed into rural Surrey ran into a camp of "Egyptians." These gypsies, having their own troubles with the local inhabitants, chased the plague-fleeing Londoners from their campground.[34]

If one had to stop over on the way, it was best to travel as far as possible the first day on the road. Even wearing one's best clothes did not guarantee hospitality, though villagers kept their sights on ill-clothed beggars and drifters thought to be most susceptible to carrying the contagion. "How fearful people were thirty or forty if not a hundred miles from London," a Puritan preacher ruminated.[35]

Up in Leicestershire, Lucy Hastings worried about the whereabouts of her relatives and friends, expecting their approach any time. They, in turn, were concerned about rushing to Donnington Park with the infection still on their belongings. These reactions were sharply at odds with the self-absorbed fleers and unwelcoming country hosts described in plague tract literature.

Anne Stavely, for example, had set out for Donnington Park during the mass flight of late June. She was eager to rejoin her oldest daughter and relieve Lady Lucy of caring for her. After the first days on the northern road, Anne felt relief that no tokens or buboes had appeared on her or her children. Still, she was determined not to risk frightening the young earl and his sisters by arriving with her other children within the quarantine period assigned to infected households. So she sought out a safe haven in the Midland countryside and stayed there for forty days.

But after the forty days, Anne was too weak to travel the last leg of the journey northward. She took up her pen to say with profuse apologies that she was "unable to rise to so long a journey." Recalling Lucy's many favors "both formerly and latterly," she expressed her hopes of soon being able to relieve her of caring for her daughter.[36]

The countess's son-in-law had a different dilemma. Sir James Langham and his children had stopped halfway to Donnington Park, in Northamptonshire. Unfortunately, the damnable plague followed them and surrounded the town. "We here enjoy (thanks be to God) a good health," he informed his mother-in-law. "But do with some trouble think we are like to be confined to this place." What could he do? Lucy Hastings would want to see him and the grandchildren, but they would all have to wait out the contagion. "The sickness dayly [increases] in and about London," Sir James lamented, "and there is scarcely any county [in] wh'ch the venome of that disease is not scattered."[37]

The young London playwright John Dryden, who had climbed the social ladder through theater contacts with nobility, was in the right place at the right time. Through a fellow playwright, the sixth son of the earl of Berkshire, Dryden had met the earl's daughter, Elizabeth, and married her at the end of 1663. After royal orders closed Westminster's theaters because of the plague, the newlywed Drydens left their rented lodgings near the Strand for the west-country estate of Elizabeth's father. John roamed the idyllic countryside outside Charlton, Wiltshire, and Elizabeth gave birth to their first child. He wrote copiously and elegantly—but not about the contagion or his flight from its path.[38]

The Puritan revolutionary iconoclast John Milton, whose lodging in Cripplegate was threatened by plague, lacked Dryden's social connections. A Quaker friend, Thomas Ellwood, who was preaching clandestinely in Buckinghamshire, rented a cottage for the blind poet and his children. By the time the Miltons reached this temporary haven, Ellwood was in jail for flouting the laws against dissenter worship. When Ellwood was released from prison, Milton proudly showed him his completed work, *Paradise Lost.* Surprising the author, Ellwood responded, tongue in cheek, "But what hast thou to say of paradise found?" When the two met again after the Great Fire of 1666, Milton showed Ellwood his *Paradise Regained,* written during his idyllic stay at the country cottage. Milton thanked Ellwood for his hospitality and for suggesting the book with his query.[39]

Other Londoners with material and spiritual resources vital to the city's functioning were also in headlong flight. Among them was the dean of Saint Paul's cathedral, William Sancroft. Like Symon Patrick's early flight from London's plague to a fashionable Midlands spa, Sancroft's southward journey in July to one of the king's favorite spas was prompted by concern for his health. His personal physician, Peter Barwick, had been urging that health cure for some time. Sancroft had remained at the cathedral long enough to draw up a special service book for use in the churches of London and the surrounding countryside and to arrange a plague relief fund for the infected and unemployed poor around the cathedral. Then he set out for Kent, reaching his destination without any hostility from country persons, for who would challenge a man of his rank on the possibility of his carrying the deadly infection?[40]

Every week Dean Sancroft received assurances from his staff that they were managing in his absence. But they also reported appalling sickness and suffering in Saint Gregory's parish, which served the cathedral's neighborhood. People were beginning to criticize the dean's prolonged absence, they admitted. Dr. Barwick tried to quell the unrest by maintaining that he had told his patient to go long before the plague, and it was not "in the skill of everyone" to judge the circumstances behind someone's flight from contagion.[41]

Emotions ran high as families decided whether to split up. The normal course for a middle-income tradesman who hesitated to leave his trade but could afford to rent lodging in the country was to remain with the danger while the rest of the family left, especially the young ones, who were thought to be most susceptible to the infection. But some citizens' stratagems defied conventional wisdom. The wealthy London dealer in lead, John Moore, feared for his nephew John's health and chances of getting an apprenticeship because of the plague. He wrote to his brother Charles up in Leicestershire, telling him of the dangers and asking if he wanted his son home, a reasonable idea. But John also offered to keep his nephew on if his father approved. "I shalbe as carefull of him as myself," John informed Charles. Whatever happened, the nephew survived. John Moore died in 1704, passing on his estate to his nephew John.[42]

Another privileged Londoner returned to London after an early flight. Two months after leaving Covent Garden for that Midland spa in Northamptonshire, the Reverend Symon Patrick decided to go back to his parish. By this point, his parish clerk was no longer hiding plague fatalities. They came in twos and threes, and these numbers would soon triple and then quadruple. "Notwithstanding" these factors, Patrick wrote in his memoirs, "I resolved to commit myself to the care of God in the discharge of my duty." Refusing to be talked out of returning by Dr. Willis, Patrick accepted his advice on how to fend off the contagion, visited his mother and fast-failing father on the way south, and preached his first sermon back in his pulpit on July 23.[43]

Samuel Pepys' inn-keeping cousin, Kate Joyce, and her husband, Anthony, faced their own quandary. As the plague in their poor, infected parish came closer and closer, Pepys grew more and more anxious for Kate's safety. During the third week in July, the plague carried away 141 persons in Saint Sepulchre—the fourth highest toll within the metropolis. In a single night 40 persons had expired, "the [church] bell always going," Pepys moaned. Despite his fears of hackney coaches and the Holborn Road, he took that route to their inn. He argued with Anthony to let Kate go to the Pepys' homestead in Cambridgeshire. Anthony balked. His arguments were "profit, minding the house—and the distance, if either of them should be ill." He simply could not afford to have his wife leave. Pepys was beside himself, and Kate "troubled." Finally, Anthony agreed to let Kate go a short way, to Hampton Court, where she had friends near the palace.

Pepys returned home, limp with exhaustion, relieved, and yet fearful of what lay ahead, "believing that it is great odds we shall see one another again." He, the daredevil of all daredevils in the city, was staying on—so long as his navy suppliers were around to sign contracts and add a gratuity. He did not say so, but he also knew that, for the present, food and drink and transportation remained available at prices someone of his class could afford. His butcher, baker, and favorite waterman had not fled, nor had the great mass of persons in these trades. They were trapped in the city, unable to leave their livelihood, yet knowing that their trades, along with those of tavern owners and innkeepers, were among the most vulnerable to the contagion because of their constant contact with people and potentially infected goods.

Some others involved in commerce in the city were also staying, including persons much higher on the economic ladder than Pepys. His goldsmith associates had remained at their business addresses on Lombard Street. So had the prominent London scriveners Clayton and Morris, at the Flying Horse in Cornhill. They were keeping current with property lease payments to their clients, many of whom were in the country, and they would soon draft a will for Lord Loughborough up in Leicestershire.

Albemarle was alone at the Cockpit in Whitehall, and his deputy Craven was nearby on Long Acre. Inside the wall Mayor Lawrence carried on with a shrinking Court of Aldermen, among them Sir William Turner. Dr. Hodges was staying on inside the wall, and the apothecary Boghurst remained at Saint Giles in the Fields. In Southwark, John Allin provided physick and prayers illegally but quietly to English and immigrant dissenters.

Samuel Pepys saw his wife safely into their temporary downstream quarters and returned to London, he manning one boat and Will another. They rowed silently against the tide, keeping their thoughts to themselves. Pepys entered his empty apartment in Seething Lane, "very alonely."[44] He had every reason to feel sorry for himself. Despite his philandering, he loved his wife and missed her company dearly.

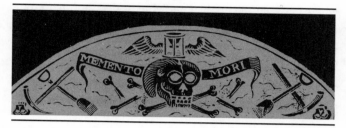

The Medical Marketplace

Get Rue and Wormwood now into thy house
To drive away the Fleas, the Moth and Louse.
Be sure no Physick take, nor do not bleed
Without the Doctor see an extreame need.
And as abroad thou in the streets doest go,
Bare Rue to keep thy self from stinks also.

—*Poor Robin, An Almanack after a
New Fashion* (1665), advice for July

As the days grew warmer and the infection spread faster and farther, everyone who couldn't flee was turning to the medical marketplace. At Saint Bartholomew's Hospital just outside the western wall near Smithfield market and Aldersgate, crowds routinely gathered around an overturned box from which a "mountebank" proclaimed his "tested" potions and "guaranteed" cures for plague.[1] Throughout the suburbs and city, a wide variety of popular healers, called cunning men, wise women, white witches, conjurers, and other appellations, offered an herbal plaster for buboes, a soothing elixir, and antidotes for the feared pestilential poison.

The medical establishment, consisting of physicians, apothecaries, and surgeons, called all of these promoters "quacks," warning the public of dire consequences from their poisonous potions. The three elite groups thought of themselves as the only true practitioners of the healing arts and tried to maintain monopolies on their branches of medicine through their respective organizations: the College of Physicians, Society of Apothecaries, and Company of Barber-Surgeons.

Somewhere between the popular and elite healers, another group of care-givers were carrying on a brisk business, as they always did. Medical astrol-ogers used the stars and seasons to advise clients on everything from when to be bled to when to conceive. Their almanacs included prognostics on pesti-lential epidemics, complete with recipes for plague preservatives and cures. Closely allied to them were alchemists and other unlicensed devotés of ap-proaches to medicine frowned on by orthodox physicians. John Allin secretly practiced medicine in Southwark, hoping for a breakthrough in curing all disease with his combined knowledge of alchemy and astrology.

The Great Plague had brought forth a quiver full of antidotal arrows, but who among the many self-proclaimed experts on plague should be listened to? The invasion of the sickness was a golden opportunity for swapping or stealing one another's notions and potions, all packaged in attractive medical jargon. In the most healthy of times, it was said that there was "scarce a piss-ing-place about the city" that didn't have posters advertising the services of a medical quack, so what must the situation have been in a time of plague? In-side the wall, attractive books were displayed in the bookstalls at Amen corner near Saint Paul's, fresh from the print shops around Saint Bartholo-mew's. Some medical tracts, recently translated, had found their way from Holland, Germany, and France. Each week's editions of the *Newes* and *Intel-ligencer* carried ads for promising potions. For the illiterate carter, a cheaply printed sheet of advice to the poor "in time of plague," read aloud by a pass-erby for a penny or two, offered some hope.

Any potential treatment was embraced as the death toll rose. One week it was 2,000 dead; the next week brought 3,000 to their graves. Gone were the low death reports of the previous year, which during the same two weeks to-taled 402 and 348. In the delightful book titled *Quacks,* the medical historian Roy Porter makes a guarded suggestion that many sellers of popular med-icine "were less cheats than zealots: if we speak of delusion it is primarily self-delusion." His colleague, Bill Bynum, when asked "what was a quack?" replied: "Quack is what Quack does."[2] When a tempting preservative or cure didn't prove effective, many Londoners tried something else (and something else and something else) until the hoped-for relief was found—no recrimina-tions. In the culture of Protestant England, there was also a right—even a duty—to self-help.

In May, when it looked like the disease might become a major "visitation," an emergency public health subcommittee of the king's council called on the most elite body of London medicine, the College of Physicians, "to put a stop to that evil as far as [they] could by some remedies." Several of the college's members dusted off their manuals from earlier epidemics, revising their contents slightly as "Certain Necessary Directions for the Preservation and Cure of the Plague." The king and mayor had their special copies, and citizens could find the work in any apothecary shop (see map 3) and most bookstalls around town. Listed were foods to be avoided (raw cucumbers, melons, and cherries were considered particularly dangerous) and foods to eat and directions on how to raise or prevent fevers (depending on the stage of the sickness) and how to balance the humors.

The belief in four "humors" in the human body—blood, phlegm, yellow bile or choler, and black bile had been passed down from the great Greek physician, Galen (A.D. 130–201), to the seventeenth century. Medical students, after passing their B.A. and M.A. at Oxford or Cambridge, studied classical medical texts for seven years to earn an M.D. (Some shortened the process by getting a quick degree at a European university.) To practice, most doctors sought a license, typically from the College of Physicians, through a perfunctory examination or from an Anglican bishop (whose licensing authority was based on a belief in the close connection between spiritual and physical healing). The members of the College of Physicians in London were a very select group, numbering about fifty.

According to the Galenic medicine practiced by these physicians, every individual had a particular "constitution" with its own humoral variation. One's humors could be altered by diet, exercise, sleep, elimination (including sexual activity), the emotions, and the quality of air—known to medicine as the six "nonnaturals" because they covered everything necessary to health over which a person had some control. A patient could run up a sizable bill as his or her doctor fine-tuned humors with a regimen suitable to the patient's individual condition. The standard regimens included bleeding, purging, sweating, and vomiting. The seasons came into play as well. In spring a person might have more blood, and bloodletting could restore a healthy balance. The onset of an illness, which presumed a corruption or putrefaction of the humors, called for evacuation to eliminate the putrid matter.[3] To an orthodox Galenist, the poison of plague called for an especially strong application of all the eliminating tools, including bleeding.

These aristocrats of the medical establishment looked down on everyone else, including the apothecaries and surgeons, whom they asserted were mere "empiricks," plying their trade like any artisan without the theoretical knowledge that alone made medicine intelligible. They did not have the last word, however, even within their own doctors' ranks. For some time a breakaway group of academically trained caregivers, calling themselves "chymical physitians," had challenged traditional medical wisdom in a pamphlet war of words. They spoke of a curative "vital spirit" inside the body that responded to the right chemical combinations. The plague offered them a splendid opportunity to gain a competitive edge over their old-fashioned rivals. Although about forty of the fifty doctors in the College of Physicians had fled to the country, many chemical physicians and their chemist associates were staying on. They claimed to wish to help the poor. If a desperate Londoner wanted to try something new and had the purse to do so, this group offered cures with salts, sulfur, mercury, and liquid gold. "Fight fire with fire," these avant-garde doctors declared, meaning that one should attack an ailment with an antidote as potent as the symptoms rather than following the Galenist use of opposites (e.g., a cooling substance such as beer for a fever).

Immediately below the physicians on the medical ladder were the apothecaries, who were pushing for a new royal charter to gain the right to treat patients as the physicians did, not just hand out remedies prescribed by them. Apothecaries had learned their trade mainly through apprenticeship, yet most had acquired a basic understanding of academic medicine along the way. Many already practiced medicine on their own, combining traditional medical advice and regimens with herbals, antipestilential pills and potions whose efficacy was borne out by a loyal following.

Apothecaries could easily be found about London. Thomas Spooner had a shop at the Red Lion, and Roger Dixon's house was close to the Thames in Water Lane near the Customs House. There were apothecary shops in Cheapside and around the Royal Exchange, and several were on main thoroughfares in Westminster. In Saint Giles in the Fields, William Boghurst dispensed medical advice and drugs at the White Hart.

Next down the ladder were surgeons, whose services were less costly than were doctors' treatments or apothecaries' drugs. The Company of Barber-

Facing page

Fig. 5. An ADVERTISEMENT from the Society of Chymical Physitians touching MEDICINES . . . for the Prevention, and for the Cure of the PLAGUE. Broadside licensed for printing on June 28, 1665. The eight chemical physicians listed in this ad used God's presumed blessing of their "search into . . . the mysterious nature of diseases" and the king's command to prepare plague remedies to attract clients and advance their campaign to organize as a rival to the College of Physicians. By permission of the British Library, shelfmark C.120.h.5

AN
ADVERTISEMENT
FROM THE
Society of Chymical Phyſitians,
TOUCHING
MEDICINES by them prepared, in purſuance of his
Majeſties Command,
For the *Prevention*, and for the *Cure* of the
PLAGUE.

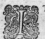

IT Being a matter avowed by the moſt laborious *Phyſitians* practiſing in this famous City, yea and now openly acknowledged by thoſe alſo in ſeveral Prints, who are principally addicted to *Galenick Doctrines* and *Medicines*, that Remedies made by *Chymical preparation* are of greater Excellence than any other, for preſervation from Diſeaſes, as well as for the Cure of them, and that the other failing, the people are to have recourſe unto *Chymical Medicines*, whereby it is clearly given and granted, that they are the moſt powerful and efficacious *Means*, and thereupon have been by thoſe worthy Perſons particularly recommended for publick uſe, in this ſad time and deplorable Eſtate of *Peſtilential Contagion*; We cannot but with all our hearts congratulate our Brethren, touching this their ſo ſeaſonable and ingenuous an acknowledgment, rejoicing to ſee the day, that the unhappy Controverſie betwixt us and them, touching the efficacy of *Medicines*, is now at an end : ſo that we look on it as a good *Omen* towards a more full and free coming over to us in the future, even of the moſt averſe of thoſe that till of late have been otherwiſe enclined ; and it gives hope, that we may one day come to a more Brotherly correſpondence, and unanimouſly endeavour to reform and rectifie the ſtate of Medicine, both as to Principles and Practiſe, according to the *Chymical* and more ancient way.

We therefore, the *Society of Chymical Phyſitians* of *London*, being deeply moved with commiſeration of the calamity befallen this great City by the *Peſtilence*, and perceiving it every day to encreaſe, notwithſtanding the uſe of thoſe *common Galenical Medicines*, which have been recommended to the people by others, have thought fit, in obedience to his Majeſties command, to hold ſeveral meetings, and have thereupon deliberately conſulted about the preparation of ſuch Medicines, both *Preſervative* and *Curative*, by Art Chymical, as are not borrowed out of former *Authors*, but agreeably deviſed and fitted to the nature of the preſent *Peſt*, which in many things differs from the *Peſts* of former times, or in *Forreign Countries* where thoſe Authors lived. Which Medicines ſo prepared we here offer to our Countrymen, not doubting but that the great God, who hath given us a heart and light to ſearch into the myſteries of *Nature*, and the *myſterious nature* of diſeaſes, will ſo ſecond our endeavours by his ſpecial bleſſing, as to make us and our *Remedies* as his own hands, to ſecure the ſound, and ſave the ſick from this devouring Maladie.

In purſuance whereof, it is thought meet to ſignifie the places, to which all perſons concerned may repair and be furniſhed with the *Antidotes* ſo by us prepared, at reaſonable Rates, with *Directions* how to uſe them in order to *Preſervation*, and in caſe of *Cure*.

Viz. at the Houſes of

Dr. *William Goddard*, in *St. John's Cloſe* neer *Clarkenwel*.	Dr. *Everard Manwaring* next door to the *Blew Boar* at the foot of *Ludgate* Hill without *Ludgate*.
Dr. *Marchamont Nedham* in *St. Thomas Apoſtles*.	Dr. *George Thompſon* next to the *Blew Boar* Inn without *Algate*.
Dr. *Edward Bolneſt* in *Jewen-ſtreet* neer *Cripplegate*.	Dr. *Thomas O Dowde* at his Houſe againſt *St. Clements* Church in the *Strand*.
Dr. *Thomas Williams* in *Two-Cranes Court* in *Fleet-ſtreet*.	Dr. *Richard Barker* in *Barbican*.

Theſe Places are named, becauſe our *Society* is not yet provided (as we intend ſuddenly to be) of a Publick Houſe or Colledge, with publick Officers, to whom the people might be directed to reſort for the *Medicines* ; and there is a neceſſity of doing ſomewhat immediately, becauſe of the preſent diſtreſs of his Majeſties Subjects.

Licenſed 28 June 1665.

London Printed for *John Starkey*, and are to be ſold at his Shop at the *Mitre* near *Temple-Bar*.

Surgeons and College of Physicians both were "well entrenched oligarchies dominated by self-perpetuating cliques," but surgeons had skills doctors didn't possess. They could cut for stones in bladders and kidneys, remove tumors, and fix dislocations and fractures. They were noted for their fine instruments—which no physician used, believing surgery to be beneath his calling. The outcome of a surgeon's treatment was easy to judge, unlike that of a doctor's fine-tuning of humors. Surgeons could be found around the hospitals for the poor—Saint Bartholomew's and Saint Thomas across London Bridge—and near many apothecaries. Their company hall was near the western wall and drew medical professionals as well as the interested public, such as Samuel Pepys, to their anatomy demonstrations and lectures.[4]

An estimate can be made of how many surgeons, apothecaries, and doctors offered medical care in London. Licensed practitioners connected to the three professional organizations numbered around 250, all of them men; an additional 250 persons, including 60 women, may have offered similar therapies without a license. The normal ratio was roughly one caregiver for every six hundred persons inside the old city, according to Andrew Wear, a specialist of early modern medical care in England.[5] Since most of the members of the College of Physicians had fled from the city and far fewer licensed caregivers practiced in the poor suburbs, the ratio in this sickly time was hardly encouraging. A merchant who had stayed on was unlikely to find his family doctor still in town. At any time working-class families in the suburbs were far less likely to see a male caregiver because there were fewer around than in the city and their fees were beyond reach. Parishes provided emergency medical services to their poorest residents, and during plague epidemics a few suburban parishes paid a doctor, apothecary, or surgeon to treat some of the infected poor with medicines or lancing of buboes.

Women caregivers were widely sought after for their special skills and nurturing ways. Furthermore, midwives and many nurses were believed to be immune to the plague, having already been in the thick of the epidemic and not touched. These female medics often knew as much as if not more than the theoretically oriented men when it came to practical health care. Some people high and low were skeptical of London's nurses, accusing them of thievery or even murder, but nurses were the major source of medical care for poor families on parish relief. At Saint Margaret Westminster, they were paid two shillings a week to care for a child and five shillings a week to nurse an adult. Once a family was shut up with the plague, a live-in nurse was likely to be its only caregiver.

The line between all these "professional" caregivers and the rest of the medical marketplace, always blurry, virtually disappeared in the face of the mysterious plague, which treated Galenist theory and bogus cures with equal indifference. Quacks, according to Dr. Hodges (who was staying on), "thrust into every hand some trash or other under the disguise of a pompous title."[6] Yet who was the "legitimate" practitioner and who the quack, when the answer depended on effectiveness rather than the origin of the therapy? Dr. Willis, a paragon of medical professionalism and friend of Reverend Patrick, had his own "when all else fails" cures for standard ailments. To treat jaundice the doctor combined fresh urine with ashes from the ash tree and reduced the mixture by heating to a paste. As it dried and hardened, the patient's jaundice vanished. Willis related that this cure was known by the "vulgar sort," which can be translated to mean that he looked to popular medicine when his learned remedies didn't work.[7]

Dr. Cocke touted himself as the doctor of the poor. Fair enough. Most of his plague manuals and emergency recipes were priced just right for them. Many well-worn herbal recipes prescribed by doctors like Cocke, however, probably originated with a white witch lacking the university education he considered necessary for the practice of medicine.[8] A white witch was known to try honest, "good" cures and had quite a closet full of medicaments, usually herbal, the result of trial, error, and folk tradition. These cures worked their way up the social ladder via the household maid of a noble lady in the country, for example, and then passed on through a male relative in the city to his university-trained physician. Perhaps the countess of Huntingdon's healing acumen, well known among her Leicestershire neighbors and her relatives in London, originated in these upward-bound remedies. Out in Essex, Lady Mary Luckyn had much the same reputation as a conduit of medical wisdom.[9]

Medical knowledge could work its way in the other direction, too. Almanacs and books of herbals were accessible to the literate and through them to others who could not read. Home remedies were jotted down in a family "receipt" or "recipe" book containing information about cooking, health, and run-of-the-mill cures for distempers. People treated family members when illness came their way. Friends swapped recipes. For remedies, someone could just as easily go to the garden as to Galen.[10]

Antidotes Spiritual and Material

When I wake up I thank God for preserving me the night past, then I gargle my throat, wash my mouth, nostrils, temples, ears, and forehead with vinegar and water.

—DR. THOMAS COCKE, *Cautionary Rules and Directions* (1665)

Ask God for his blessing, Dr. Cocke affirmed, "without which neither Master Paul nor Apollo, Galenist nor Chymist, Food nor Physick can do anything." The belief was common, especially for plague.[11]

In 1664, a son of Rev. Ralph Josselin fell gravely ill, passed through the "crisis," and recovered. Josselin gave God credit for the miracle of his child's recovery and was also grateful that a physician friend could stay with the family through the ordeal. When Ralph fell ill himself and took to bed with a fever, he again found relief from a physician's hand. But most of all he relied on prayer. His diary often began with prayer and then ended with thanks to God. He inspected his own urine, read the odd medical book, and used herbal concoctions made by his wife or a noble lady friend while also believing that, through God's mercy, his wife's prayers had saved the life of a village woman. Faith healing was as natural to these villagers as breathing good country air.

From his parsonage and farm on the outskirts of Earls Colne, Josselin gazed at the flat fields broken by blue-black, gently rolling hills on the horizon. The stifling air brought no signs of rain, and his crops were wilting. The plague had been in Yarmouth for some time and was spreading like wildfire around London. But more disturbing thoughts were on his mind. As the holy days approached, he asked his congregation to search within themselves for what might be displeasing to God and "rectify it [so that] His anger might be averted." He did not object to his parishioners or anyone else reaching for medical potions; he did the same. But he pondered their limited efficacy in healing. "God in mercy preserve us, and heal the city," he wrote in his journal concerning what he had heard about the response in London to the pestilential taint. "Medicaments used, but no publique call to repentance."[12]

Closer to London, Reverend Patrick's old friend from his first parish settled into her sister-in-law's home outside Brentwood, Essex. Though she missed her husband, Denis, who was continually on the move as head of the Royal Navy's victualing operation, Elizabeth Gauden was relieved to be away from their mansion across the river from plague-ridden Westminster. She had just received a letter from Symon Patrick, who had buried sixteen victims of the plague during the past week, five times the weekly burials from all causes before this visitation. He was discussing, in his roundabout fashion, ways they could protect themselves from the plague—he in the infected capital and she just off the main road that connected London to the Essex countryside.

"There is some danger no doubt in this place," he wrote from his Covent Garden lodgings. "But I am not in any feare, which will make the danger lesse." Symon and Elizabeth were writing letters once or twice a week. Writing to her helped him relax after preparing his Sunday sermon and again after the long midweek services the king had mandated "so long as it pleaseth God to visit the land with the pestilence." The pastor had just finished writing a homily on the Ninety-first Psalm. "It is apparent from what physicians write concerning preservatives against this pestilential disease," Patrick added, "that they can prescribe nothing like trust in God, which contains the virtues of them all. It expels fear [and] calms the passions and stops the rage of the boiling in the blood."[13]

But no one was free of worry at this time. Reverend Patrick's relative medical sophistication might have made him more anxious about being alone in the daytime and going out into the distempered air at night to pray at interments. As a precaution, he had brought in a supply of medicaments, which distinguished him from Reverend Josselin. "I forgot to tell you," Symon informed Elizabeth, "that instead of the plague drink you writ of they have sent me plague water." The mix-up does not seem to have bothered him. The new plague water, he informed her, "is distilled and nothing like what I had before; but never trouble them to send mee more." To Elizabeth's worries he responded reassuringly: "Dr. Michael Thwayte directed me to make and drink presently of London treacle and Lady Allen's water." Then he admitted the truth: "I bought both presently, but forgot still to mix them: only now and then I take a little treacle."

Patrick paid more attention to diet than to drugs. He knew the classic regimen, from choosing the right meat and drink to maintaining a calm disposition and regular evacuation, including semen. He referred offhandedly to sex, teasing Elizabeth about an imaginary mistress. Symon was more concerned about their emotions, especially hers. The doctors said emotional stress could invite the infection and maybe even bring it on by unbalancing the humors. His favorite emotional antidote was his trust in God, but there was a close second. Elizabeth's love for him, he declared, would keep him alive by making him long for it. He called this love between them a strong antidote. "In what dispensary did you find it? Its a medicine of your owne making."[14]

Prescribing Physick

To Break the tumour [bubo]: Take a great onion, hollow it, put into it a fig, rue cut small, a dram of Venice treacle; put it in a wet paper, and roast it in embers; apply it hot unto the tumour.

To Draw: When it is broken, to draw and heal it, take the yoke of an egg, one ounce of honey of roses, turpentine one ounce, wheat flour a little, London treacle a dram and a half; mix these well, spread it upon leather. Change [the poltice] twice a day.

—College of Physicians, *Certain Necessary Directions for the Prevention and Cure of the Plague,* 1665

Physicians had long employed bleeding, sweating, purging, and vomiting to treat a wide range of physical ailments including fevers.[15] Apothecaries had special juleps for thirst and opiates for sleep; these concoctions could relieve much of the misery of a plague patient as he prepared his mind and soul for death. Surgeons were in demand with their lancets or long-handled cauteries; they knew how to draw out the poison from a bubo after softening it with a plaster. "You will find it less cost, paine, or trouble to go to a chyrurgeon [surgeon] to make an issue," it was claimed, "than to have him come to you to dress a carbuncle."[16]

Times were changing. The College of Physicians' new plague manual cautioned its members not to use bleeding, purging, or vomiting as therapies for plague. Too many patients died afterward from loss of blood or a weakened condition. But old habits die hard. After all, ancient Egyptians and Greeks had found bleeding to be therapeutic, and so did their European successors.[17]

Dr. Thomas Sydenham mixed the old ways (bloodletting and sweating) with the new (aggressively attacking an abnormality with a like quality). A caregiver, he advised, should rely on "heating medicines even though plague is an inflammatory disease." By producing a sweat, he continued, the body would exhale the infectious particles from the blood. If this failed and the blood became more inflamed with heat, bleeding would be in order. If the patient's pain became unbearable, the doctor resorted to a favorite tonic used by the chemical physicians—opium. If all these devices failed, he recommended relying on nature's therapeutic powers and hoping for the best.

The plague drug of choice was theriac, a mixture of viper's flesh, garlic, rue, vinegar, walnuts, onion, and (to leave nothing to chance) opium. For the very poor an onion could be applied directly to a plague sore to draw out the venom. The ancients of Alexandria and Rome had discovered the perfect antidote to plague poison: viper's flesh, "like attracting like."[18] They tested it on criminals with apparent success, and it took on a mythic reputation.

Chemists on the canals of Venice developed their own theriac plague water, which was widely merchandised as Venice treacle. The English rushed into the market with a variation, London treacle. All the middling and upper-class people staying in London seemed to have a supply, and those who fled took it with them. For increased marketability, plague waters and powders were named after famous users like Sir Walter Raleigh and were advertised with grandiose claims in Roger L'Estrange's semiweekly newssheets. The duchess of Kent's powder was "in the hands of a Person of Quality that had the honor to wait upon the said countess until her death" (seemingly a counterproductive statement).

Exclusive shops enticed the well-to-do purchasing public. Dr. Waldron's electuary against the plague was sold by Richard Loundes at the White Lion near the little north door of Saint Paul's cathedral, at Mr. Magnes' shop in Russell Street, Covent Garden, and at Mistress Blundel's in Westminster Hall under the Court of Common Pleas—"and nowhere else." There were no better locations to reach the richer sort. Incidentally, all three retailers were booksellers. The latest plague literature could be purchased in tandem with the newest edition of a guide to healthy eating, *The Art of Cookery*.[19]

Families' all-purpose "receipt" books often contained cures for plague and other medical disasters. "Keep this above all worldly treasure and under God trust it," wrote the proud possessor of a plague recipe, "for there never was man, woman nor childe that ever this disceived if it were taken in time." It was also good for smallpox, purple fever, measles, and surfeit.[20]

It was now two months after Samuel Pepys had first run across people sharing their knowledge of plague remedies at London's Great Coffee House in May, "some saying one thing, some another." His own plague remedies included some plague waters. When abroad he cheerfully imbibed those his guests offered. The sight of red crosses on the doors in Drury Lane sent him scurrying for another kind of prophylactic: "It put me into an evil conception of myself and my [foul] smell, so that I was forced to buy some roll-tobacco to smell and chaw—which take away the apprehension." He had no doubt heard the legend that tobacconists did not die from the pestilence. Schoolboys at Eton that summer were caned if they missed their daily smoke before matins, and gravediggers were never without their pipes. Two centuries later, workmen excavating the London Underground discovered clay "plague" pipes along with a cluster of human skeletons.[21]

Tobacco and plague water put Samuel in a better mood, but he was casting about for more pleasurable prophylactics. By July, his rabbit's foot, which had warded off colds during the bitter winter, no longer seemed an adequate talisman. On his rounds, he stuffed his nose with sweet-smelling herbs. On occasion, however, he went about in hackney coaches that might not have been disinfected after transporting the sick to the pesthouse, as public orders required. Still more puzzling was the increase in his dalliances as the plague claimed more and more victims, since many of his trysting grounds were rife with infection. Afterward, Pepys recorded the encounters with a playful mixture of foreign words in his private diary—in shorthand, like the other entries, to escape detection if his wife should chance upon his journal.[22]

Pepys arrived home late one night after traveling up and down the Thames on business. He was bone tired yet relieved to see his assistant Will, whom he insisted on putting up despite fears of catching the infection from him. The next day also promised to be busy, but he didn't intend it to be completely taken up with his navy colleagues and suppliers. At the Harp and Ball, Samuel made a "bargain" with Mary to go to the good air up in Highgate and Hampstead. At the appointed time, he returned to the tavern by boat, and they took a coach northward, he "much pleased with her company, pretty and innocent," while he had what pleasure "almost" he would with her.

That night, Pepys was too tired to put this reckless tryst into his quaint multilanguage code. "And so at night, weary and sweaty, it being very hot beyond bearing," he wrote, "we back again and I set her down in St. Martins Lane." He had gone on to the Royal Exchange, written some letters at his office, and finally turned in for the night. "So away to bed," he ended his diary note, "shifting myself and taking some Venice Treacle, feeling myself out of order."[23]

A standard procedure for keeping a home plague-free was to burn tar, pitch, niter, frankincense, and rosin in the room most frequented and also before the doors and on the rooftops. For the poorest families, brimstone or vitriol was recommended. A typical recipe reads: "Place green vitriol, beaten well, over coals in a chaffing dish, and keep for use; or pestilential vinegar thrown on a hot brick."

No one was more adept at capitalizing on the popularity of fumigation than was James Angier. Flushed with self-proclaimed success in Paris, Lyons, and Toulouse, his London practice took off in June, helped by a shrewd publicity stunt. Angier chose the perfect site for his demonstration: an infected house in Saint Giles in the Fields that had claimed four plague victims and left two others sick out of twelve lodgers. Members of the king's inner circle eagerly accompanied Angier to the home. He came through the test with flying colors (no more deaths). His ads multiplied, as did the shops and taverns stocking his fumigants. A receipt for his fumigation of Mrs. Southwall's home in Saint Giles in the Fields has survived. He netted ten pounds for that one call—more than the average household's annual income of seven pounds. In 1921 Angier's accomplishments were proudly chronicled in a commemorative booklet by the Angier Chemical Company at 86 Clerkenwell Road.

Dr. Cocke instructed householders that it was safe to throw saltpeter, oil, or a bag of gunpowder into their outdoor braziers to ward off the infected air. He also recommended ringing bells and firing off guns. Was he serious? At least he was offering the poor a chuckle or two, as these costly prophylactics were as elusive for them as was the horizon.

Something for the Poor

The swelling under the ears, armpits or in the groins . . . require the care and skills of the expert Chirurgeon. But do not leave the poorer sort destitute of good remedies:

Pull off the feathers from the tails of living cocks, hens, pigeons, or chickens, and holding their bills, hold them hard to the Botch or Swelling and so keep them at that part until they die [the birds that is]; and by this means draw out the poison.

—College of Physicians, *Certain Necessary Directions for . . . the Plague*

Poor Londoners felt trapped by the plague in a way that Samuel Pepys and Sir William Turner could scarcely comprehend. The poor were less mobile, less able to pay for "physick," less trusting of academic medicine, and far more distant from medical texts because few of them could read.[24] If the *Certain Necessary Directions* reached these unlettered folk by word of mouth, they may have laughed painfully at its naiveté. Could anyone possibly find a reasonably priced live fowl in the local markets during this visitation? And what nurse could be conned into grasping a squawking bird and pressing it against the running sore of a bubo while her patient squirmed in pain and fright?

Again Dr. Cocke was helpful. His little paper on plague preparations for the poor was placed in bundles at the doors of suburban churches by order of the duke of Albemarle.[25] Housewives could go to their kitchen cupboards and find all the necessary ingredients: salt, London treacle (two or three pence worth would do), vinegar, and saltpeter, plus broths, ales, and the run of household herbs. At the top of every list stood garlic, the essential poor person's medicine in many folk traditions. Cocke included advice on sweating and keeping down the fever, how to induce vomiting and when to stop it, as well as how to prepare homemade lozenges and plasters. At the Pestle and Mortar in French Lane or the Queen's Arms in Fan Church Street, his "blistering plaister" sold for a penny or two. These plasters were to be placed on buboes for up to six or eight hours, after which the swellings broke and were anointed with oil of roses. Cocke grew enthusiastic as he ticked off the items one could use: unguent of althea, cordials, and posset drinks made of sage to aid in breaking and draining the buboes. But here he was forgetting his audience, slipping back into the rich man's balms that these poor people would never see.

Daniel Defoe said that there had never been so many people consulting astrologers and their almanac advice as during the plague epidemic, and he may have been right. It cost a poor peddler only a penny or two to have someone read *Poor Robin* aloud, and the almanac's tips were laced not only with outrageous humor but also with advice from astrological signs for plague treatments. This pestilential season, the advice ran, will not cure mad persons. The summer's fleas "will lie with women without asking any leave," the almanac continued, and the noose at Tyburn will remain an "eye-sore" to highwaymen and cutpurses. Only the last quip was a bit of a stretch; trials had ended with the coming of the infection, and murderers were more likely to die in a plague-infested jail waiting for the courts to start up again.[26]

The celebrated astrologer William Lilly had been an artful dodger of both Revolution and Restoration censors and had amassed a considerable fortune along with making two profitable marriages and publishing sensational prognostics containing vivid illustrations suggesting a great pestilence and fire. His fame among the rich and poor spread throughout the land, and not just for his almanac's medical advice. His hands-on therapy attracted a steady stream of patients to his rented lodgings on the Strand.[27]

As early as April, Lilly had been fearful of a pestilential summer, yet he remained in Westminster through May and into June, leaving only at the request of his landlord, who panicked at the sight of sick patients who might be carrying plague on their bodies.[28] Lilly and his family moved to their country home upstream in Surrey, generously taking the landlord's children along for safekeeping. The landlord and his wife died in the city, but Lilly's newly extended family all survived, and he continued his medical practice in his rural neighborhood.

The poorer sort "flockt to him from several parts," bringing along their urine for inspection just like rich people. Lilly did well by doing good. He treated rich and poor alike with his standard Galenic treatments, adding a cordial and something to sweat the poison out for plague patients. Occasionally, a courtier waiting out the plague in the country pressed a shilling or half a crown into his hand for advice and for treating the local poor "freely and without money." His purse swelled with these windfalls.[29]

Lilly walked the blurry line between traditional academic medicine and magic. In a typical year he took on two thousand clients, including nobles and gentry (124), seafarers (104), female servants (254), and trades and crafts persons (128).[30] Like most astrologers, Lilly was consulted on missing husbands and pregnancy (was she or wasn't she?) and to determine under what astrological signs and climatic conditions the conception of a male child and heir was likeliest. Lilly, Gadbury, and other medical astrologers read stars and planetary conjunctions to see when the air would become corrupted, and they told their followers in what season they should be bled, purged, or left to nature.[31]

Belief in witchcraft had just passed its peak a generation before, when it had been written: "Tis a common practice of some men to go first to a witch, and then to a Physician." Skeptics abounded now, yet white witches (mainly women) and other popular healers who might tap into the supernatural for their cures were as popular as the astrologers who read the signs of the zodiac. The line between magic and religion itself was somewhat indistinct. Wasn't the devil driven out of the newborn at baptism? Monarchs laid their hands on scrofula patients to the sound of an old incantation: "The king touches thee; God heals thee." The historian Keith Thomas, in his classic *Religion and the Decline of Magic*, tells us moderns: "If magic is to be defined as the employment of ineffective techniques to allay anxiety when effective ones are not available, then we must recognize that no society will ever be free from it."[32]

The white witch was surely busy this plaguetime, even if she was all but invisible in the written records. Her patients came, as they always had, for a balm or charm, perhaps a cure for sick cattle, even a corrective for sterility in a newly married couple. Did she really know "medicine"? And did it matter? Those who sought her or a male conjurer believed in the magic. Possibly she offered plague preservatives and cures not too different from those offered by doctors on the Strand. The odd witch may have died of plague, but no one accused witches of causing death from this disease.[33]

Like the witch, the contemporary doctor believed in the efficacy of the cures he was offering. The noted chemical physician Dr. George Thomson offered a special cure for the pestilence derived from an emulsified "Buffo frog." Thomson's treatment called for killing the toad by hanging it by a leg, drying it, and then grinding it finely. "The venomous Idea of hatred and terror in the Buffo," he wrote with total confidence, "annihilates the Image of the pestilential poison"—another case of "fighting fire with fire"[34] or "like with like."

Who in this time of testing was the false physician, the purveyor of useless magical cures, the outright quack? For that matter, who in the medical marketplace was in a position to judge?

Wonder Drugs

I am looking out for new quarters, where I may have two roomes, and one for stills to work in, in the winter, if the lord give life, where I intend to sett up divers chymical stills, if the lord please, and one furnace amongst the rest for the maine worke if you can furnish mee with *Materia Prima*.

—JOHN ALLIN, Southwark, to Philip Fryth in Rye, September 14, 1665

As the dog days of summer approached, the devoted alchemist John Allin was prowling the plague-infested streets of Southwark in search of a rare plant that he called his *prima materia*, otherwise known as *coelifolium* or *trammels nostoc*. This was not the ideal time for such an undertaking. An open plague pit was visible from his window, and death was "approaching nearer and nearer." In case he died, the widower Allin sought care for his three young children in Rye and also safekeeping of his writings on plague and other valuables. But his real obsession in these days was distilling his precious *prima materia* into a dark, oily substance that would transform gold into the ultimate wonder drug, known to the ages as *aurum potabile*, the secret to long life and health.[35]

Allin was following in the footsteps of distinguished herbalists, astrologers, and alchemists from the previous generation.[36] He was not alone. By Middle Temple Gate in Fleet Street, one could obtain an ounce of the pre-

cious potion for five pounds. A stone's throw away, a rival stationer offered a
better deal: for only one pound, one could have *aurum potabile* distilled from
"a pure christaline and innocent spirit, and known consequently to be the
universal medicine and an antidote against all pestilential and contagious
distempers."[37]

What no one dared say was that every substance ever used as a gold sol-
vent had failed. Allin pressed on in quest of his special plant, asking his
friends Fryth and Jeake in the country to be on the lookout for it. The elusive
spores or seeds must be collected under perfect conditions, he warned. They
were to look for them on sandy soil in the dead of night after a rain accompanied by a southwest wind. If they waited until dawn, the precious specimens would be shriveled up and ruined. With all the excitement of a chemistry pupil, Allin scribbled a postscript to a letter to Fryth: "I saw this day
some *prima materia* in the streets."[38]

The competition between rival wonder drugs intensified as the population
in the capital thinned. Those who remained could choose between powdered
unicorn horn, phoenix egg yolk, and an Arab cure-all from stones in camels'
intestines. A popular herbalist from the previous age had touted the medici-
nal benefits of eringo root, or sea holly. It cured yellow jaundice and dropsy;
relieved wind, colic, and pain in the loins; provoked urine; and expelled the
kidney stone.[39] Now it was turning up in Samuel Great's apothecary shop in
Colchester, whose inhabitants were caught in the epidemic that Ralph Josselin had been dreading in spite of all his faith. Great's pharmaceutical practice
flourished. He made a special candied eringo from sea holly found on the
nearby coast. The local people were convinced it would protect against the
pestilence and even cure it.

Dr. Hodges thought these exotic cure-alls were hoodwinking the gullible
public, who in desperation tried anything as the plague toll climbed from
2,000 to 3,900 in just two weeks. The hottest weeks of the summer were still
ahead; the plague was far from peaking. Hodges tested the camel stones for
their alleged effects, increasing the dose tenfold to give them a fair trial. As
he suspected, the stones were a dud, just like the poisonous toad and myth-
ical unicorn![40] Half a century before, the Great Plague commentator Thomas
Dekker had been equally scornful of quacks and mountebanks "sucking the
sweetness of silver (and now and then of aurum potabile) out of the poison
of blains and carbuncles."

But behind most doctors of physick loomed the shadow of a white witch.
Remove ourselves from Thomas Sydenham and we find echoes of John Allin's rhetorical claims, for their medical worlds overlapped in practice and in

theory. To be sure, there were some outright charlatans this summer, deliber-ately deluding the frightened and gullible trapped inside the capital city. A remarkable con story from this terrible time bears repeating. A London con-stable caught four thieves robbing a pestilential corpse in a London street and asked why they weren't afraid of contagion. They replied that their pro-tection came from rubbing themselves with vinegar mixed with various herbs, a sure prophylactic. Word of this conversation spread quickly and in a few days London apothecaries announced the latest curative for plague, "Four Thieves Vinegar." It enjoyed a brisk sale and was marketed long after the plague disappeared.[41]

There is another perspective on this manipulation of the market. During one of his walks in an infected section of town, John Allin noticed people wearing amulets. His curiosity drew him closer. Dr. Cocke, academic physi-cian that he was, would have nothing to do with these "deleterious and poisonous things." But Allin studied the effect of the toad poison in these amulets. "Upon any infection invadeing from time to time," he reported tri-umphantly to his friends in the country, they raise a blister, "which a plaister heales, and so they are well." Perhaps he might "get the true preparation of it," he told Philip Fryth, hardly able to contain himself. If successful, he promised to send a sample in the mail.[42]

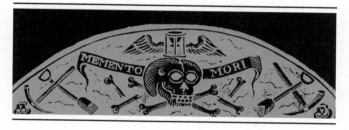

Plague's Progress

It is now day. Let us look forth and try what consolation rises with the sun. Not any. For before the jewel of the morning be fully set in silver, a hundred hungry graves stand gaping and every one of them, as at a breakfast, hath swallowed down ten or eleven lifeless carcasses. Before dinner in the same gulf are twice so many more devoured. And before the sun takes his rest those numbers are doubled.

—THOMAS DEKKER, *The Wonderful Year* (1603)

The Rising Toll

"The most extraordinary hot that I ever knew," Samuel Pepys recorded in his diary in mid-July. The intense heat seemed to be drawing the infection right out of the ground, just as people said happened in a pestilential season. "Plague grows hott," Ralph Josselin penned in his journal two weeks later. "Persons fall down in London streets." In two short weeks the official plague count had doubled, from 1,089 to 2,010. Plague victims were dying in all the suburban parishes and almost half of the parishes within the walls. And with the hot, dry weather came the specter of another disaster. Farmers were reporting an extremely meager hay crop, the lifeblood of healthy livestock. Shortages of vegetables, fruit, dairy products, and meat loomed. Even if the summer harvest were normal, what farmers would dare bring their vegetables and fruits and livestock into the infected capital? "The country feares all trade with London," Josselin observed. Fortunately, there was a break in the weather. Showers cooled the city air, and in the countryside crops grew far better than anyone expected. By early August Josselin wrote: "God good in the season. Harvest comes in well. A great rain which the earth needed."[1]

The relief was short-lived. In London the heat and sickness began striking every parish.[2] Saint Margaret Westminster's situation was among the worst. In the best of times, this parish had too few manufacturing jobs for its large number of workers, making them overdependent on employment with the courtier and professional service classes. The wholesale flight from plague of courtiers had collapsed the job market and placed an extraordinary burden on the parish's poor-relief funds and voluntary donations.

The preeminent courtier parish of Covent Garden could probably cope, thanks to its smaller population and money from absent peers and tradesmen sent in to Reverend Patrick. But sickness and death were about to devastate the heavily industrialized suburbs outside the courtier district. Smelly, messy trades like brewing, glassmaking, tanning, and printing outside the walls and down at the riverbank had attracted plague in past epidemics. Porters, who carried goods from the wharf to manufacturers throughout London, were also susceptible, as were servants, whose tasks could take them almost anywhere. Saint Giles Cripplegate alone accounted for 130 trades and 14,000 jobs; if past patterns held, mortality in many of these groups would be high again. Cloth making was at the top of the vulnerable trades; in previous epidemics, weavers, cord winders, buttonhole makers, tailors, and glovers had fallen in droves.[3]

Inside the wall, still the safest place to be, another dangerous situation loomed. Merchants and financiers were the heart and soul of the old city, and many of them were staying after that first mass exodus. But how long could the goldsmith Vyner continue trading money at the Sign of the Vine on Lombard Street, or the scriveners Clayton and Morris keep managing the dwindling volume of legal papers and property rentals at the Flying Horse near the Royal Exchange, or Alderman Turner stay with his unsold bolts of cloth at the Golden Fleece in Saint Paul's churchyard? The merchant guilds were closing their halls, with no meetings planned by their members "as long as God's displeasure lasts." Individual guildsmen were left on their own.

Parishes close to Dr. Hodges' home and Alderman Turner's shop near the cathedral were shutting up their first infected houses and inns. The clerk of Saint Olave Hart Street was recording the first plague fatalities a street away from Pepys' apartment and the navy office on Seething Lane. Throughout the metropolis stood shut-up houses with their red crosses. A nurse was always within, and outside a warder zealously guarded the door except when buying "necessaries" for the inmates. A bearer with his dead-cart stopped in front of a newly cross-marked door calling out: "Bring out your dead." The bearer, often an unsavory looking individual (for who would take such a job?), strapped down the body to a board, or if there were two bearers, they might carry out a body on a sling and place it in a dead-cart. Eventually, the sad cargo was deposited in the nearest churchyard or plague pit.

One by one neighborhood lanes emptied of traffic as the epidemic spread. Residents stayed indoors as much as possible, sealed their windows, and kept braziers or pots of fumigants burning to clean the air. The shrunken core of courtiers and professionals in Westminster and the members of the city's merchant guilds knew they would be handed a gigantic bill for relief of the sick and unemployed in the coming weeks. The king was no help. His mind was on the war at sea, the contagion approaching the royal assemblage up the Thames at Hampton Court, and, when possible, on distraction (having brought along every diversion from court musicians to his favorite mistress). Pepys had gone to the king's temporary residence on navy business on the tenth of July and was taken aback by the degree of panic, worse than in the city: "It is, I perceive, an unpleasant thing to be at Court, everyone being fearful of one another; and all so sad, inquiring after the plague—so that I stole away with my horse."[4]

Changing Street Scenes

That none be suffered to sing or cry ballads in the streets, to sell by way of hawking any goods or commodities whatsoever.
—Proclamation of the Lord Mayor, July 4, 1665

Silence enveloped the city. Gone were the hawkers of wares; they had been forbidden to serve the public. The city's criers—"Buy brumes, almanacke; mackrill and mussels; aqua vitae! Buy any milk?"—were mute. Missing was the familiar voice of the ratcatcher:

> Rats or Mice! Ha' ye any rats, mice, polecats or weasels?
> Or ha' ye any old sows sick of the measles?
> I can kill them, and I can kill moles,
> And I can kill vermin that creepeth up and down and peepeth in holes.[5]

Rather than rats and mice, the Guildhall focused on killing their enemies— cats and dogs. Neighborhood beadles and constables had gone through the streets at the end of June telling householders to kill "all their dogs of what sort or kind soever before Thursday next at ye furthest." The deadline passed and negligent pet owners faced prosecution, if the arm of the law could reach them.[6]

A flurry of controls on human movement came next. Public gatherings were forbidden. Schools for boys and girls closed down, including dancing and French schools. To the detriment of justice, the city's law courts also stopped their normal functioning. Old Bailey was shut with spectacular abruptness. A man was indicted for blasphemy, but when he appeared before the judges he looked very sickly. A physician from the pesthouse was called in and searched him, discovering a plague sore. The justices suspended trials, and the penal system limped along with occasional arrests and interim detention.[7]

Dissenters holding illegal "conventicles" in private dwellings were prime targets for arrest, for they might be plotting an uprising against the absent king and cathedral dean under cover of plague. Quakers were well represented at Newgate prison, where jail fever and plague broke out. Debtors were more likely to be put into Ludgate prison or a secondary jail, called a "comptor." Prisoners were provided with food and running water from the city conduits by order of the Guildhall, though supplies were not dependable.

Watches were mounted at the gates and landing places on the Thames "to restrain and prevent the ingress of all vagrants, beggars, loose and dangerous people." Watermen were forbidden to carry into the city any obviously infected or suspicious-looking person. The mayor ordered the high parish authorities to clamp down on disorderly tippling, gaming, rowing on the river, "and other offenses," especially on Sundays. Here was a multipurpose decree, linking existing laws against profaning the Lord's Day with punishment of licentious behavior that spread the infection and further provoked God's righteous anger.

Taverns and inns were also suspect. All vintners, inn holders, sellers of strong water, and alehouse and coffeehouse keepers were forbidden to "entertain" citizens (though citizens could still order food and drink sent to their homes). Only traveling guests were to be accommodated on the premises—"with sobriety and moderation." This was just one regulation too much for city dwellers with precious few avenues left to allay their jitters. Samuel Pepys had already chafed at the ban on fairs, maypole dancing, and cherry bobbing. He was especially inconvenienced by the closing of the theaters—his favorite nonamorous entertainment. In noncompliance he continued to use the taverns and inns of London and Westminster, both for flirting and for arranging contracts with navy suppliers. These establishments closed only when a proprietor died or finally gave up and headed to the clear country air. To his delight, Pepys found some of his favorite coffee houses off Cheapside still open.

By order of the privy council only one type of public gathering was permitted, even encouraged: special plague services at the cathedral, abbey, and parish churches. These rituals had begun in June, with an official day of celebration after the Royal Navy's victory over the Dutch off Lowestoft. Sunday and midweek services continued with a litany against the plague and prayers of contrition, supplemented with special Fast Day services on the first Wednesday of each month. These services, held in all London churches and throughout the realm, doubtless gave solace to worshipers and brought in money for infected households and citizens out of work. Though many rectors had fled to the country, their assistants or temporary replacements courageously filled many of the gaps. No one seemed to mind that popular dissenting preachers ejected at the Restoration were slipping back into their pulpits and exhorting their old congregations to repent their sins and wait on the Lord's mercy.

The popular fairs around London and in the countryside were cancelled one after another until God's avenging hand was lifted. There would be no Bartholomew's fair outside Aldersgate this year. Its carnival-seeking habitués, from noble dandies and masked ladies to cutpurses and painted women of fortune, were scattered to the four winds.[8]

Alderman Turner looked at his unsold bolts of fine cloth and pondered the controls he and his colleagues were placing on the city and its liberties. "I have little to say at present," he told his Paris partners, "there being nothing to doe by reason of the sicknesse." Perhaps with divine assistance, the Guildhall's regulations might check the progress of the plague, he wrote unconvincingly. "But in ye interim every one hastes out of towne which causes that there is no sale for goods and merchants pay ill."[9] Of course, the "every one" he referred to were the "better sort" with country places or family to depend on.

Sir William's luxury trade was uncertain, and the other merchant guilds were in trouble. He could scarcely fathom the plight of the working-class people on whose health the well-being of the city and suburbs ultimately depended. Though the poor had no way of voicing their needs directly to Mayor Lawrence at the Guildhall or Captain General Albemarle at the Cockpit in deserted Whitehall, one door was open to them. In the weeks to come, the neighborhood parish would be their primary source of spiritual comfort and material support.

Parish Responses

The prayers of the church are continued and ye persons attending as yor worship
was informed . . . Great complaint there is of necessity [among the poor].
—STEPHEN BING, petty canon of Saint Paul's cathedral,
to Dean Sancroft, July 27, 1665

From the outside, these neighborhood churches appeared idle between services. But often someone was busily engaged inside. The governing body of
priest and vestry had met several times in May and June to set up relief and
burial procedures and to establish the weekly wages for searchers, nurses,
warders, and buriers. After that, the vestry rarely met as a body; it was too
risky to come together, and the churchwardens would know how to carry on.
They had the parish account books and cash and the authority to improvise
if the needs outgrew the means.

Bells had to be repaired and broken ropes replaced from the constant ringing for deaths and burials. Sheds were needed in every churchyard to house
the buriers and searchers away from the public. The parish clerk attended
burials and kept a running account in the register of all deaths, occasional
christenings, and even less frequent weddings. The collection of poor taxes
by "collectors of the poor" and their disbursement by the overseers of the
poor at the command of the churchwardens were crucial lifelines. Gifts from
inside and out of the parish provided further aid. Most of the money, in one
way or another, was linked inexorably to dying.[10]

In July the contours of death emerged all too clearly in the Bills of Mortality posted each Thursday morning in parishes and many public places.
The most widely infected parishes were now the densely populated Saint
Giles in the Fields, Saint Giles Cripplegate, and Saint Margaret Westminster (table 4).[11] During a normal, nonplague year, the clerk at Saint Margaret's recorded 10 to 20 burials a week. In 1665 the toll climbed from 14 the
first week of the outbreak to 411 by late summer. By the year's end the official
total would be 4,710. Many more residents died without being registered, and
another 78 succumbed to plague the next year. Hearth tax accounts identify
3,061 heads of household in Saint Margaret's. At the plague's peak, the poor
tax and other means would pay for the care, feeding, and/or burial of up to
1,700 persons in a single week.[12]

In Saint Margaret's churchwardens' account book for 1665,[13] every item of
expense was tabulated, down to the candles that lit the night for the grave-

diggers, new bell ropes and shovels, axes and burial shrouds—the closest that many of the departed had to a coffin. The watchers' names and the locations of the houses they guarded provide a shadowy map of how the disease spread. The cat and dog catchers were paid for disposing of stray animals— three to four hundred at a time! Apothecaries were paid for physick, sur- geons for lancing and dressing buboes, and doctors for their therapies. Sev- eral of these medical providers, sadly, found their way into burial records. The existing pesthouse was expanded by ten "rooms," and supplies were brought in for eating, sleeping, and burying (see appendix B).[14] These ex- traordinary steps in plague relief were reenacted time and again in every par- ish within Greater London—and beyond.

Warders at the red-crossed door of dwelling after dwelling in alleys and lanes were visual proof of Saint Margaret's plague burden. Close to the grand King Street, which stretched from Whitehall to the abbey, stood a checker- board of uneven suburban housing with fitting names like Long Ditch, Bell Alley, and Thieving Lane. Beyond them lay a ramshackle hamlet called Knightsbridge. When the pestilential fever came, it overwhelmed these places.

Bills of Mortality list plague victims in Saint Margaret's beginning the third week of June.[15] The churchwardens' accounts tell a different story. In May several members of two neighboring houses in Long Ditch became in- fected. On the tenth Alice Gale was interred, the cause of death not listed in

Table 4. Greater London Bills of Mortality: Plague Burials and Total Burials, June 27–August 1, 1665

| Week | Number of Burials (Plague/Total) | | | |
	St. Giles in the Fields	St. Giles Cripplegate	St. Margaret Westminster	All 130 Parishes
June 27–July 4	140/203	32/98	26/50	470/1,006
July 4–11	213/268	49/103	34/58	725/1,268
July 11–18	218/268	114/232	56/79	1,089/1,761
July 18–25	329/370	208/421	98/120	1,843/2,785
July 25–August 1	229/282	302/554	101/133	2,010/3,041

	£	s	d
Anne Knight	0	2	4
Jam: Hamilton		2	4
Marie Woodfeild		2	4
Robt Mills & his wife		4	8
Mary Jones		2	4
Anne Cave		2	4
Mary Perrie		2	4
John Humes		2	4
Joane Reade		2	4
Eliz: Litson & her child } at the	3		
Kath: Perry Pest Hou		2	4
Anne Vines		2	4
Izabell Kennaday		2	4
Phelis Pearce		2	4
Thom Browman & } his Wife 3			5
Kath: Fennell		2	4
Anne Watson & her Ch:	3		
Jam: Whateley & his } wife for warding 3			5
Nath: Snow & his wife			5
Elizab: Thomas Nurse			5
Marie Cole Nurse			5
Freeswood Manwaring Nurse	7		
The Gravemaker		10	
The Searchers for 2 weekes		16	
John Wood & Willm Hewell } at ye Posthouse 3		2	6
For drinke for ye Bricklayers } & Labour at ye Posthouse 3			5
A Trusse of Straw			8
Maryt Butler Nurse			5
Martha Ravenow		1	
Hanah Browne 2		2	
Wm Feilding		1	
John Moseley 4		3	
Elizab: Moore		1	
Jane Gladstone		1	
Jane Mare 4		4	
Joane Westcombe		1	
Grace Dennis 2		2	
Elizab: Greene 4		4	
Thom: Perkins 4		4	
Maryt Williams		1	
Jane Page 2		2	
Joane Merrideth & Elizab: } Horton		2	
Sarah Aldritch 4		4	
	7	5	8

	£	s	d
To Doro: Morgan 3	0	3	0
Anne Perry 2		2	
Luke Hand 1		1	
Maryt Gibbons 2		2	
Mary Spentow 2		2	
Kath: Cattletons		1	
Mary Snow		1	
James Lane		1	
Susan Humphreys 2		2	
John Lee 3		2	
Anne Taylor 2		4	
Izabell Lamb 2		2	
Sarah Hill 4		3	
Marie Calway 2		2	
Maryt Barrow 5		5	
A Nurse in Sea Alley		1	
Doro: Cunningham 5		5	
Marie Gardner 7		7	
Joane Rowte 2		2	
Anne Downes		1	
The Const: & Clerc of } Knightsbr: for ye Visited } there	0	17	4
For Carrying a Bed from } St Steph: Ally to ye Pest H: 3		1	
Sworn Order of ye Justices		1	

9th Weeke: July: 24th

	£	s	d
Kath: Boston }	0	2	6
Her Nurse		1	
A Padlock & some drinke } for ye People shutt up		1	
John Petty		1	2
Edw: Everead		1	
Sarah Skudamore			4
Jones his Wife			6
The Dog Killer for burying } 500 doggs		3	
Widd: Collyer		1	
The Dog Killer		1	

Expended by
Joseph Bonner & } Exam
Christoph: Sheene }

	£	s	d
To John Hudson	0	4	0
3 Visited Persons in } Smyths Alley 3		2	
	4	5	10

the parish register. During the week of the twenty-ninth, Marie Gale, presumably of the same family, was sent to the pesthouse along with her neighbor Nicholas Snow and his wife, followed by Margaret Gale. A porter was paid three shillings ten pence for removing them.[16]

A warder was promptly dispatched to Long Ditch to guard its infected houses. People above the servant class who fell sick were permitted the dignity of dying at home. The Gales did not qualify; they may have been boarders in a rooming house. The Snows were probably also on a low rung of the social ladder. After surviving the infection, they became keepers of the pesthouse, at five shillings a week.

The parish printed a map to the pesthouse after the first acknowledged victim, Mary Fennel, was interred on June 14 at the parish's expense. But the week before Mary's death, Alice Fennel had also been buried (the cause not stated in the parish register), leaving Katherine Fennel, who was taken to the pesthouse with an allowance of two shillings for her expenses for the week. Katherine's home was in Bell Alley, today the site of beautiful Parliament Square, but then a stifling cul-de-sac of decaying wooden houses.[17] Knightsbridge was also burying plague victims, with thirteen falling in five days. Examiners went out in pairs to check on run-down houses suspected of being infected; wealthy residents a few streets away did not want to think about the nearby danger.

During the week of Mary Fennel's death, June 13–20, seven plague burials were listed in the parish register. The next week, plague claimed twenty-six of a total of thirty-eight fatalities—officially. The real death toll that week must have been close to fifty or sixty. The infection had spread heavily through Long Ditch, Bell Alley, Thieving Lane, and Knightsbridge. The pesthouse already had a score of inmates—mostly women and their children.

Facing page

Fig. 6. A page from Saint Margaret Churchwarden Plague Accounts for 1665, showing expenditures for the weeks of July 17 and 24. This sheet lists pounds, shillings, and pence given for persons at the Westminster pesthouse and many individuals and families shut up or otherwise in need; for drink and work of bricklayers, straw and a bed at the pesthouse; to nurses, searchers, and a gravemaker; to the constable and clerk of Knightsbridge "for the visited there," the Westminster justices of the peace for a plague order, and the dog killer for burying five hundred dogs. City of Westminster Archives

By the end of June, the pesthouse was painfully overcrowded, as whole families joined solitary souls. Some people were fortunate, among them Katherine Fennel, who escaped the fate of the rest of her family. She remained at the facility with weekly rations until released on August 14. Later she was paid for nursing. By the end of the calendar year, nearly three thousand indigent residents of Saint Margaret's had been buried at the parish's expense.

Like a stealthy shadow the infection moved on from its dismal entry points to equally unattractive Saint Stephen's Alley, Bowling Alley, Mill Bank, Horseferry Banke, Tuttle Street, and Smyths Alley. In July the inevitable happened: The great yards and broad streets, on the one hand, and the congested lanes and alleys where the poor dwelt, on the other, became an interlocking network of contagion. Oddly enough, this development brought new hope as well as death, especially on King Street. Its fifty-seven householders had been assessed substantial poor-tax sums, and forty-nine met their assessment. Most of them had undoubtedly fled, but word of the plague's ever-increasing toll followed them, and they sent money back. A similar response came from the absentees of Dean's Yard. Dr. Busby, who had transported his Westminster School boys to safety in the country, paid fifteen pounds to his parish and added twenty pounds for a surgeon's services to the infected poor.

All told, Saint Margaret's two churchwardens gathered in more than £1,650 this year, with gifts accounting for £1,117. These receipts almost covered expenditures for the infected poor, which totaled £1,715. The churchwardens advanced the difference, expecting to be reimbursed when the parish returned to normal. Even these figures masked the enormity of the undertaking. Wealthy householders who lost family members to plague sometimes made donations, in addition to their own burial fees, to cover simple burials for hundreds of poorer persons. This separate budget showed an income of £132 19s. 6d. Another truly touching entry states that Robert Crosse left £1 13s. 7.5d. at his death to the parish for care of his two children. It was obviously all he had left, right down to the last halfpenny; he had been unable to pay his own burial fee.[18]

As the crisis deepened, the two churchwardens, Richard Arnold and Nicholas Upton, struggled to keep a semblance of sanity and order. A survival of the spirit at work here can be measured by the peers' donated pounds and by an elderly man's offering of bodices, stockings, and shoes for two little girls at the pesthouse whose mother had died there destitute. The churchwardens' pen strokes, neat and precise deep into the plague year, betokened a life-affirming respect in the midst of death.[19]

Two parishes away, Symon Patrick coped in his own way with the help of a solitary churchwarden and his faithful clerk, whose wife and children were dying of the common sickness. At night Patrick read the rites of the dead, his clerk and a gravedigger at his side. Even though public funerals were banned, he still accompanied the body to a last resting place, calling it a "funeral"—an unusual act for this sad season.

Inside the wall, Saint Paul's staff carried on gamely without the dean. The cathedral did not have the poor relief burdens of a regular parish, but the poor of neighboring Saint Gregory's clamored for help, and the dean's "peculiars" beyond the walls (parishes which he was legally bound to help) were in dire straits. John Tillison and Stephen Bing and Dr. Barwick became more and more anxious as Sancroft's relief money dried up. Several minor priests on the cathedral staff died; others slipped away to the countryside. "I intend, God willing, to keep close His work in the church except great hazard should befall me," Stephen Bing informed the dean as July drew to a close. "The Lord in mercy look upon us."[20]

Pepys' Predicament

Thus we end this month, as I said, after the greatest glut of content that I ever had; only under some difficulty because of the plague, which grows mightily upon us, the last week being about 1700 or 1800 of the plague . . . So God preserve us all friends long, and continue health among us.

—PEPYS, *Diary,* July 31, 1665

Samuel Pepys had his own special predicament. His business took him continuously across town and up and down the river as the linchpin between the wartime navy's voracious appetite and its far-flung suppliers of victuals and other necessities. To maintain his normal frenetic pace seemed sheer madness, putting a dangerous strain on his constitution and inviting the infection wherever he went. On July 12 he attended the first monthly Fast Day service at his church "for the plague growing upon us," giving generously for the care of the infected poor. Luckily, Saint Olave Hart Street was still free of the infection, but that could not last. On the twenty-fourth, the parish clerk recorded the burial of Mary Ramsey, daughter of a poor man living in one of the draper guild's almshouses, the first plague death recorded in the parish. In fact, a sister of this girl had been laid to rest the day before—without the telltale *P* after her name in the same register. The next day a poor parish boy boarding with the Ramseys died from the sickness and joined these two girls in the lower churchyard of the parish.[21] The burial grounds seemed ample for additional bodies.

The scene at the far reaches of Westminster was sobering. On the eighteenth Pepys approached Hyde Park, where Albemarle's soldiers were camped in tents in case a riot should break out among citizens protesting the shutting up of houses or dissenters should plot an uprising. Pepys was startled to learn that these troops had been pressed into plague work and were burying the dead of Westminster in the open Tothill Fields, "pretending want of room elsewhere." He thought the act dehumanizing. During the last visitation the New Chapel churchyard had been walled in for public burials; now only those who paid a burial fee could be interred there. On his way home he passed through King Street, shocked at how the plague had spread throughout this main thoroughfare, shutting up its taverns and inns, including the Axe on the cul-de-sac where Elizabeth and Samuel had lived before they moved to Seething Lane.

The next day Pepys paused at the Spring Garden down by the river, expecting to mingle with the crowd. But instead of the usual throng of townspeople and visitors dressed provocatively and sipping wine and flirting, Samuel saw not one guest, "the town being so empty of anyone to come thither." A solitary woman out of her mind scolded the proprietor for letting her newly dead kinswoman be thrown in a plague pit instead of using his influence to arrange her burial in the churchyard.[22]

Pepys doggedly kept to his rounds at the Exchequer and the Royal and New Exchange, stopping in at the Customs House tavern. There was no activity here. He borrowed an alarm clock at his watchmaker's while his was being repaired and donned his black silk suit for an appointment with his distant cousin, an upholsterer on Cornhill. But these were petty tradesmen— small fry. What about the high-society people whose consumer tastes fueled much of London's economy and who were frequently shopping and making merry on the Strand? Pepys had been at the Cockpit for instructions from Captain General Albemarle (who was not only in charge of the local troops but also a key player in naval supplies as admiral general of the fleet). Pepys had become cautious about how he traveled, going by boat as often as possible. Taking a coach back to Seething Lane, he couldn't help seeing the dramatic change, "not meeting with but two coaches and but two carts from Whitehall to my own house" and few pedestrians.[23]

There was another change about which he spoke less frequently, though it could hardly escape his notice: working people losing their jobs as their masters closed up shop and left the city. The early modern world of capital and labor—each dependent on the other—was in danger of coming unglued. Fortunately, the banker-goldsmiths who exchanged his credit from the Exchequer for money to pay his suppliers (the bankers getting their money eventually from the Treasury, with 6% interest) were still in the city. Without Vyner and Blackwell and Colvill, he would be lost. And suppliers for the navy were still holding on in the city.

Pepys was performing an intricate balancing act amid the unraveling of the economic fabric. While others were scattering or hanging on for dear life, he was making money in large amounts because of the pressing war needs of the navy. He was the right person in the right place, arranging contracts and receiving sweeteners from both sides—his friend Denis Gauden as head Navy Victualer at one end and eager shipbuilders, outfitters, and suppliers at the other end of the contracting business.

Then there was the "Tangier business" as an extra plum, a newly acquired royal way station in Morocco promising great profits to those who could turn it into a premier port for warships and commercial vessels plying the Mediterranean. Pepys was on the Tangier board along with such notables as the duke of Albemarle and the king's own brother. Eager contractors were pressing him with *douceurs*, making Tangier "one of the best flowers" in his garden.[24] He could not stop, or would not—it was not entirely clear what made Pepys run these days. He risked death with every trip on Fleet Street. Even travel on the river was dangerous, for the lightermen were dying in droves. These men were also becoming particular about where they would take people and what price they charged. Pepys was fortunate when he could hire a ride at ten shillings instead of the inflated rate of twenty shillings.

Despite the increase in shut-up places and infected areas, Samuel Pepys had definitely not eased off from his risk-taking adventures.[25] One forbidding night he sought a rendezvous at the port of Deptford. The skies were dark and the rain unrelenting—a welcome break in the weather, if not conducive to trysting. "I had un design pour aller à la femme de Bagwell," he wrote tantalizingly in the lingua franca he reserved for erotic entries in his diary, "mais ne savait obtenir algùn cosa de ella." Pepys had played Mrs. Bagwell's shipwright husband for the fool by dangling hopes of lucrative carpentry work with the navy before him while dallying with his wife time after time. On this occasion he was not lucky in love, however, and he took the river home through pelting rain, falling into bed "in a most violent sweat." On another night's adventure, returning in pitch dark from Hampton Court, he docked at the heavily infected tapestry-making village of Mortlake for some pleasure with his friend Nan.[26]

Pepys' most death-defying adventure happened late that night after carousing with Nan. He steered a wherry homeward, and as it approached London Bridge he chose the narrow route through the middle two supports. Here the water rushed in a torrent; the supports had been built up at the base many times during the past century, narrowing the passage and increasing the force of the water. The rider would go through at breakneck speed, with a sudden drop as the water pooled out on the farther side. The sane way was to go through the widely spaced supports on either side, where the water moved gently. This night Pepys chose the fast way and maneuvered his boat through successfully—no easy feat, for many had perished in the attempt—making it home safely by 2:00 A.M. He recorded the event without revealing why he had chosen the route or acknowledging the risk of dying.

As July ended Pepys reflected on what had passed since the great exodus from his city. The parish church bells tolled five or six times a day, he said. "I begin to think of setting things in order, which pray God enable me to put, both as to soul and body." He missed Elizabeth, yet when he visited his wife he was troubled "that this absence makes us a little strange instead of more fond." There were reports that the Exchequer office, which handled royal finances, would soon be moved to the country. Navy officials sometimes met at Deptford, but that port town had also become infected. John Evelyn, commissioner for the sick and captured sailors, lived very close to shut-up houses.[27]

Regardless of the encroaching epidemic, Pepys had enjoyed spectacular successes these past four weeks and was able to compartmentalize his pluses and minuses. "But Lord," he said with detachment from his own perils, "to see what fear all the people [removed to the country] do live would make one mad." How different it was for him: "Thus I end this month with the greatest joy that ever I did in all my life, because I have spent the greater part of it with abundance of joy and honour, and pleasant Journys and brave entertainments, and without cost of money."[28] This euphoria was brought on by his profits this month—greater than at any time in his life—and there was still more to come if all his negotiations were successful. He had been received by the king several times at Hampton Court and once down at Greenwich, to his great pride (though he was crestfallen at having to stand while his superiors sat at a sumptuous dinner). He was equally pleased with his part in brokering the marriage of the shy daughter of his patron and distant relative, Lord Sandwich, to the awkward son of the Carteret family. The negotiations took place in the nearby Sussex and Essex countryside, where these noble families and their relations were waiting out the visitation in London.

Pepys' initial reception in the country startled him. He had managed for weeks in the infected city, and he found it absurd that all these escapees and the local residents were terrified at the slightest chance of someone bringing in the infection. Samuel had to fib, saying he was living entirely with Elizabeth in Woolwich and had not gone near London. The chaplain who was to marry the young couple had fallen into a fever and died, thoughtfully, a "long way off," Pepys said. Fearing for her daughter's financial security, Lady Sandwich moved up the wedding date in case the groom should die of the plague. Pepys, being a distance from them, hired six horses to get to the ceremony, only to find the wedding party emerging from the church. They had been joined in their "old clothes . . . the young lady mighty sad." At dinner, the guests celebrated, "yet in such a sober way as never almost any wedding was in the great families."[29]

A darker shadow fell over this month's pleasures. Pepys took a last boat ride to Hampton Court on July 27. He dispatched all his business and then lingered to see the king and queen speed off in their carriage to a new haven—far from this riverside retreat, for the plague from London was closing in. Charles had chosen splendid quarters in the cathedral city of Salisbury, safely removed from his infected capital but with access to his beloved sailing ships on the Channel. Albemarle and Craven were now completely on their own in Westminster. Although they had a small horse guard to maintain order, the distance of the monarch made it harder to threaten working people in the suburbs with punishment by the king if they broke open shut-up houses or gathered at their favorite alehouse in defiance of plague regulations. At the Guildhall, plague controls fell squarely on the shoulders of Mayor Lawrence, assisted by the few aldermen still in town, a handful of justices of the peace, and a few dozen soldiers at the Tower of London.

August's Bitter Harvest

> Now in some places where the people did generally stay [on], not one house in a
> hundred but is infected, and in many houses half the Family is swept away . . . The
> nights are too short to bury the dead; the long summer dayes are spent from
> morning into the twilight in conveying the vast number of dead bodies unto the
> bed of their graves.
>
> —THOMAS VINCENT, *God's Terrible Voice in the City* (1667)

Late in July a Cambridge student went by house after house shut up in London, "all over the city almost," he reported back to his college tutor. He had
come down to check on his father's house in Saint Giles in the Fields but
could not get in. The family home had been shut up for a week, and the servants left in charge by his absent father were dying along with hundreds of
neighbors. If Saint Giles's sexton tolled the bell for every death, "the bell
would hardly ever leave ringing," the son moaned, "and so they ring not at
all." The contagion had spread beyond the suburbs into the villages and
towns along the Great Northern Road. Outside the city, he saw people lying
sick in a thatched cottage "all most starved, so great a dread it strikes into
people." The only thing that was keeping healthy people in London now, he
exclaimed, was fear of thieves ransacking their houses if they joined the tens
of thousands who had fled during the first mass exodus a month before.[30] By
the end of August, only four parishes in Greater London had escaped the infection. The figures reveal the extent of the sickness (table 5).[31]

Death marked the calendar of the month, week, and day now. The week
began with Sunday prayers of repentance and propitiation, and church bells
tolling each new death in the parish punctuated the hours of the day. On
Thursdays citizens braved the open air to consult the latest Bill of Mortality,
and on the first Wednesday of each month they ate sparingly at home and
went to their churches for the Fast Day worship and collection for the infected poor. On Wednesday, August 9, Symon Patrick knew only too painfully what day it was: "There dyed, as you will see by tomorrow in the bills,
20 in this parish, whereof 16 of the plague," he wrote to Elizabeth Gauden.
His sermon earlier that day was the draft of a tract for parishioners shut up
with the plague.[32]

At the infected seaport of Deptford, John Evelyn made a special diary
entry to mark August's Fast Day: "A solemn feast throughout England to
deprecate God's displeasure against this land by pestilence and war." The

preacher's text was from Leviticus, calling his parishioners to submit "humbly" to God's punishment. Samuel Pepys got up early the same day, "being the first Wednesday of the month, for the plague," he duly noted. Nor was Sunday to be forgotten. In the heart of the old city, the crowds were so great for a fiery dissenter who had taken over a vacant pulpit that people climbed over each other's backs to find a seat.[33]

The voice was Thomas Vincent's, ringing through the crowded sanctuary of Saint Katharine Creechurch.[34] He knew how to set the mood in this desolate city. "No rattling coaches or prancing horses, no calling in customers, no offering Wares, No London-Cryes found in the Ears," he lamented. "If any voice be heard it is the groans of dying persons." He exhorted the congregation to compassion by telling them of seeing a crying woman, resting against a wall with a little coffin wherein lay a child. He believed it was her last one, "coffined up" by her own hands. There are others, he said, who are so frenzied by the fever and pain of their sickness that they run near-naked in the streets, some throwing themselves into the Thames River to cool their bodies.

Frightening images like this do not appear in Samuel Pepys' diary. As August unfolded Pepys' parish reported a mercifully small number of plague deaths, there being twenty-one listed in the bill for the full four weeks. Most wealthy parishioners had left, including the entire family of William Penn, navy commander and father of the founder of Pennsylvania. Yet Samuel knew there were far more plague fatalities in many parishes than were listed

Table 5. Greater London Bills of Mortality: Plague Burials and Total Burials, August 1–September 5, 1665

	Number of Burials (Plague/Total)			
Week	St. Giles in the Fields	St. Giles Cripplegate	St. Margaret Westminster	All 130 Parishes
August 1–8	259/290	356/691	173/199	2,815/4,031
August 8–15	242/277	521/886	228/269	3,880/5,319
August 15–22	175/204	572/874	191/220	4,237/5,568
August 22–29	148/170	605/842	309/345	6,102/7,496
Aug. 29–Sept. 5	178/202	567/690	321/348	6,988/8,252

in the weekly Bills of Mortality. In mid-August, the city parishes started burying their dead at day as well as night. The mayor warned householders to stay indoors after 9:00 P.M.; shut-up households were being allowed to go out to get a breath of fresh air—and presumably to keep them from breaking out of their homes at other times. As the bill for the last week of the month was being prepared, Pepys chanced upon Saint Olave Hart Street's clerk and asked how the plague went in the parish. The clerk replied candidly, "There died nine this week, though I returned but six."[35]

For the first time, Pepys expressed his deep fear. "I am as well as can be," he wrote hopefully. "When I come to be alone, I do not eat in time nor enough, nor with any good heart." His thoughts turned to making out a will—twice: "for my father and my wife." He finally admitted the truth: "A man cannot depend upon living two days to an end." Relieved to be in a "much better state of soul" if he died suddenly, Pepys turned to the unpleasant prospect of moving his papers to the temporary headquarters his superiors had arranged at Greenwich. The new venue "by no means pleases me," he wrote, "being in the heart of all the labourers and workmen there, which makes it as unsafe as . . . London."[36]

Samuel Pepys drifted off to sleep dreaming of an erotic encounter with Lady Castlemaine, the king's mistress. Waking to the real world, he told himself it was but a dream. Yet he fell back to musing on the following day: "What a happy thing it would be, if when we are in our graves (as Shakespeere resembles it), we could dream, and dream but such dreams as this— that then we should not need to be so fearful of death as we are in this plague-time." It was an interesting twist to Hamlet's soliloquy on dying.[37]

Pepys reached the end of August far less sanguine than he had been the month before. "Thus this month ends with great sadness upon the public," he admitted. The contagion was now "everywhere through the Kingdom almost." Twice he had come upon plague-infected bodies: once in the dark of night as he climbed the stairs from the riverbank to his London home, and the other time in an open coffin he passed on foot between Greenwich and Woolwich. The sight of a body being taken from a ketch at Deptford triggered mournful thoughts about his physician, Dr. Burnet, who had died after surviving his home quarantine. Pepys was so unnerved by these thoughts that he forgot to take care of business at the office. "Everyone's looks and discourse on the street is of death and nothing else," he noted. He made his final preparations to move in with Elizabeth and the maids at Woolwich to be near the Navy Board's temporary Greenwich headquarters.

The death toll rose relentlessly. "In the city died this week 7496; and of them 6102 of plague, but it is feared that the true number of the dead this week is near 10,000, partly from the poor that cannot be taken notice of through the greatness of the number, and partly from the Quakers and others that will not have any bell ring for them."[38] The poor who were found dead in the street were surely not listed in the death counts. Dr. Hodges and the duke of Albemarle estimated that unreported deaths might have increased the actual death count by 25 percent. Among the dead were victualers, brewers, neighborhood bakers, and wealthy tradesmen and financiers on Lombard Street. Others had quietly closed their businesses and joined those fleeing London. The thinning of their ranks finally drove even the devil-may-care Pepys out of his city in search of navy suppliers who had moved farther away.

Ten long weeks had passed since Pepys had seen privileged citizens hurtling through the Cripplegate exit, too frightened to think of the laboring people they were passing by. Pepys remained determined to keep in contact with his banker-goldsmiths who were still holding out in Cheapside and with Albemarle at the Cockpit. There had been only one meeting of the mayor and aldermen this month; Mayor Lawrence and Alderman Turner were working quietly to keep emergency services in operation. "The sicknesse encreaseth and the towne is empty," Sir William lamented.[39]

The greatest crisis remained in the suburbs. A remark in a private newsletter early in August gives an inkling of the depth of this catastrophe. "The total of ye Burials this week according to ye Bill is 3014," the report began. "In St. Giles Criplegate alone dyed 554." But the real toll could not be measured. The Guildhall was still managing to shut up homes in the portion of this parish under its jurisdiction, but "the infected of the outer parts go about at their pleasure."[40]

The Crisis at Cripplegate

Ye miserable condicion of St. Giles Cripplegate, which is one of your peculiars, is more to be pittied than any parish in or about London, where all have liberty least the sick and poore should be famished within dores, the parish not being able to relieve their necessityes.

—JOHN TILLISON to Dean Sancroft, August 15, 1665

Outside the ancient "cripple gate" at a bend in the northern wall sat the plain church of Saint Giles. Red Cross Street, built over the old Roman road out of town, and White Cross parallel to it, ran northward. Fore Street stretched eastward, and Barbican ran to the northwest. West of Red Cross Street resided wealthy families with stately mansions and fine gardens. To the east the neighborhood became progressively more crowded and poor until one reached Moorfields and the hospital for the insane, Bethlehem or Bedlam.[41] Cripplegate may have been the largest of all the metropolitan parishes, with its forty-four acres and twenty thousand inhabitants on both sides of the northwestern wall. Nearly half would be dead before the end of the year. Cripplegate's disaster was greater in sheer numbers than anything occurring in Westminster or the city, and the losses struck at the heart of its economic life, decimating one local trade after another and creating a ripple effect throughout the metropolis.

Daniel Defoe was born to a butcher on Fore Street just before the Great Plague. The Puritan poet John Milton, author of *Paradise Lost,* had seen to it that his daughters learned a trade under the direction of Cripplegate weavers. Cloth making was a major industry, and victualers, brewers, and vintners supplied food and drink on both sides of the city wall. Tanners, glovers, and pinmakers flourished. In the homes of these skilled workers' well-to-do employers, five or more servants were busy with household chores and errands. Other merchants with businesses in the city (the founder of the Vyner goldsmith firm, for example) lived in Cripplegate with large household staffs.

One source of wealth was sadly missing in Cripplegate. Most of the great families that once had lived in palatial estates in Cripplegate's western half had relocated to the best parts of royal Westminster. The parish poor-tax roll was badly shrunken, an ominous sign for a community dependent on the health and employment of working people. The earl of Bridgewater was one of the last noble holdouts, feeling secure in his thirty-six-hearth mansion with its prized gardens and thick walls. But Red Cross Street lay just to the east, with its 645 dwellings and inns averaging a modest three hearths. That spring, as plague approached his parish, the earl heard that his goldsmith neighbor had died of suspicious causes. Before the old man was buried with pomp and ceremony by his nephew, Robert Vyner, who ran the goldsmith firm, Bridgewater took the Great Northern Road to his country estate in Hertfordshire. The earl's letters to his Cripplegate house manager barely mentioned the plague and then only to make sure that a nephew who had slept in an infected London house didn't visit him.[42]

The parish that Bridgewater left behind kept a remarkable register of its experience with the infection, opening up the world of London's workers like no other written account.[43] Alone among parish clerks, Nicholas Pyne rou-

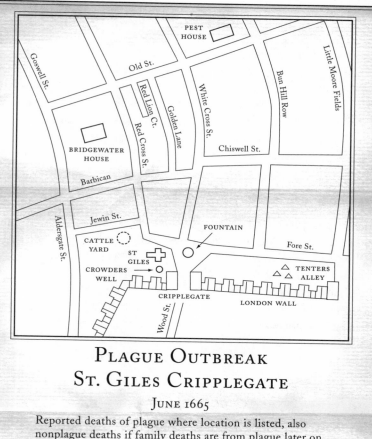

PLAGUE OUTBREAK
ST. GILES CRIPPLEGATE
JUNE 1665

Reported deaths of plague where location is listed, also nonplague deaths if family deaths are from plague later on.

June 2	John Barber, Old St.
2	Wife of Phillip Puller, Goswell St.
5	Servant of Earl of Bridgewater, dies of dropsy
5	Ann, dau. of Samuel Lewis, glover, White Cross St.
12	Richard Green, dies of surfit
17	Nathaniel Stirrup, needlemaker, Old St.
17	Jane, widow of John Barber, Old St.
22	John, son of James Viner, silversmith, Red Lion Court
26	Elizabeth, dau. of James Frenchborn, Old St.
27	Anne Cunningham, single woman, Barbican
28	Suzanna, dau. of N. Stirrup, Old St.
30	Alexander Watkins, weaver, Barbican
30	Ann, wife of A. Watkins, Barbican
30	John Clark, taylor, Checkers Alley off Golden Lane

A total of 19 plague deaths were entered for June.

Map 2. Plague Outbreak at Saint Giles Cripplegate in June 1665.
Parish Register and Hearth Tax for Lady Day (March 25, 1664) for locations

tinely added to the deceased's name the cause of death, noting frequently his or her occupation and place of residence. In August 1665, the parish clerk painstakingly recorded twenty-three hundred individuals as dying *ex peste*. Of this number, he identified 31 percent by profession or trade. In death these 723 common laborers, skilled artisans, tradespeople, members of the professions (doctors, lawyers, scriveners, etc.), and servants of merchants and peers represented a cross-section of fallen Londoners. The sixty corpses that a city boy witnessed as he galloped through Cripplegate to see his younger siblings boarding out in the plague-free countryside—and many other plague victims—momentarily become human beings in this register of the dead.[44]

The Cripplegate vestry took the usual measures: putting a wall around the churchyard, impounding wandering pigs and other livestock, and ordering householders to sweep their streets. Other rules applied specifically to the parish. Residents near the churchyard were warned not to use Crowder's well. All taverns closed down except Castle tavern by the churchyard, which was reserved "for the use of the parish."[45] A curate held Sunday services with the help of a courageous chaplain who preached and visited the sick in the absence of the rector, who had joined his patron, the earl, in flight.[46] Three churchwardens succumbed to the infection.[47] Mr. Pyne managed to keep going.

June passed, and July. In August, that terrifying month when mortality at Cripplegate climbed from 500 to 600 and then topped 800 a week, Pyne carried on with his meticulous entries until the third week, when his own name entered the register along with his wife's. The cause of their deaths was "dropsy," a favorite entry during the last few weeks. An observant parishioner recorded a different story: "August 20 Mrs Pyne, Wife of Mr Pyne our parish clerke . . . died *ex peste*."[48]

Although underreporting plague fatalities seems to have been common throughout Greater London this summer, Cripplegate's ratio of "plague burials" to "total burials" in the printed Bills of Mortality was exceptionally low. Because Pyne specified the cause of death in his register, we can analyze Cripplegate's nonplague fatalities in a way that is not possible for any other metropolitan parish and also compare these findings with the register's figures during previous years. This comparison reveals far greater mortality from many diseases other than plague in 1665 than seems likely, given seasonal and other patterns of mortality revealed in the parish register's records for the previous ten years. In June 1665, only 29 of Cripplegate's fatalities were attributed to plague, while 29 were linked to consumption—a high number for that time of year. Fever and spotted fever, commonly confused with plague, were claimed for 21 and 25 deaths. Gradually, the gap between plague deaths and all fatalities narrowed as the total of recorded burials approached eight hundred a week. In July the ratio of plague to total fatalities rose from one-third to one-half—still highly suspect. During August the figure approached the three-quarter mark. But these figures are also suspicious. It is possible that two or three other diseases may have been at epidemic levels, but a dozen shadowing the death curve of plague is beyond belief (see figs. 7 and 8 and appendix C).[49]

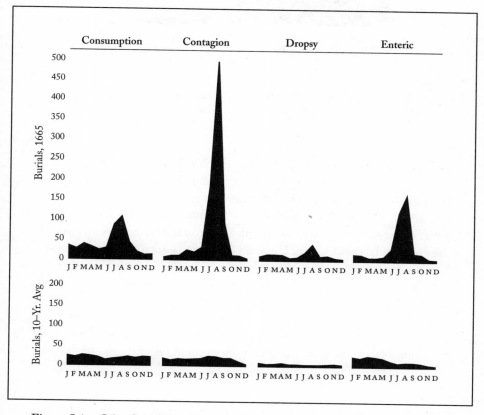

Fig. 7. Saint Giles Cripplegate Parish Records: Nonplague Burials in 1665 and the Previous Ten-Year Average. For an explanation of the categories of death from the Bills of Mortality, see note to table A.1. Saint Giles Cripplegate Register, GL, MS 6419/5–7

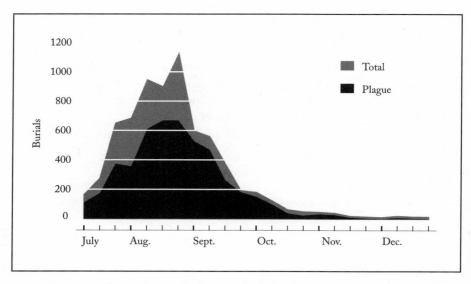

Fig. 8. Saint Giles Cripplegate Parish Records: Total Burials and Plague Burials, July 8 to December 30, 1665. Saint Giles Cripplegate Register, GL, MS 6419/7

There was little doubt about the demographics of death that August as the epidemic peaked at Cripplegate and continued to increase in many other parts of the capital. Plague had disrupted every aspect of life, from health and welfare to family bonds and other relationships, as well as religious faith. Every night during the terrible month of August, Reverend Patrick recited the last rites of the Anglican Church in Covent Garden's small churchyard. During the last three days of the month, he interred six, then another six, and finally five former parishioners. An unnamed child was found dead in someone's cellar. Several maids fell to the infection in their master's house. Then Patrick's faithful churchwarden and a widow pressed into service as a parish nurse both succumbed.[50] As September began Symon Patrick and Elizabeth Gauden were debating their views on life after death.

PART III

The Abyss

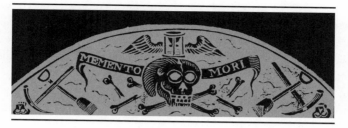

The Doctors Stumble

Never let any man ask me what became of our physicians in this massacre. They hid their synodical heads as well as the proudest and I cannot blame them. For their phlebotomies, lozenges and electuaries, with their diacat-holicons, amulets and antidotes had not so much strength to hold life and soul together as a pot of Pindar's ale and a nutmeg . . . Galen could do no more good than Sir Giles Goosecap.
—THOMAS DEKKER, *The Wonderful Year* (1603)

Almost in every church in London or Vestry, there is to be found a Printed Memorial of [the doctors'] pains and care in [past] sickness-time.
—WILLIAM JOHNSON, *Agurto Mastix* (1665)

House Calls

Nathaniel Hodges, now in his thirty-sixth year, had come far for a village vicar's son. At Christ Church, Oxford, he had read widely in the liberal arts and the medical classics that informed everything from physiology to anatomy. He had received his M.D. from Oxford University on the eve of the Restoration and then opened a comfortable medical practice at Red Lyon Court in the heart of London. Like Symon Patrick and Samuel Pepys, Hodges had risen quickly within the ranks of his chosen profession, and he was now a member of London's College of Physicians, England's most elite medical organization.

Hodges' parish of Saint Stephen Walbrook seemed the perfect place to live and work, a well-to-do enclave of sixty-nine households with a very high median of 6.7 hearths. Assuming that the average family had six members, including two or three servants, the population would have been about four hundred persons. In the fifteen years before 1665, Walbrook had experienced on average eighteen deaths a year from all causes. Even after plague entered the parish that summer, fatalities from all causes remained low: three in August, eleven in September, five in October, and three again in November.[1] Yet the pestilence hemmed in the tiny parish on every side. Saint Mary Woolchurch, where the infection first surfaced inside the city walls, lay just to the north. "The disease, like the Hydras heads, was no sooner extinguished in one family, but it broke out in many more," Hodges observed as the contagion overwhelmed London's cadre of physicians, apothecaries, and surgeons. "In little time we found our task too great, and despaired of putting an entire STOP to the infection."[2]

Dr. Hodges trusted the college's traditional Galenic way of fighting diseases by adjusting the individual's "humors" through bleeding, purging, sweating, and vomiting. He did not always practice strictly by the book, but he participated heartily in the college's defense of traditional therapy and of its own medical monopoly against two ambitious rivals, London's apothecaries and upstart chemical physicians.[3] Both the apothecaries and the chemical physicians were engaged in a pamphlet war with the college, asserting their own ability to test patients as effectively as any Galenic physician, if not better. Hodges matched the upstarts' erudition and invective word for word, asserting the need for academic training in medicine and trumpeting the college's claim to control all medical practice within a seven-mile radius of the capital.

To ordinary citizens this medical turf warfare must have seemed arcane and almost irrelevant to their daily struggle to stay healthy. But for Dr. Hodges and his professional rivals, the stakes were high.[4] Plague raised the stakes even higher, for it posed the supreme test of the rival medical groups' competing claims to heal the body of all disease. Their reputation and wealth as well as the lives of their patients hung in the balance as they battled over which approach to the plague worked.[5] Haunting memories of the college doctors' pitiful performance during previous great plagues added to Hodges' burden. In 1603 they had fled en masse from the pestilence, prompting the medical writer Thomas Dekker to compare their ineptitude to that of a popular stage buffoon of the day, Sir Giles Goosecap.[6] Adding salt to the wound, James I had rewarded the empirically minded apothecaries for staying on in 1603; they were chartered as the Society of Apothecaries, freeing them from membership in the Company of Grocers.

Unfortunately for Hodges and the rest of the College of Physicians, the pathology of plague did not fit well with Galenic theory. While this mysterious malady might involve some corrupting or putrefaction of an individual's internal humors, its origins seemed to be external because the disease struck down citizens regardless of their different constitutions. Hodges took out his frustration with academic medicine's limited understanding of plague by criticizing popular remedies. It irritated his professional pride to hear people saying that exposure to the French disease (syphilis) protected against the plague. What an antidote! He wondered why one would ever endanger body and soul with such recklessness.

Caught between imperfect medical theory and dubious popular cures, Nathaniel Hodges relied on his traditional training and personal instincts as he treated his plague patients. "I think it not amiss to recite the means which I used to preserve my self from the Infection during the course of my business among the sick," he later recalled. Rising early in the morning, Hodges placed a nutmeg in his mouth as a precaution, and in the course of two or three hours saw all of the patients who crowded into the waiting room of his house.[7] He paused for breakfast and then went out to see the housebound. To ward off the infection, he brought along chafing dishes with coals. He ignited them and placed them at the entryway, before the windows, and under the beds if there was enough space. Quicklime, thrown onto the coals along with various spices and herbs, produced a penetrating steam "to destroy the efficacy of the pestilential miasmata."

On his rounds, Hodges held lozenges in his mouth and took care not to go into sickrooms when he was sweating or short of breath, thinking his resistance might be low. By midday he needed to fortify himself before seeing any more infected patients, and he returned home for a glass of sack "to warm the stomach, refresh the spirits, and dissipate any beginning Lodgment of the Infection." Then he partook of a generous amount of boiled meat with pickles, which he felt helped prevent the distemper, before resuming work. "I had always many persons come for advice," he recalled. "As soon as I could dispatch them I again visited [patients] until 8 or 9 at night."

Drawing on Galenic therapy, Hodges advocated opening the pores and calming the spirits of his plague patients with liquors and soporifics to achieve a balance of the humors, replacing their "dis-ease" with a normal healthy "ease." He also prescribed a moderate regimen of purgatives and sweating to rid the body of any impurities. He held back from bleeding someone with the plague, however, heeding the College of Physicians' warning that bleeding was dangerous for a constitution weakened by the infection.

West of Hodges' neighborhood, in the shadow of Saint Paul's cathedral, the poor of Saint Gregory's parish huddled in ramshackle rental properties owned by the absent Dean Sancroft and other substantial citizens. The parish was heavily infected. Peter Barwick, Sancroft's personal physician and a member of the College of Physicians along with Nathaniel Hodges, could see an unending need for food, fumigants, and faith. He used the dean's relief fund to meet these needs, but Dr. Barwick did not himself attend plague patients. "Though I have little to do," he wrote to the dean at his spa in Kent, "I wishe I had lesse. I thank God I am well and have not come yet that I can suspect within harmes way." Four days later he added a revealing detail: "I hope you will pardon me for writing to you, which I would not have done but that I have not been in any house that I could as much as suspect of contagion since I saw you."[8]

Dr. Barwick's belief that the distemper could be passed by contact with an infected person or place would explain his hesitation to go into infected houses. He was known to visit places where the danger was almost as great, however. A committed Christian and the brother of Dean Sancroft's predecessor, Barwick passed through a throng of worshipers at the cathedral three times a day to assist the clergy. Possibly this traditionally trained practitioner was experiencing a loss of faith—not in his religion but in his therapy.

Shut-up households abounded in the alleys behind the cathedral, a disheartening prospect for any physician. Plague had emptied residences next to Barwick's home in Angel Court, their inmates having died or fled. "We have noe neighbours left in ye court besides a goldsmith," he wrote grimly to Sancroft, "but Mr Fleetham locks up ye avenues every night." He ticked off the infected houses around Saint Gregory's and one of the dean's rental properties where two lodgers had been found dead of the plague. Dr. Barwick's hand would administer no vomits, sweatings, or blisterings to the cathedral's infected poor.

While most of Barwick's and Hodges' colleagues did not stay around to test their rational humoral therapy, the rival group of apothecaries remained in considerable numbers. By the end of July, plague reached a peak in Saint Giles in the Fields, with 323 plague fatalities in the week's official bill plus 47 of "other causes." Advertisements appeared in L'Estrange's weekly newssheets offering help for a small fee to anyone in the city, suburbs, or countryside. "William Boghurst, Apothecary at the White Hart hath administered [drugs] a long time to those infected with the plague, to the number of 40, 50, or so patients a day." Boghurst trumpeted his medicines as the very best "with wonderful success by Gods blessing," including an excellent plague water, soothing lozenges, and (at only eight pennies an ounce) his special electuary antidote.[9]

This advertisement stopped just short of offering to treat patients rather than simply selling medicines. William Boghurst was much more than a dispensing chemist, however. Indeed, it would be virtually impossible to distinguish his caregiving and diagnosis from that of Nathaniel Hodges. "I commonly drest 40 soares in a day, held their pulse [and remained] a quarter of an hour to give judgment and informe myself in the various tricks of it," he recounted.[10] Nor was he satisfied with one visit. "I most commonly gave judgment whether people would live or dye at the first visit, almost always at the second, and whether they would have carbuncles, buboes or blains; whether they would have a fever or noe."

In his journal Boghurst recorded that he was not at all afraid and documented a tale of service unlikely to have been made up. He visited people inside their infected homes, as well as seeing patients in his waiting room, and "commonly suffered their breathing in my face [as they were dying]." Backed by experience, he refrained from bleeding his patients. He ate and drank with them and sat by their beds until the end. Even in their final hours, Boghurst would not desert them, lingering until they breathed their last and closing their mouth and eyes. If no friends or relatives were around, he would help coffin them up and see them to their graves.

As though immune to disease, Boghurst "passed through a multitude and continuall dangers . . . being engaged throughout the day until 10 at night, attending patients in one house after another." Recounting his caregiving acts, he wrote of "dressing soares and being always in their breath and sweat without catching the disease." This self-testimonial rang true; he praised plague nurses he encountered "who were in like danger."

Serving the Public

Their memory will doubtless survive time, who died in the discharge of their duty, and their reputation flourish who (by Gods providence) escaped [death].
—DR. NATHANIEL HODGES, *Letter to a Person of Quality* (1666)

How many brave spirits had stayed on to fight the infection with their herbal or chemical cures, therapies handed down from the Black Death's caregivers, and anything else they could think of? How many of them would outlive this fright of the mind? With four-fifths of the College of Physicians and an unknown number of apothecaries and surgeons in flight from the capital, perhaps between 250 and 300 doctors, apothecaries, and surgeons remained out of a normal cohort of some 500 to 600 licensed and unlicensed practitioners claiming professional skills.[11]

Watching the plague's toll on practitioners soar in early September, the unlicensed doctor John Allin passed on the grim news: "I heare also yt above 7 score Drs, Apothecaryes and Surgeons are dead of this distem[per] in & about the city." A few weeks later, Samuel Pepys was shocked by the ongoing toll among medical practitioners in Westminster who had refused to join the exodus of their courtier clients back in July. Now it was all suffering and silence: "They tell me that in Westminster there is never a physitian, and but one apothecary left, all being dead."[12] John Allin's estimate of 140 fatalities when the epidemic was at its peak suggests that 50 percent of those who stayed may have fallen in private or public practice—25 percent of the total cohort of licensed and unlicensed practitioners serving London in normal times.

Despite this appalling mortality some parishes kept finding a doctor, apothecary, or surgeon to treat their infected poor. The need for these caregivers was especially great in the suburbs, which had no central guildhall to coordinate medical services. There were also public medical servants at Saint Thomas Hospital in Southwark and Saint Bartholomew's outside the western wall, the old pesthouses of London and Westminster, and the three additional facilities in the suburbs.

In mid-June, when it was clear that the epidemic could not be contained, the mayor finally asked the College of Physicians to recommend six or more doctors who would be willing to serve London's poor. Of eight college doctors who volunteered, the mayor and aldermen chose only two, Nathaniel Hodges to serve inside the walls and Thomas Witherley, a resident of Saint Andrew Holborn parish, to care for the sick poor in the western liberties of the city. They joined an emergency health committee headed by Sir William Turner, another alderman, and two sheriffs.

The city fathers were dragging their feet and pinching pennies. Money was tight and the city's treasury was perilously low after the unusual winter expenses. The mayor and aldermen were holding on to their emergency funds for more pressing needs, such as buying fresh burial grounds and preparing for mass graves. The two doctors were to be paid handsomely, however, though without a "life stipend" and survivorship to their widows if they fell in the line of duty—provisions that the college had earnestly requested.[13] Should Hodges and Witherley survive to September, each was promised a stipend of one hundred pounds "for the prevention and cure of the plague

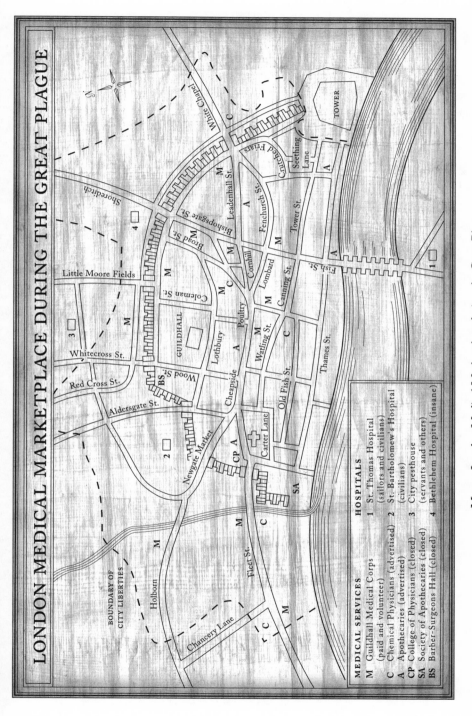

Map 3. London Medical Marketplace during the Great Plague

within the city and liberties." Additional salary payments would be made if their services continued through the fall.

The emergency medical committee approved a single surgeon to assist each of these physicians. Dr. Hodges chose Thomas Harman, whose Finch Lane house lay in one of the most infected areas inside the walls. Dr. Witherley selected Thomas Grey, whose residence at the juncture of Fleet Street and the Strand placed him close to many infected parishes west of the wall. Recognizing the extreme danger faced by these surgeons, the Guildhall gave Harman and Grey each an advance payment of £30, promising an additional £30 at Michaelmas in September and £40 at Christmas—if they lived.[14]

When Lady Day (March 25) arrived in 1666, the city chamberlain paid Elizabeth Grey seventy pounds for the work of her husband, "late citizen and chirurgeon of London, deceased." Three months later Ellen Harman received thirty pounds for Edward Harman's "care and paines in looking after the visited poore the last year." Harman had succumbed during his first quarter of public service, and the amount paid to his widow did not come close to the life pension that the college had requested.[15] The law of averages had not been kind to the Harman and Grey couples. In lancing a bubo, a surgeon risked a deadly infection, leaving his companion a widow and possibly beholden to their parish for financial relief.

Grey and Harman were the first in a brave line of surgical defense. As the plague moved through the metropolis, the Guildhall appointed two more surgical assistants and published appeals for additional medical workers. Isolation wards were nonexistent, and many local residents near Saint Bartholomew's Hospital were induced to take in infected patients at high risk and reasonably attractive remuneration.

As the contagion spread, the supervising doctors looked for help from their fiercest institutional rivals. Four apothecaries were appointed. Because of their dual skill in diagnosing illnesses and preparing medicines, they could do more than a physician, and Dr. Hodges knew it, though he treated them as assistants rather than full-fledged colleagues. Their bills for physick were double the stipends for the physicians and far in excess of the surgeons' salaries. The explanation was the high cost of their medicines: whereas a surgeon received £30 and a doctor £100 quarterly from the Guildhall's coffers, an apothecary could be paid up to £300 for "physick" for the same period.[16]

In August two newly appointed doctors asked for the public's patience, claiming that the city "is not as devoid of physicians as generally reported." In reality the system was overwhelmed, and these public physicians required six hours' notice for appointments from plague sufferers.[17] Boghurst was appalled at the thin coverage by the public medical corps, seeing the poor people in his part of London in dire need. He lamented that two or three young doctors were appointed to "handle 30 or 40 thousand sick people, when two or three hundred was too few."[18]

Four private doctors took pity on the city's infected poor and began treating them free of charge at various locations. Dr. Humphrey Brookes covered the area around the eastern wall. Another Dr. Brookes cared for the poor in Saint Bennett Gracechurch parish, where there were fifty-seven fatalities in sixty-five households. The central wards were covered by Dr. Glover. Dr. Parker offered his services at Saint Stephen Coleman and Saint Giles Cripplegate. He was a brave man, for these two parishes on either side of the northern wall were overwhelmed with massive weekly death counts when he made his offer. Cripplegate would reach a mortality count seven times that of a normal year.

Dr. Barbone offered his services just beyond the western wall. He wished to serve the plague-infested parishes by the Fleet stream and Thames riverbank, which included Saint Bride's and Saint Dunstan in the West. The court of aldermen at the Guildhall demurred, for Barbone was both a foreigner and a dissenter. Instead, Barbone was assigned to medical service at a pesthouse, where he eventually died of the plague.[19]

Such stellar acts by individuals contrasted sharply with the institutional response of the medical establishment. Sadly, the College of Physicians closed its doors after updating its printed advice for the public and offering the Guildhall that small cadre of its members to serve the infected poor. A scant few financial entries were made in its books for the rest of this great plague. The building's custodian, Dr. Merritt, left town with his family. Thieves had free entry to the empty headquarters and absconded with one thousand pounds in silver and money from the college's treasure chest. There was the added blemish of the departure of all but ten or eleven of the college physicians, who fled for their lives rather than remain to fight a hopeless, perhaps suicidal, battle with plague.[20]

From all available evidence, it seems, nevertheless, that London's medical corps acquitted itself more bravely in 1665 than in previous plague epidemics.[21] Those who remained offered devotion and compassion, important components of healing in any age. In these respects Hodges, Boghurst, and many others who had braved the infection had not stumbled. Unfortunately, they were tripped up by professional infighting.

The Pamphlet Wars Prolonged

Certain scurrilous, lying pamphlets have been vented abroad against me, under disguised names . . . to shelter [the Galenists], being Conscious that if they should come to a chymical Tryal they should be found most Dross.

—GEORGE THOMSON, *Loimotomia, or the Pest Anatomized*

That reasoning [is] absurd, which pleads for the Empiricks to be countenanced as if their experimentings might very much further this pretended Reformation in Physic.

—NATHANIEL HODGES, *Vindiciae Medicinae et Medicorum*

A boiling cauldron of acidic disputes benefited no one. The neighborhood apothecary of Saint Giles in the Fields, William Boghurst, was not too busy with the infected poor to cast a few stones. Many of the doctors, he proclaimed, "because of their fearfulness came not to close practice, but stood shivering at a distance, and profited the less both themselves and their patients, and commonly lost their lives to boot."[22] Perhaps Boghurst was unaware of Dr. Hodges' hands-on therapy in the heart of the city or of Dr. Thomas Wharton, holding fast to his station across the bridge in Saint Thomas Hospital despite an influx of infected sailors from the high seas and sick soldiers from Hyde Park barracks? But Boghurst's sights were trained on less heroic medics, especially those who had fled.[23] The Gresham professor of physick, Dr. Goddard, had disappeared. So had the "English Hippocrates," Dr. Sydenham, along with Reverend Patrick's personal physician, Dr. Micklethwaite, and his colleague at Saint Bartholomew's Hospital, Dr. Terne.

After the flight of Saint Bartholomew's two physicians, the resident apothecary Francis Bernard remained at his post along with the ill-fated surgeon Edward Harman and several nurses. The hospital board said little about the doctors' absence, although they reprimanded a nurse for inviting a male friend into the hospital for the night. Had the two been caught together, she might have been summarily dismissed or paraded around in a cart at noon and placed in the stocks. As compensation for the absent doctors, the governors provided Bernard with a furnace for compounding medicines and winked at his practicing physick. Eventually, they authorized him to treat patients "until further order therein" (meaning until the two doctors returned).[24]

When the plague began, William Johnson, the college's dispensing chemist, suggested that the doctors and their arch rivals join forces, with the apothecaries and surgeons taking orders from the physicians for the duration of the visitation.[25] The apothecaries responded, disingenuously, that they never went beyond prescribing medicines "unless in charity or where the physician refuseth or cannot be called in." Dr. Hodges fumed that this "special service" of the apothecaries was an excuse for poaching on the physicians' territory.[26]

The full fury of both sides descended on the hapless chemist. The apothecaries viewed Johnson as a turncoat for supplying the doctors with plague medicines for the handsome sum of one hundred pounds. And when Johnson died suddenly, after allegedly attending an autopsy performed by the chemical physician George Thomson, the college doctors reacted with deep suspicion.[27]

The college's fellows had already lost ground to the chemical physicians just before this epidemic, when some of Charles II's closest advisors voiced support for incorporating this rival group as a separate medical body. The king himself became interested in chemical experimentation, setting up his own laboratory at Whitehall Palace. Now the college's own chemist had attended a gathering of apothecaries and renegade chemical physicians and watched them dissect a plague-infected corpse! To Dr. Hodges, anatomy lessons were rational discourses drawing on essential medical truths handed down by the "ancients" to the "moderns," not experimental acts devoid of theoretical grounding. Examining a plague-ridden cadaver's innards simply to see what could be seen was the ultimate medical folly, Hodges declared, and Thomson the worst kind of "empirick," verging on quackery.[28]

Dr. Thomson, a member of the College of Physicians as well as an experimental chemical physician, was not one to back away from a fight. Indeed, he may have started this latest round in the ongoing turf war. "Chymical physitians were no empirics," he asserted in his pamphlet, *Galeno-pale*. Thomson and his group were as grounded in theory as any Galenist, he argued, and far better at improving it. He claimed the Galenists were holding back knowledge and worse, killing more humans with their bleedings and blisterings "and such like butchering tortures" than the sword ever had. He knew because he had practiced every kind of medicine, beginning with a Galenist teacher and culminating in collaboration with chemists and surgeons. Throwing down the gauntlet, he challenged Hodges to compete in successfully treating sick persons at a local hospital before impartial judges. Should Hodges refuse this challenge, Thomson warned, he would expose him as "a meer sounding piece of vacuity."[29]

The Anatomy Lesson

I was left destitute of two of my dearest friends in my saddest condition.
—GEORGE THOMSON, *Loimotomia or the Pest Anatomized* (1666)

For Thomson, the defining trial of this plague epidemic turned out to be his ill-fated dissection. A patient in Petticoat Lane in the eastern suburb of Whitechapel had recovered from the plague thanks to Thomson's cures, but two of his servants were not so lucky. Against his better judgment the grateful man handed over for dissection the body of his fifteen-year-old servant. Thomson's plague dissection was far from the first exploration inside a plague victim's body, though such dissections were not common. During the Black Death, a Perugian professor had dared to open up the body of a plague cadaver. Finding a poisonous boil near the vicinity of the heart, he concluded that from this boil the plague venom passed throughout the body. Later autopsies suggested the stomach or spleen as the seat of the infection.[30]

As Thomson opened the body and placed his hand into the still-warm abdominal cavity, he was startled to discover an unnatural color and pitchlike fluid within the spleen. This had to be the seat of the infection. Then he encountered black juice in the stomach, which he associated with the body's defense mechanism—its "archeus." The dark liquid, he said, "shows the luminous spirit or archeus is deprived of light. The shadow of death must needs follow."[31]

This talk of an archeus was part of Helmontian orthodoxy. At the turn of the seventeenth century, the Flemish nobleman-physician and devout Christian Johannes Baptista van Helmont had combined medical, chemical, and moral theories in a synthesis that greatly influenced England's budding chemical physicians. Among his major tenets was belief in a chemical and spiritual governor and sentinel of the healthy body, which he had called the *archeus*. He also theorized that this archeus could be overwhelmed by seeds of disease entering the body.[32]

Unable to explain everything that he saw during his plague autopsy, Thomson, by resorting to the body's failing "archeus," had taken as great a leap of faith as had the Galenists, with their notion of an internal putrefaction of the body's "humors." On a personal level, he feared that his own archeus was failing him after he had cut his hand during the dissection. Could this protector have been caught off guard and let in the infection from the cadaver?

Thomson said he stopped to wash his hand and hold it over a dish of burning brimstone. But he worried that he might not have acted in time to aid the defending archeus in checkmating the powerful poison. On an earlier occasion, when he had cut himself while dissecting a spotted fever cadaver, he had saved himself with his patented Buffo frog treatment and strong liquors, culminating in draining by applying leeches. This time, being alone in his patient's house except for a surviving servant, he rushed across town to consult two of his physician friends. The first one, Dr. Dey, was of no help, since he was suffering a relapse of the plague he had thought he was rid of. As night set in Thomson called on his closest associate in the pamphlet wars, Dr. Starkey. But this friend was more in need of a cure than himself, with the fatal signs being visible on his body. Starkey, the best plague doctor of all, in Thomson's opinion, had made the mistake of trying to bring down the plague's fever with cold beer (in line with the Galenist notion of curing a condition with its opposite quality). This inexplicable deviation from the sound chemical cure of applying a hot antidote to a feverish condition, Thomson said, had cost Starkey his life.[33]

Some other medically informed individuals in London had a different opinion about what had taken place on that fateful day, based on the suspicion that Thomson had not been alone during the autopsy. John Tillison got wind of the rumors at the cathedral and breathlessly passed on his version to Dean Sancroft: Drs. Burnet, Glover, and O'Dowde, along with one or two fellows of the College of Physicians, the chemist Johnson, and some surgeons and apothecaries had all died suddenly. What a grim harvest of disparate souls. Burnet was Pepys' personal physician, Glover one of the doctors treating the sick poor for the city, O'Dowde a prominent chemical physician, and Johnson the chemist of the Galenist College. The cathedral canon ventured an explanation that the corpse had been full of tokens and "being in hand with ye dissected body some fell downe dead immediately and others did not outlive ye next day at noon."[34]

Across London Bridge, the religious dissenter and unlicensed doctor John Allin declared the death of these men sheer folly. These medical visionaries had insulted the Galenists and tempted God with their overweening pride. Confident that their chemical cures would conquer plague, they had seen the sickness as a disease more than as a divine judgment. From what Allin heard, they had bought the most infected corpse they could lay their hands on for dissecting. "Upon ye opening whereof, a stench ascended from the body and infected them every one, and its said they all are dead since, the most distractedly madd."[35]

What really happened? The educated public was left to speculate from existing knowledge about plague and the few irrefutable facts of the case. On the one hand, even if the deceased persons had been at the autopsy, they might have been infected before it. On the other hand, the stench from the cadaver could have conveyed the poison to their bodies, causing their demise within twenty-four to forty-eight hours.

An impartial person might have judged Thomson's autopsy a success of sorts. He had come across a "glandulous substance like a lamb's stone" in the right ventricle of the heart. Drawing on William Harvey's discovery of the circulation of blood, he offered an ingenious explanation of the plague victim's pathology. The obstruction in the heart, Thomson reasoned, prevented the archeus from circulating the blood properly and thus ridding the body of the disease. What an intriguing combination of medical theories this was, mixing Harveian circulation and the spiritual life force that the English chemical physician had adapted from the empirical continental experimenter van Helmont and his precursor, Paracelsus.[36]

Thomson's defense of his controversial dissection, written after the epidemic passed and included in his *Loimotomia* of 1666, failed to silence his critics. Nevertheless, it gave him a printed forum for laying out in exacting detail his observations and explanations of how this deadly disease affected the human organs.[37] Going further into the physiological responses of the body to plague invasion would require progress on many medical and scientific fronts. At the Royal Society, an eclectic group of scientific investigators was making some halting steps in that direction.

The Virtuosi

I reckon the investigation and divulging of useful truths in Physick . . . among the greatest and most extensive acts of charity.

—ROBERT BOYLE, *The Usefulness of Natural Philosophy* (1663)

The fledgling Royal Society, chartered by Charles II three years before this Great Plague, claimed the entire physical and biological world as its laboratory. Its working members (called *virtuosi* because they experimented in a wide range of subjects) were much more open than were members of most institutional groups of the day. Interested laypersons like Samuel Pepys (the "curiosi") eagerly attended their public demonstrations. The virtuosi's inspi-

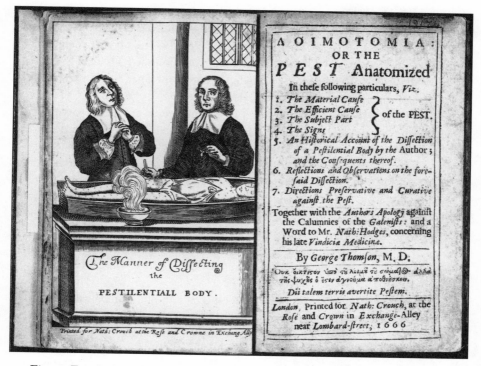

Fig. 9. Frontispiece and title page of George Thomson, *Loimotomia: or the PEST Anatomized* (1666). The frontispiece depicts the dissection of a cadaver covered with plague tokens, illustrating Dr. Thomson's controversial plague autopsy in 1665. The title page indicates the breadth of Thomson's medical interests, ranging from the signs and sources of plague to the analysis of his plague dissection, suggestions of plague preservatives and cures, and his pamphlets against his arch-rival Galenists, especially Dr. Nathaniel Hodges. The Wellcome Library, London

ration came from Francis Bacon's electrifying call, after the Great Plague of 1603, to reexamine the wisdom of the ancients, from Aristotle to Galen.[38] Since then, a constant drumbeat for "renovation," "reform," and "renewal" had sounded from their chosen place on the medical frontier.[39] This language sent shudders down the backs of most members of the College of Physicians, but some individuals in the medical establishment welcomed the attempt to integrate medicine and the new science.

Among the leading lights of the Royal Society's scientific inquiries were Christopher Wren, Edmund Halley (of comet fame), Richard Lower, and

Robert Boyle and his onetime assistant, the microscopist Robert Hooke. A few physicians were also members, including Thomas Willis, whom the ever-inquiring apothecary William Boghurst hailed as "that great ornament" of Oxford University.[40] Curiously, the empirically minded Thomas Syden-ham, although a friend of Robert Boyle, was not a member, nor was he supportive of much of the virtuosi's agenda.[41]

At the society's beginning in 1662, its leading members were too young and ambitious to bow to tradition. Halley was a mere twenty-seven, Wren thirty, Boyle thirty-five, and Willis forty-one. Pepys observed some of their demonstrations that were almost comical. "So out to Gresham College and saw a cat killed with the Duke of Florence's poison," he wrote in his diary. "And saw it proved that the oyle of Tobacco . . . [has] the same effect." Many experiments, however, had a high level of sophistication and possible applicability. England was fast achieving prominence in experimental science: Boyle proposed his signature gas laws, Hooke observed animal and plant cells with a microscope, and Willis charted fevers and blood circulation in the brain.[42]

There had been setbacks, to be sure, especially in blood transfusion from animal to animal and once from animal to human, which caused life-threatening thrombosis and embolisms. Richard Lower transfused blood between dogs, though not many survived. In a lighter vein, Pepys chuckled over the prospect of transfusing blood from a Quaker to the archbishop of Canterbury. A later attempt by a Parisian experimenter to exchange blood between an animal and a human resulted in the latter's death, and such transfusions were not tried again for two centuries.

Despite these failures the urge to explore continued, with anatomy high on the list of experimental subjects, although its usefulness for advancing the art of healing was controversial. Dr. Thomson believed that his own dissections helped the fight against disease, even as he castigated the Galenists for wasting their time in "impertinent and superfluous searches in stinking carcasses." Their academically oriented anatomy, he charged, was meant only "for ostentation and to get fame abroad."[43] That was certainly not true of experimental dissections in the Baconian spirit. New treatments for kidney stones and a better understanding of the role of the spleen in digestion unfolded. Wren's precise anatomical illustrations aided Willis in pinpointing the brain's arterial blood supply. Hooke saw "insects and worms" in body fluids, tissues, and organs through his lens and joined Lower in blowing "ayre" into the lungs of dogs whose blood had become blue from asphyxiation. They observed that the blood turned bright red and sustained life when air entered. This led to debates on where to find the healthiest air for the blood and the other humors.

Within a few weeks of the plague's entry to London in 1665, the members of the Royal Society had scattered to the four winds. But distance didn't hamper their communication. From Oxford, Robert Boyle corresponded with the Royal Society's secretary, Henry Oldenburg, who stayed on in Westminster, and greeted such fellow refugees from the capital as Sir William Petty, John Graunt, and several doctors. Boyle offered hospitality at his residence, and unofficial meetings of the society were held.[44]

Though neither a physician nor a professor of medicine, Robert Boyle had become an authority on the human body and disease. He combined old and new medical concepts and forged connections between epidemic illness and the environment. To replace the Galenic emphasis on fine-tuning the body humors, Boyle adopted a new mechanical-corpuscular philosophy, which assumed that all nature was composed of interacting particles, many of them chemical in nature. By this theory subtle plague corpuscles penetrated the body, corrupting or putrefying its own corpuscles. He suggested that chemically activated effluvia in the soil could be a prime source of these plague particles. And he engaged chemical physicians in exploring the possible role of fermentation of the blood. Perhaps, he said, this raised the body temperature, opening pores and releasing the poison.

Boyle's ideas percolated in the medical marketplace. The apothecary Boghurst hailed him as "that illustrious Virtuoso" and spoke of chemical plague corpuscles invading the body from the "foeces of the Earth extracted into the Ayre." These plague seeds, Boghurst concluded, explained the horrific toll from the infection better than did the weakness of an individual's constitution or the air that people breathed: "The whole kindred [of a family] dying of the Plague, were commonly taken all alike, affected alike, proceeded in their sickness alike, lay the like tyme and dyed alike."[45]

Boyle talked to popular male and female healers and bent the ear of his academically trained medical friends.[46] Reports reached Oxford of Valentine Greatrakes, "the stroker," who cured persons long afflicted with convulsions by his touch. Boyle wondered if cures like this might be produced by way of chemical substances on Greatrakes's hands. Perhaps, he speculated, these substances prompted the evacuation of morbific matter from the sufferer's body.[47]

The intuitive Boyle left no stone unturned. He ran across an out-of-print catalogue among his books, entitled "Of all the Simples and other easily preparable medicines that had been found successful against the plague," dated

1605. He suggested that Oldenburg have it reprinted in London to help doctors treating plague. To the end of his days, Boyle continued probing into the natural causes of epidemic diseases.[48]

Thomas Willis came closer to a breakthrough on plague, perhaps because of his medical experience.[49] William Harvey's demonstration of the rapid circulation of the blood had helped to turn him against bloodletting except in certain treatments (e.g., cutting off an artery supplying a tumor, thereby depriving it of life-nourishing blood). Willis believed that the body attempted to cure itself through fermentation of the blood, and in his work on fevers he had speculated that this was the body's way of expelling pestilential poison. But at a crucial point in proclaiming his new vision of fermentation, Willis returned to a traditionalist view that the body humors should be kept at an "equal temper and motion of fermentation." This strictly Galenic interpretation flew in the face of his previous work. Perhaps he felt constrained by his acceptance into the College of Physicians in 1666.[50]

The microscope was just coming into use, promising unprecedented discoveries in medical science. A generation before, Galileo's telescope had opened up a new world of sunspots and revealed the moons of Jupiter. Experimental scientists on the Continent and in Britain reported seeing "animacules" in the human body through their crude microscopes, following up on Fracastoro's theory of the seedlets of disease. "The seeds of most [animacules] are so small," one observer said, "that 190,000 of them laid together in a straight line, did not exceed the length of a barley corn."[51]

By chance, two studies on the uses of the microscope appeared in London's bookshops as plague was advancing into the suburb of Saint Giles in the Fields. The ever-enthusiastic Pepys was captivated by Hooke's treatise, which he picked up in Saint Paul's churchyard. He missed a timelier message in the companion volume by Hooke's friend Marchamont Nedham. Spurred on by Fracastoro, Nedham had looked for visual evidence of "certain Atoms, Corpuscles or Particles, sometimes animated into little invisible worms as in the case of Pestilential infection." Athanasius Kircher had seen these creatures through his microscope, Nedham said, and had postulated: "Upon the opening of buboes and tumors, they have been found full of innumerable vermicules indiscernible by the eye."[52]

Only one person at this time had a microscope powerful enough to detect the small "atoms" that Kircher discussed. Using a self-made microscope with a magnification of 400×, the Dutch draper Anton van Leeuwenhoek saw human sperm and "animacules" that resembled the long-sought-after "seeds" of plague. He wrote the Royal Society about his findings, but the English virtuosi were unable to follow up on his work with their microscopic range of 20× to 50×.[53] In the real world of plague patients, Boghurst, the ever-observant apothecary in Saint Giles in the Fields, could see only the effects of Kircher's animacules, though he was pretty well convinced they existed.[54] Inside the city wall, Dr. Hodges was also edging away from Galen and toward Kircher's "animated matter." Regrettably, neither he nor his "credible authorities" could tell "if such minute insects caused the pest." Hodges drifted off into speculation about a "nitrous Spirit" arising from the earth and a saline quality of plague that caused fermentation of the blood.[55]

The brightest and best of Restoration England's medical theorists and practitioners penetrated into some fascinating areas, reaching the outer limits of contemporary scientific knowledge with the tools at their command.[56] What they attempted to understand in a variety of physiological unknowns was impressive—especially in the case of plague, which frightened away many a potential investigator because it was unique, mysterious, and lethal. The depth and breadth of this contemporary exploration merit respect and admiration.

Lacking a clinical understanding of the pest, however, medical practitioners were at sea as to how to conquer it. The professionals fell back on mostly standard treatments. They knew that they could comfort the stricken and save a few patients with the help of God, a scalpel and plaster, and nature's curative powers. That was something to be proud of, for what age can cure all its diseases? Of course, these medical specialists did stumble on the pathway of the Great Plague. The most destabilizing stumble was the warring among proponents of rival therapies and medical groups and the lost chance to combine their talents against the most fearsome disease of their time. Yet the kindly Nathaniel Hodges, the daring Dr. Thomson, and the fearless William Boghurst formed a common front, whether they admitted it or not; they bent over sick and dying patients and tried to ease their suffering, without apparent concern for their own lives, as the contagion showed no signs of letting up.

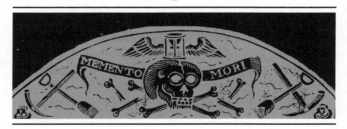

Business Not as Usual

Everyone hastes out of town, which causes that there is no sale for goods, and merchants pay ill.
—Sir William Turner, London, to M. Pocquelin of Paris, June 29, 1665

In the early hours of July 22, 1665, an elegantly dressed man could be seen passing through the city. His silk shirt, well-tailored doublet, and flouncy breeches made him stand out as he stopped at the goldsmiths on Lombard Street and paused at Saint Paul's churchyard near the tenements of Saint Gregory's parish. Resuming his travels, he sped along Fleet Street and onto the Strand, crossing the river to the archbishop's palace at Lambeth before heading back to Westminster and the old city. Here was someone who appeared to be thriving in spite of the sharp drop-off in trade and manufacturing in the city and suburbs. The attire of the self-confident Samuel Pepys was all the more surprising because the downturn had left few sectors of London's economy unaffected. It reached into the great merchant families and leading financial circles of Cheapside and Lombard Street—the pillars of the guild economy and mainstays of financial operations by the Guildhall.[1]

"The sicknesse encreaseath and the towne is empty," Alderman Turner informed his partners in Paris two weeks later. He had just returned from a brief trip to the country, and the capital looked more deserted than ever. To be sure, some fellow guildsmen in the major trades inside the walls were still carrying on but, in addition to most of Turner's noble customers, many of his wholesale buyers were now out of town. "I am not in any condition to make any considerable advances," he informed Pocquelin père et fils. "When

I cann I shall advise you." By the end of August, his situation was no better. Customers in the country remained delinquent on past accounts; merchants holding on in the city had no money to buy anything new. In October, commerce in the capital was still at a standstill, contrary to predictions by astrologers of an approaching end of the epidemic. "The sicknesse continues much notwithstanding the coldnesse of weather," Turner lamented to the Pocquelins. "I pray God stay it. It makes a miserable trade."[2]

Sir William's personal plight mirrored the public one. Soaring naval costs for the war and plunging tax receipts because of the plague placed the private and public sectors of London's economy in jeopardy simultaneously. The navy's head victualer, Denis Gauden, had purchased huge quantities of naval supplies on his own credit. At the rate he was going, he would soon owe his contractors half a million pounds. Unfortunately, the goldsmith-bankers, Vyner and Colvill, who usually covered these debts in the expectation of getting their money back with interest from the Crown, balked at helping him because the plague's effect on trade had virtually halted repayments of their existing loans and left them low on cash.[3]

Yet Gauden's navy colleague Samuel Pepys was managing to stay afloat and prosper by working the same victualing market with his skillful personal relations and attention to detail. Pepys' ability to connect suppliers with the navy's never-ending needs and his influence with the Royal Treasury and Lombard Street had increased his profits with every passing month of an epidemic that was snatching purse and life from entrepreneurs far more wealthy and powerful. The leading goldsmith-banker of the age, Alderman Backwell, was "in greats straights for money," having bailed out the king once too often, Pepys wrote in his diary, and now Backwell's assistant was sick with the plague![4]

Pepys' triumphant travels about town on the twenty-second of July capped protracted financial negotiations. For weeks he had been stopping at the Royal Exchequer in hopes of procuring one of its antiquated payment devices. These were hazelwood sticks, notched to show the thousands, hundreds, and tens of pounds that a creditor of the royal government was due. It was a coup for Pepys to secure these coveted tallies. But knowing that official payments always ran in arrears, he used the sticks to work the credit system of the state as a consummate insider. His goldsmiths, John Colvill and Robert Vyner, gave him notes worth fifteen thousand pounds for his sticks, an amount they could carry, even in the current debt-collection crunch, until eventual reimbursement by the Royal Treasury with 6 percent interest plus 4 percent for the extra delays and risk.[5]

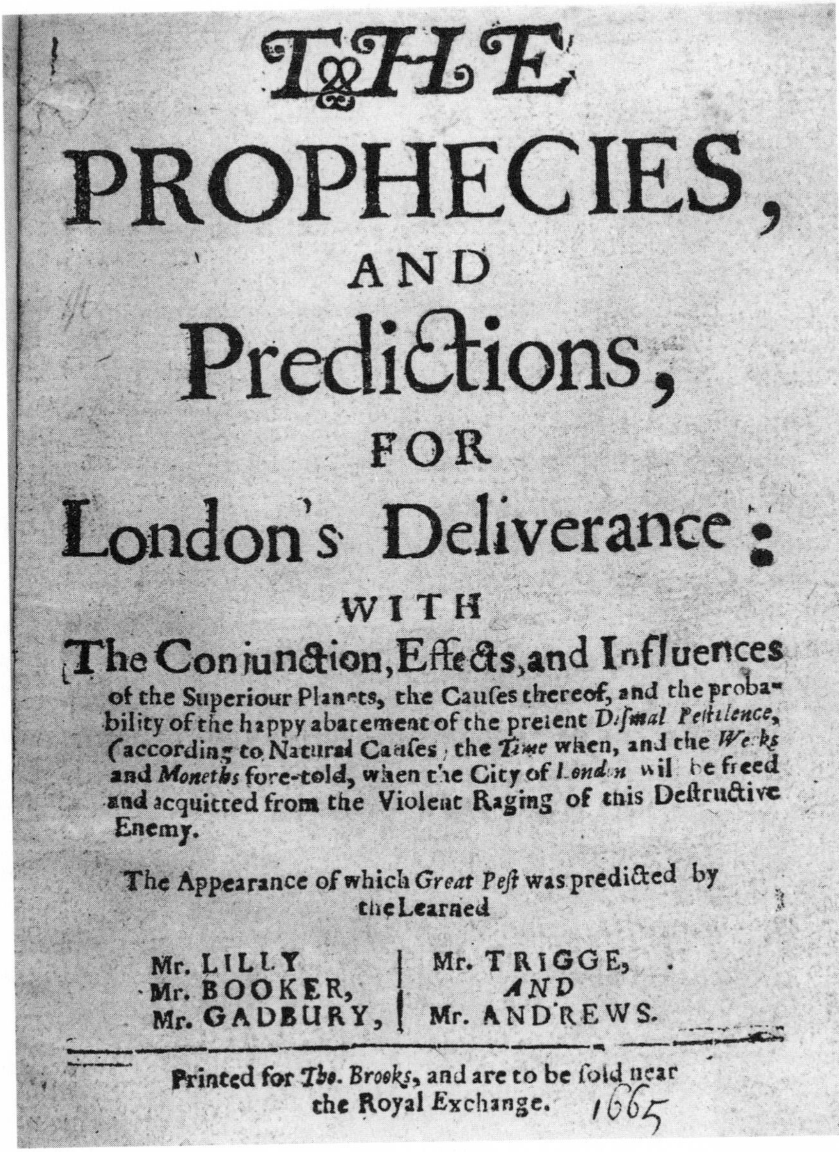

THE PROPHECIES, AND Predictions, FOR London's Deliverance:

WITH

The Conjunction, Effects, and Influences of the Superiour Planets, the Causes thereof, and the probability of the happy abatement of the present *Dismal Pestilence*, (according to Natural Causes) the *Time* when, and the *Weeks* and *Moneths* fore-told, when the City of *London* wil be freed and acquitted from the Violent Raging of this Destructive Enemy.

The Appearance of which *Great Pest* was predicted by the Learned

Mr. LILLY	Mr. TRIGGE,
Mr. BOOKER,	*AND*
Mr. GADBURY,	Mr. ANDREWS.

Printed for *Tho*. *Brooks*, and are to be sold near the Royal Exchange. 1665

Fig. 10. Frontispiece of *The Prophecies, and Predictions, for London's Deliverance*. This tract, published sometime after the beginning of the Great Plague of 1665, purported to foretell the ending of the epidemic and listed five prominent astrologers whose almanacs for the year could be interpreted as predicting the calamity. Courtesy of the Museum of London

With this windfall, Pepys continued on his merry way through the city and the better suburbs to pay down his debts and maintain his reputation as a person worth doing business with, even in this worst of times. Savoring the luxury of a pullet dinner at home that night, he recalled the pleasure of stopping at the Golden Fleece. "I called upon Sir W Turner," he said proudly, "so I may prove I did what I could as soon as I had money to answer all bills."[6]

Counting the Loss

[I] stayed in the city . . . till I could find neither drink nor meat safe, the butcheries being everywhere visited, my brewer's house shut up, and my baker with his whole family dead of the plague.

—SAMUEL PEPYS to Lady Carteret, Woolwich, September 4, 1665

Silence marked the struggle for survival by poor working people, whose services were helping Turner and Pepys ride out the plague in comfortable style. No diary entries were recorded in the city's cheapest rented quarters in pestered alleys. Here unlettered hands of textile and leather workers performed their stage of the manufacturing process for a merchant-employer. If they were extremely lucky, they would receive a weekly subsistence wage right through the epidemic on material that for some unknown reason was extremely contagious. All too frequently their luck ran out. Many merchants fled to the country, leaving their workers at the mercy of parish relief and any odd job they could find. The fear of starvation would follow them, week after week, unless death from plague released the entire household from that specter.

Master craftsmen in the metal and wood trades were more secure financially because they controlled the entire production of their line of work and sold directly to the public. But their work involved risks to life and livelihood that were far beyond those that Turner reported in his correspondence and Pepys in his diary. No blacksmith hammering utensils on a forge took up a pen to mark the dwindling number of customers who ventured down his forbidding, narrow lane as July gave way to August and the death count among his fellow craftsmen neighbors soared. Nor was it likely that a city carpenter, after arriving home with bread and beer from a day of emergency labor on a churchyard shed to house the parish buriers, recorded the windfall of a few pennies that had staved off dipping into his small savings for another week.

The family might pause over their sparse supper to offer a prayer of thanks-giving to God, their version of Sir William Turner's handwritten "Praise to God" that continued to adorn the top of his ledgers despite the pestilence.

Even after Pepys moved down to Woolwich in September, when he re-turned for business in the city he found a waterman to bring him upstream to his old office and a tavern to quench his thirst and give him food and cheer. Yet he never mentioned the dangers that dealing with the public brought to these occupations. Without fares, boatmen could not survive, but with fares might well come the deadly pestilence on a customer's body or clothes. When his brewer's place was shut up, Pepys recorded the fact with-out mentioning the obvious: workers in the hot, smelly brewing trade were dying en masse from the plague. His cousin's husband, a tallow chandler by trade, was hard pressed to supply gravediggers with candles for their night-time labor, yet the man undoubtedly considered himself lucky to have any trade at all.

Sir William Turner's mail was shuttled in and out of London every week by carriers on horseback. He said nothing about letters carrying the infection and endangering the lives of the carrier and receiver. Other persons depend-ent on that service expressed their anxieties. William Boghurst's wife re-ceived packages for her apothecary husband, thankful that the messenger at-tached them to a long pole. "I blesse God that I have one friend left at Rye yt will communicate with me in receiving and answering of letters," John Allin wrote with relief to Philip Fryth. The postmaster at the main London letter office let the king know of the dangerous yet crucial role his staff played in keeping the lines of communication open. The post office was thick with smoke from constant fumigation, and the fifty sorters and several window men suffered from the smoke and a drastic cut in income because fewer people were using the public post these days. A score of the workers had al-ready succumbed to the infection; the rest were carrying on.[7]

A few persons were keenly aware of the importance of these working-class Londoners to those above their social station. Among them was a visionary thinker, Sir William Petty, the economic counterpart of Thomson and Boyle on the medical frontier. After the plague had died down, Petty wrote "that the late mortality by the Pest is a great loss to the Kingdom," whereas others looked at it as only a temporary displacement of people and goods.[8] Petty's fellow demographer and friend John Graunt had just published another tract, reinforcing his view that the loss of workers from plague was unimpor-tant. Property values and other assets, he contended, would rebound quickly after the visitation. But Petty was of a different mind. On the basis of goods and services produced by the nation's three million workers, he concluded "that 100,000 persons dying of plague, above the ordinary number, is [£]7 millions loss to the kingdom."[9]

While Petty was calculating this economic waste at his country retreat, the parish clerks of London were counting the human losses. Chance seemed to play a role in determining who caught the infection and who struggled on. But increased risks came from running errands, visiting market stalls, working near the city waterfront in the brewing and victualing trades, or laboring as cloth workers and tanners in the city's blind alleys and shabby suburban lean-tos. On the Strand and in Little Britain by Cripplegate, large numbers of workers in the printing trade succumbed. Watermen and their families by the Thames in John Allin's Southwark parish suffered appalling mortality. The inmates of crowded tenements near Saint Paul's churchyard were dying by the dozens, while the dean's staff and Sir William Turner in far better quarters nearby were virtually unscathed.

Near the Tower stood the comfortable city residences of Pepys and Gauden. Their families and servants were safe in the country. But many of their neighbors' help were not so fortunate. Their masters were the middling sort of professional people, members of the merchant guilds, and navy administrators—persons who could afford three or four servants and maids. These domestic servants and apprentices were the unfortunates for whom the Saint Olave Hart Street church bell was tolling five or six times a day, each toll giving Pepys a shudder of fear. They were not alone, however, as July gave way to August and August to September. An accountant right on Seething Lane was among the plague fatalities, and a few streets away the aspiring assistant to Backwell, London's premier goldsmith, died.

Working-class Cripplegate's burial register reveals the stark contours of death in the occupations listed for 723 of the parish's 2,300 plague victims in August (see appendix C).[10] William Pratt, left behind to mind Bridgewater House, was followed to the parish churchyard by 288 other servants. The clerk acknowledged plague as the cause in many cases; other victims succumbed in households with many fatalities, suggesting contagion as the likely cause. Widows also sadly represented working-class vulnerability. Elizabeth Pike was the first of 163 widowed women to succumb to the pestilential distemper during August. Forty single women and two spinsters were also listed, among them maids and nurses. In the household of an absent deputy alderman of the ward, seven of his maids and servants died keeping watch over his empty abode.

Knowing the danger they left behind, some fleeing masters gave detailed instructions. "I pray you use all possible care to preserve yourself and my house," a departing auditor of the Exchequer told his clerk after fleeing with the court on the fifth of July. The clerk was to keep the porter out, to see that every morning the servants took some London treacle or a kernel of walnut with salt and rue roasted in a fig, and to let no one out of doors on an empty stomach. The warning ended with instructions to exterminate rats, keep the household's small cats inside, and kill or cast off the large cats.[11]

The vulnerability of servants tested the limits of a master's compassion. Dr. Burnet sent his servant to the pesthouse and then shut himself up with his household, setting an example of social responsibility that others of his class found difficult to follow. Pepys panicked when his trusty assistant and former servant Will Hewer dropped by in the middle of the day and lay down on a bed complaining of a headache. A vision of Will visiting his ailing father in infected Saint Sepulchre put Pepys "into extraordinary fear." He finally got his household help to ease Will out of the house without upsetting him too much. The next day Will was back with Pepys, working on navy business; it had been a false alarm.[12]

Servants suffered the most, but a large number of skilled trades were also vulnerable, led by cloth working. Almost everyone knew stories of plague entering communities via cloth, especially light-colored fabric. Every aspect of cloth making had its dangers. In August 208 persons listed as cloth and clothing workers died in Cripplegate, including 90 weavers, 28 glovers, 18 buttonmakers, 17 tailors, and 10 printmakers or needlemen. A few early plague fatalities in a cloth-working family might be misdiagnosed, but when children, parents, and servants succumbed one after another, the parish register acknowledged pestilence as the cause of the last fatalities. John Barber, a weaver, died along with four others in his household. Another weaver, Richard Green, died of "surfeit" according to Mr. Pyne. Five days later one of his servants succumbed, and the next day another servant, probably all of the plague. Usually, the servants fell to the infection first (probably because their errands took them into dangerous haunts), followed by the family. Some plague tracts accused masters of deserting their servants, but this was certainly not the case with these artisan masters, who stayed on as one servant after another succumbed. The one constant dread among the cloth workers of Cripplegate was that the entire household might expire. Six weeks after the passing of the Green family's head, that household's toll reached eleven: seven family members and four servants.

Workers in the building trade also faced extreme danger because their jobs took them into many plague-infested areas. Carpenters, joiners, bricklayers, nailers, plumbers, and plasterers all fell to the common sickness in Cripplegate. Fatalities followed these workers inside the wall. The beadle-caretaker at the Carpenters' Hall died of the infection. The carpenters had kept their hall open, unlike the wealthier guilds, fumigating all the rooms for the few carpenters who occasionally showed up. The company books list several fatalities among the members.[13]

The landscape of death among the skilled working population and common laborers of Cripplegate presented a grim prospect. No craft or trade that exposed workers and their households to crowded spots or smelly, messy trades seemed safe. Metalworkers were dying in inordinate numbers. Twenty-one were listed among Cripplegate's dead in August, after plying their trades as wiredrawer, twister, and cooper. Blacksmiths and porters, tobacconists and vintners, even a few dissenter ministers who had settled into the parish of the Miltons and Defoes after the Restoration, succumbed.

Unskilled workers probably suffered an even greater toll. Nicholas Thrift, "labourer," lost his wife and two children, all buried the same night. The register gave the causes as spotted fever, abortive, and plague. Thirty-three "laborers" were listed in the register in August, but many more fell without a trace—the clerk having no clue of their work or their existence. Pyne's register rarely mentioned a death in Tenters Alley, a glaring oversight of a densely populated working-class living space. The city pesthouse and a gaping pit were close by its shabby housing—likely last stops in the lives of several of its residents.

Vital Services

Plague raged so much among the Poor it came by some to be called the Poors Plague.
—Nathaniel Hodges, *Loimologia*

Reverend Patrick was trying to explain his situation to Elizabeth Gauden without alarming her. "I intend to be wary about my house," he began. "But stay here I cannot, without hazard to my health, the rooms being so cold, and my landlord gone." The problem was where to go and how to function in his old place in the meantime. There were few handymen to make his rooms comfortable again. Symon knew of the danger of engaging such a person, if such could be found. Deciding to try draperies to keep out the cold, he penned a somber note: "I will content myself with hanging one room, where I lye, and let the rest alone."[14]

Here was the crux of the survival problem for professional persons like Symon Patrick in Covent Garden and the ejected minister and unlicensed physician John Allin in Southwark, who never complained of the lack of money. Both of them could afford the necessities and could get by for a while without most of the things usually made or finished by London artisans. Other material needs, however, were important for everyday living, and some were vital to their very existence. Someone had to be providing them, or else Patrick and Allin and the two hundred thousand or more persons still alive in the capital in September would be at even greater risk.[15]

Patrick never liked to dwell on such mundane things, preferring to focus on the spiritual blessings that were guiding him through this catastrophe to whatever end God intended for him. But material survival did prey on his mind. If he became sick, he did not know how to find a nurse, though he knew friends would do all they could to get a reliable woman. As for the handyman, Symon finally admitted to Mrs. Gauden, "I have inquired, I assure you, about a man to do my business here sometimes, but the towne is empty of all such persons; and he that was wont to do it is dead, I am sure, for I buried him."[16]

Food and drink were another matter. Patrick managed to find both, enough to meet his needs. But he avoided telling Elizabeth where he went except to the church and churchyard and on rare day trips across the river to see his brother and her husband, Denis, in Surrey. Then he let the cat out of the bag by describing a plague doctor on the Strand leading thirty recovered persons from the local pesthouse. "But now I have told tales of myself, and confessed that I go sometimes abroad," he admitted. He must buy stockings, though the infection might be clinging to them. For that matter, he couldn't do without beer and wine, whose vessels might also be infected. But especially bread, he added forlornly, was most attracted to the infection. There was no way out; buy bread he must, "for I know not how otherwise to have it."[17]

Where could he purchase his bread and beer and victuals when the food workers of Greater London were dying like the flies that Boghurst had seen last autumn? Twenty-four fatalities were listed as food handlers during the peak of Cripplegate's epidemic. If they were at all representative of the situation elsewhere, the crisis touched the entire victualing industry: grocers, butchers, cooks, cheesemongers, and millers are recorded in the burial register, and some simply as "victualers." How many more died without being listed?

A major brewmaster like Alderman Bucknell employed many workers while living away from the infection-prone brewing site. He negotiated a handsome new contract with the government to collect its excise taxes, profiting from the king's desperation to make up for plunging collections of the hearth tax because of the plague; Bucknell's brewery workers faced misery and death from the same disease.[18] Tavern keepers, already vulnerable from strangers coming for a drink, increased their danger if they brewed their own beer. Pepys' diary mentions one tavern after another closing down, usually due to a guest becoming infected or the death of the master and his wife. Alehouses, catering to working people, were also highly vulnerable. By the old palace yard in Westminster, "old Will," who once served ale at the Hall to Pepys and his friends, lost his wife and three children, "all dead in a day," Samuel heard.[19]

Yet bread and beer were always available, and a fresh supply of vegetables could be found at the many markets inside the wall and at drop-off spots for produce in the suburbs. For people with Pepys' taste and purse, flesh markets continued to stock poultry and other meats. Somehow, within the pool of victualers who constituted 16 percent of London's population, enough persons survived to feed the metropolis. The victualers were worth far more this year than the high value of £138 Petty placed on the average worker's labors. They were keeping Londoners alive.

They needed help, and a great deal of it, from the farmlands and gardens that surrounded Greater London. Fortunately, dire predictions that spring of poor crops had been given the lie, allaying Dr. Hodges' fear of famine making citizens all the more vulnerable to plague. There was an abundance of herbs and fruits and vegetables, from carrots and turnips to strawberries, plums, and pears, along with grapes and apples and especially cherries, all very cheap. A bumper crop of grains and other fodder compensated for the poor hay crop. And there was no shortage of cattle, sheep, and pigs. The farmers worked and ate as heartily as in any normal year. Dr. Hodges in the city and William Boghurst in the suburbs both marveled at the change of fortune from the terrible winter and early spring.[20]

Equally heartening was the way necessity and invention combined to bring all these perishable goods from the country to the capital in this economic world turned upside down. Grain was needed for the brewers and bakers; the Guildhall made sure that the grocers company and other guilds kept their share of grain to maintain a reasonable weight for a penny loaf. But how did the bulky sacks of grain and huge loads of vegetables and herds of cattle and pigs, not to mention the pullets and pasties for Pepys' table, get through the heavily infected suburbs to Pepys and Turner or even to the mass of the surviving laboring population in Cripplegate and other working-class suburbs? Many farmers who normally carted their own products to the markets inside London's walls to reduce middleman costs must have balked at going through the infected suburbs to reach their accustomed drop-off spots. Probably many left their produce at the edge of the suburbs, desperate to avoid the infection but even more desperate to unload their perishable goods at the best price offered. From there, city carters, eager for any job in this economic slowdown, probably brought most of the produce to places in the suburbs where extralegal marketing normally took place or through the walls to the major metropolitan markets clustered in the old city. Vegetables and fruit could also be barged from upstream market gardening communities. Again, economic survival outweighed the risk of death, and the transport workers opportunistically raised their fees sky high for their vital services while gambling on escaping contagion on London's plague-ridden docks. Shipping produce down the east coast to the capital was more difficult. An Essex shipowner might wish to unload his valuable cargo on the London docks, but he risked being quarantined along with his London goods on his return home. It might be better to take his local produce elsewhere and hope he could dispose of most of it.

No one wrote about this massive operation; the evidence is gleaned from rural legends and city records. Grain for the bakeries came in regularly, holding up the weight at a steady 9 ½ ounces for each penny loaf or three halfpenny loaves. A few bakers cheated on the weight, but the records show no more miscreants than usual. Samuel Pepys' baker was typical in staying at his bake oven and holding to the legal weight out of deference to his customers, the law, and perhaps a sense of honor—until he and all his family perished.[21]

Oral tradition holds that the farmers of Edmonton Hundred up in Middlesex brought their vegetables seven miles in. Whether they acted out of necessity alone or mixed with concern for other human beings in trouble, Covent Garden's victualers rewarded them after the epidemic with free market stalls. Gardeners to the west of London and Westminster are said to have left their produce at Hyde Park Corner. Their counterparts at Barnes and other places on the upper Thames barged their goods downstream to the city docks. One curious legend rings hollow. Hertfordshire's gardeners, it was said, were given the "privilege" of supplying the London markets in return for carrying corpses back to the country. It seems unlikely that gardeners would have considered acting as buriers, especially of plague victims. Perhaps the story was twisted in its constant retelling and embellishment over several generations.[22]

At the urban end of this makeshift network, London's porters and carters joined thousands of other persons eager to transport food for a few pennies. The transportation force included unskilled laborers, servants left adrift, hawkers of goods (whose famous "London cries" had been stilled and laden baskets emptied by mayoral order in June), and housewives venturing farther than usual in search of the day's needs. There are a few allusions in tracts, letters, and sermons to people starving to death, but most were of dubious authenticity. They may be tales of earlier plague times.

The bakers' hall was closed in August. But bakeries remained open until they were infected and shut up, and enough bakers survived to feed each neighborhood. Two parishes away from the Pepys, two men donated thirty dozen loaves of bread on three occasions to the poor of Saint Katherine Creechurch.[23] All of the merchant guilds kept their quotas of grain and coal for the city poor, on orders from the Guildhall.[24] The watermen and lightermen continued to ply the Thames with passengers and goods. They told their wives that, if they died of this pestilence, their survivor was to pay no further taxes. They had given their all for the survival of their social betters, their city, and the metropolis.

The Balancing Act

> As to myself, I am very well, only in fear of the plague. My late gettings have been very great, to my great content and [I] am likely to have yet a few more profitable jobs in a little while.
>
> —SAMUEL PEPYS, *Diary,* August 31, 1665

If anyone could ride out this pestilential season comfortably in the city, it was likely to be Sir William Turner. There was, first of all, his solid business base as a major trader in fine cloth and a past master of the Merchant Taylors' Guild. His public position as a leading alderman and prominent member of the Guildhall's emergency medical committee kept him on top of the deteriorating business climate in the capital. Turner's overseas resources were also a powerful anchor. His network of partners and brokers stretched from Dover and Calais to Paris, Brussels, Genoa, and Florence. Then there were his financial assets. Like Pepys, he was as good as his word, and Turner had far greater credit resources to back him up. If worse came to worst, he had the small fortune that he had already accumulated to carry him through this pestilential season.

There was another secret to Turner's success that an opportunistic entrepreneur like Samuel Pepys easily overlooked. While the Navy Board secretary's account keeping of his frenetic activities got more and more haphazard, Sir William always knew exactly where he stood. He might not be taking in much money these weeks, but he was current on paying his debts and he knew his financial worth, right down to his cash reserves and gold chain, whose links he was rumored to count obsessively.[25] Woe betide the Pocquelins in Paris when their records did not square with Turner's meticulous double-entry account books. On September 4, he testily addressed his partners in Paris that he hadn't the time to answer their letter fully but would "send you the accompt of money drawne and lett you see how much you're mistaken to say I owe you £300."[26]

His most immediate problem was a lack of cash. His account books showed a falling off of sales in June. By mid-July he could count on none of his wholesale customers, who usually bought large consignments. An entry for July 12 listed a purchase of taffeta by Roger L'Estrange, of the *Newes* and *Intelligencer*. The next entry in that account was dated eleven months later.[27]

In late July, Sir William had more than £1,000 in two new accounts, plus £400 in cash in an old joint account with the Pocquelins. A week later these reserves were gone. He had paid a French "factor" £745 on his half of a new debt for goods received and £500 on an old one. "I can advance no more," he informed the Pocquelins, "having disposed my money." He held out hope of more money coming in soon, but the continuing exodus of merchant customers from the city made that unlikely. A different way of keeping in business must be devised.[28]

Turner transferred money without handling cash, drawing on bills of exchange and letters of credit issued by persons with access to money. He was the envy of those in Gauden's and Pepys' circle; both forms of credit had become extremely scarce in the money market.[29] Equally impressive was his ability to make the most of these instruments by delaying the time when the bills or letters could be cashed. By August his accountant-relative Andrew Turner informed the Pocquelins that, besides the collapse of sales, customers had failed to pay old bills on time. The Pocquelins were no longer to draw on new bills of exchange "on sight" or even a few days after receiving them. "If you have occasion to draw on me, it will be best if you do it at 8 or 15 days [after] sight," Sir William advised.[30]

So it went into the worst of the plague season. Turner's letters to France featured constant complaints of money not coming in to the Golden Fleece. A few delinquent customers in the countryside would promise to pay their bills through the post; then nothing happened. At the end of September, Turner informed his partners: "Mr. Wade and all other [of] our debtors are out of towne. I can receive nothing." He sounded uncharacteristically apologetic: "I would bee glad to pay you some money, but I cann have none to pay you."[31]

Thanks to his extraordinary credit, Sir William Turner was riding out the storm, even if he was not making any money. Left unstated in his business dealings was the other great underpinning of his survival: the working-class people who provided the goods and services that allowed him to stay on in the city and conduct his financial operations from the Golden Fleece. There was an implicit contract, which the merchant-alderman Turner acknowledged by his public-minded deeds while keeping his motivations to himself.

A strong sense of civic duty surely lay behind Turner's continuous service on the emergency medical committee and other Guildhall assignments while most of his fellow aldermen were either in the country or closeted in their city residences. The "Praise to God" line at the top of his ledgers and his generous donations to Saint Giles in the Fields at the first sign of plague bespoke a religiously based conscience.[32] Self-survival was also at play, for if he had abandoned the Golden Fleece and the persons assigned to guard his goods had succumbed to the plague, thieves could have carried off his costly stock of unsold goods.

Pepys, too, was connected with the struggle for survival of those beneath him, though this could hardly be detected in his emotional detachment from their personal tragedies. Long after his colleagues had fled to the Navy Board's temporary quarters in Greenwich, he lingered in the city, negotiating naval contracts that employed London workers. After he left, his repeated return visits to Seething Lane and the Cockpit involved the services of watermen and tavern keepers and still more contractual arrangements that breathed a little life into the capital's moribund economy.

At the other end of the relationship between the wealthy and the poor, a few laboring persons were doing better than surviving. The cathedral's faithful assistant, John Tillison, had an unusual tale of role reversals in the metropolitan marketplace for Dean Sancroft. Tillison had gone upstream for firewood for the dean's use during the coming winter. On the upper banks of the Thames, woodcutters demanded prices far higher than usual, lightermen wanted twice the normal rate to float the faggots down to a wharf, and the wharfingers raised their prices sky high to three pounds a load for three months' wharfage on the docks, claiming the wharf area was already full with goods left unsold because of the plague. An exasperated Tillison went four miles farther upstream, finding a wharfinger who settled for five pence a load and promised to guard the wood against thieves. The dean could surely pay the total charges he had arranged for the wood, transportation, and storage, even with the loss of rental money from his tenants around the cathedral who had died of the plague. Nevertheless, Tillison felt obliged to apologize for the steep prices the pestilence had forced him to pay.[33]

Samuel Pepys was more adept than Tillison in getting good deals, and the plague was not about to obstruct his pursuit of wealth. His techniques were tailored to the situation and the class with which he was dealing. On one occasion he took two saddle horses downstream into unfamiliar territory. The local watermen refused to take him and the horses across to the other side unless he paid twenty shillings, twice the normal rate. Pepys lost his patience, swearing he would have them dragooned into the royal navy by one of the infamous impressment crews. He did not have to carry out the threat; another waterman came by and took Pepys and his horses over for ten shillings.

With his own class Pepys pressed a more civil advantage—being in the right place at the right time. Windfalls had swelled his purse ever since he entered the public-private business network, which he did while taking his cue from his kinsman patron Lord Sandwich. Sandwich had a saying that it was not one's salary that made one rich but the opportunities of getting money while in a salaried post. Pepys' current salaries of £350 at the Navy Board and another £300 as treasurer for Tangier were just the beginning of what he might take in, thanks to the Dutch naval war. Skirmishes and raids by both sides on merchant ships had depleted the Treasury while lining the pockets of commanders with captured booty and adding to Pepys' purse through his contracting for naval supplies. He navigated the shifting terrain skillfully and with better luck than did his naval superiors. Sandwich was banished from the navy to a diplomatic post in Portugal for sharing booty from two Dutch merchant ships before the king took his share, while Pepys sold off his share quickly and avoided notice. And unlike Denis Gauden, who had nothing but new debts to show for his management of the navy's vast supply network, Pepys steered his way through a sea of prospective contractors to suppliers who would reward him with handsome bonuses.[34]

The navy's need for plank and masts and rope and sailcloth was unending. Warships sailed into port for new supplies of food, drink, and clothing. Pepys was in perpetual motion, meeting suppliers at the navy office's new headquarters in Greenwich and at Albemarle's quarters in Westminster. He was up and down the Thames River and occasionally out to sea with high officials viewing the navy's needs up close. He went deep into the countryside to dine at the manor houses of business associates. He met potential contractors everywhere: shipbuilders, timber merchants, victualers, vintners, clothiers.

Pepys' elaborate procurement network kept functioning through August and well into September. Although the plague spread to the docks and shipyards of Greenwich, Deptford, and Woolwich, goods for the navy continued to reach their destination. Meanwhile, he pursued the Exchequer relentlessly, more often than not securing the tallies owed to him. Thanks to his goldsmiths, advances on these tallies reached Pepys' contractors. The gratuities that they offered in return were frequent and considerable. Captain Taylor gave him £120 for a coveted six-month shipbuilding contract. Pepys renewed a major timber concession for Sir William Warren, whose empire of wood sources stretched from the Baltic to New England. That arrangement brought Samuel a £200 gratuity.

With the plague in London at its peak, Pepys achieved his greatest financial coup. He managed to extract from the Exchequer a reimbursement of £125,000 for the head of navy victualing—a staggering sum. Although Denis Gauden remained in debt for the rest of the £474,000 that the Crown owed him, the possibility of solvency lay ahead. Gratefully, Gauden pressed a note for £500 into Samuel's hands.[35]

The line between public service and private profit was conveniently hazy, and Pepys mastered the art of going to the edge of what private and public culture considered acceptable. In his diary, he claimed that he stopped short of accepting outright bribes in advance of contracts, but his description of one lucrative deal suggests that he stepped over the line on that occasion.[36] Before the epidemic he had exulted in getting supplies to Tangier at a saving for the king of £5,000 a year, justifying his own expectation of a kickback in gifts of £300 "with a safe conscience [and] without the least wrong to the king." Neither King Charles nor Admiral Albemarle thought him rapacious, Albemarle calling him "the right hand of the navy" and saying no one but he was taking care of its needs.[37]

At the end of April, Pepys counted his "worth" (meaning total assets) above £1,400, while the average English household's annual income was £7. By the end of July, with the plague's toll climbing sharply, his wealth had swelled to £1,900. At August's end he estimated his grand total in cash and money promised at £2,180, not counting his gold and silver plate and personal possessions worth £250. But what an irony in this situation! As he started to move his things down to Woolwich, he became frightened at the prospect of having his cash stolen. Should he leave it at home or take it all with him? A friend reassured him that nobody would suspect a Londoner of leaving money when the entire household had left. Samuel left his cash in an iron chest at Seething Lane.[38]

In mid-September he returned to the city for the first time in several days. He had been out to the Exchequer in the country and was bringing his latest tallies to Lombard Street, where Sir Robert Vyner handed him a note for more than five thousand pounds. The contrast between this personal triumph and the rest of his day in the city could not have been greater. He stopped at the Bear tavern at the south end of London Bridge for a biscuit and cheese and some sack; the plague was all around. At the foot of Tower Hill, he found the Angel tavern, a favorite of his, all shut up. An alehouse by the Tower stairs was shuttered; Samuel recalled seeing a guest there a week before, now deceased. The Royal Exchange was open and full of people, but they were "plain men, all, not a man or merchant of any fashion."

Yet not all key traders were out of town. Several goldsmiths had died inside the wall of the sickness, among them the greatest merchant financier of Cromwell's time. The man's widow died shortly after, of grief it was said. The common sickness reached Pepys' outer circles of business connections—individuals high and low on whom he had depended from the beginning. He reflected once more on the death of his physician and missed his surgeon, who had fled to the country. His regular waterman's child had succumbed to the infection, and the father lay dying. Another waterman was dead; he had fallen ill a week before while ferrying Pepys on the river. And a common laborer, whom Pepys had sent out to inquire of friends in Essex, had also been struck down by the distemper.

The sickness had even invaded Samuel's extended family. The fathers of his two assistants, Will and Tom, were dead in Saint Sepulchre parish. His wife's parents were still holding out on Long Acre, but their home had been shut up. Elizabeth asked him to give them some money, and he sent a messenger from the navy office with twenty shillings.[39]

The pestilence had burrowed deeply into the patchwork neighborhoods of London. While plague deaths were dipping slightly overall, burials had increased within the wall and close to the Pepys' home. "I put off the thoughts of sadness as much as I can," Pepys wrote. The sharing of working people's grief by a growing number of professional families in the city put him into "great apprehensions of melancholy."[40]

A Cripplegate bookseller, Richard Smyth, kept his own obituary of friends, acquaintances, and customers on both sides of the city wall; several were above the artisan and middling ranks. The clerk of the vintners company had died *ex peste,* he noted. A goldsmith on Tower Street had expired, the cause listed unconvincingly as "consumption." Yet another goldsmith was dead, this one on Lombard Street; his place of residence and payment of a fine to avoid becoming an alderman marked him as a very substantial citizen and guildsman. An attorney of the Court of Common Pleas also succumbed, the death acknowledged to be plague, Smyth added. The coroner of London fell to the common sickness, and so did George Dalton, the official city remembrancer in charge of recording memorable civic acts. Smyth felt the loss of another individual doubly, as a friend and as a debtor who still owed him £150. The bell was tolling now for some of the rich and almost famous Londoners who had lost their gamble in staying in the mercantile heart of the metropolis.[41]

Smyth's circle of deceased acquaintances and friends encompassed an enormous economic, social, and occupational range—all but the peerage. He heard that a "strong water man" (seller of spirits) had died, the report reaching him the very night of his passing. A financially secure scrivener shared the ignominy of death by plague with a scrimp-and-save vinegar man who sold apples "by Mr. Ladores house." Tragedy knew no social boundaries. A short distance away, in the better area of Cornhill, a bookseller and printer, Peter Lake, hanged himself in his warehouse in Leadenhall, "reported to be distracted," Smyth wrote. The historian of the Great Plague, Walter George Bell, speculates that many persons like Lake may have been driven mad and possibly to suicide by the unfolding tragic events.[42]

Cast into this climate of material and emotional anguish, Samuel Pepys' string of luck eventually met reality. Access to new money, which had long been out of Turner's reach but pivotal to Pepys' success, finally eluded this ultimate entrepreneur of the Great Plague. On the fifteenth of October, he took a country road to Sir Robert Vyner's lavishly appointed manor house in Middlesex. Sir Robert confessed to being "in great straits." Pepys believed he was telling the truth and not just holding him off. They discussed how the fleet and sailors could be paid. Vyner did not think it possible as things stood. No money was coming in from trade or from people in the city who were still trying to carry on their businesses. Pepys endeavored to satisfy his own creditors "about bills of exchange" drawn on Tangier's profits, "but it is only words," he admitted, for he had no public money nor could he get it.[43]

How did the city keep functioning? On the first Tuesday of October, the parish clerks of London tallied the previous week's fatalities. Pepys was already unnerved, having just learned that two watermen who used to carry the navy office's letters and who had been well the previous Saturday had now been stricken. The plague, he heard, was far from over: A London merchant with an eleven-hearth city home brought the news of the bill to Pepys. Although the overall bill was down, "it encreases at our end of the town still."[44] When would it be over?

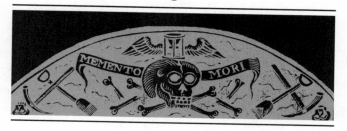

9

Requiem for London

> There was such a general calm and serenity of weather, as if both wind and rain
> had been expelled from the Kingdom ... The birds did pant for breath, especially
> of the larger sort, who were likewise observed to fly more heavily than usual.
> —DR. BAYNARD, September 1665

Nameless in Death

Londoners reflected on the disappearance from their streets of horses, carriages, and wagons—except for the ubiquitous dead-carts with their lamentable cargo. Grass was sprouting up on the streets inside the wall and in Whitehall's abandoned courtyard. Occasionally, a stylish coach conveyed a poor person to the Westminster pesthouse at parish expense.

Little rain had fallen in London since the plague's appearance with the warming breezes of spring. Death and drought held the citizens in their grasp, contrasting strangely with the bountiful harvests of the countryside that continued to feed Londoners still alive. The lack of rainfall alone mocked their effort to keep up their spirits. Why should a householder or shopkeeper continue the weekly ritual of clearing the filth from the doorway when dust and dirt piled up as soon as one's servant put away the broom? No matter what Londoners did, the capital's death toll spiraled upward with the heat as if there was no limit to the number of persons who could die. Almost 7,000 of the 8,252 burials during the first week of September were acknowledged to be the result of plague. In desperation, Captain General Albemarle and Lord Mayor Lawrence ordered public fires to be lit on every street in the vain hope that the smoke would banish the poisonous miasmas and effluvia from the doomed metropolis. The experiment lasted almost three days, until a chance downpour extinguished the flames.

During the following week the total fatalities in the Bill of Mortality were down by 562, but plague still claimed more than 6,500. The exact figures no longer mattered, since hundreds of burials were not listed in the bill that week. Hundreds died daily with no names recorded, and nonconformists and Quakers were not listed. Then came the week of September 12–19—the grimmest week for burials in London's long history.

Albemarle had the figures from the Guildhall on Tuesday evening, an incredibly fast delivery. Pepys was at the Cockpit the next day, making yet another visit from his temporary downriver abode. The city scene was a worse assault on his senses than anything he had experienced thus far: "But Lord, what a sad time it is, to see no boats upon the River—and grass grow all up and down Whitehall-court—and nobody but poor wretches in the streets." Not even a sudden dip in the temperature and more showers had muted the death scene. "Worst of all," Pepys declared in total astonishment, "the Duke showed us the number of the plague this week, brought in the last night from the Lord Mayor." The increase was about six hundred over the previous week, "which is contrary to all our hopes and expectations from the coldness of the late season." The total was 8,297, and of the plague 7,165.[1] Dr. Hodges in the city and Albemarle at the Cockpit estimated the total count at perhaps as many as fifteen thousand. Between one and two thousand bodies were being disposed of every night into the waking hours of the morning.

The parish clerks tried to record all names of residents who were lowered into a grave in their churchyards. Individual graves were in great demand, however, and in shockingly short supply. The euphemism in parish registers—"buryed in the lower churchyard" or, in Cripplegate's case, the "upper churchyard"—hid mass burials in cavernous holes dug under cover of darkness. If people living near Saint Bride's lower churchyard peered over the brick wall, they could see pieces of wood and bones from old coffins strewn about. The gravediggers had dug through existing graves to create pits large enough to hold fifty, sixty, or even seventy bodies.

In densely populated Saint Botolph Bishopsgate, just outside the northeast wall, a tidal wave of plague fatalities engulfed the parish clerk, who for years had kept one of the best registers of christenings, marriages, and burials in all of London. On June 26 he put down the fifty-third fatality for the month, double the usual June toll at Bishopsgate. The clerk's name should have been next in the register, for he was fatally struck by the plague. But the listing of fatalities stopped that day and did not resume until the next year.

For the next six months, an uncertain hand recorded (or rather misspelled) the few christenings and marriages of this barren season, but the substitute clerk gave up on inscribing anything on the burial pages of the register. Still, he did not shirk on his most important duty of the visitation: he kept a running count of all the fatalities known to him. What is more, he noted the causes of death reported by the searchers, probably tabulating them with strokes of his pen next to the columns of causes of death on the backside of the metropolitan Bill of Mortality broadsheet. Every week, as the parish's plague toll mounted, crested, and then declined, he trudged through the Bishopsgate to the central office of the parish clerks to report his figures for the printed metropolitan bill and returned to the church to receive the searchers' latest reports.

The stark figures of Saint Botolph Bishopsgate's fatalities in the weekly bills reveal all too clearly the enormity of this clerk's task. In mid-July, the week's toll of all causes was 65; the next week it reached 105. Two weeks later it soared to 180, peaking at 368 during the last week of August and 354 during the first week of September. For the entire year of 1665, the total number of fatalities for Bishopsgate was 3,464, according to the metropolitan bills. Modern demographers calculate this as 6.7 times the average mortality in the parish over the previous decade according to the same bills. But the increase in 1665 surely far exceeded that figure. The total number of fatalities for Bishopsgate reported to the metropolitan bills for the year was eight times the annual average of fatalities recorded for the previous ten years in the parish's register.[2] Even that figure masks the immensity of the parish's mortality crisis. The reported mortality count of 3,464 persons represented two-thirds to three-quarters of the parish's total population, if one could trust the tax assessors' count of 898 households, suggesting a population of 4,000 to 5,000 persons. Assuming that the tax officials missed many families and individuals in this extremely poor parish (with a mean of only 2.6 hearths), its plaguetime mortality was considerably less than total but far greater than listed in the printed Bills of Mortality.[3]

At Saint Margaret Westminster, the clerk made many individual entries without names and some family listings without the number of deceased. Ann Smith "and her children" were buried. Someone was identified only as "buried in the morning," an ignominy reserved for bodies left over after nighttime burials. On June 21 three unknown bodies were interred, and on July 20 eight more, all plague deaths. On July 30 fifteen unknown souls were put to rest, and on August 5 the body of Hannah Lawrence was lowered into the ground along with twenty-three nameless plague victims.

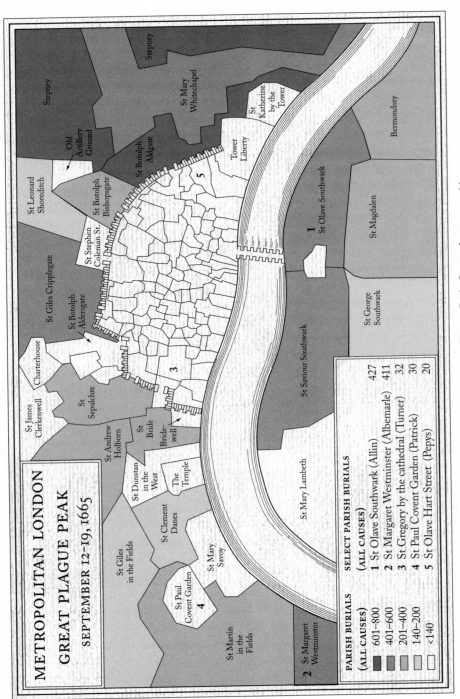

Map 4. Metropolitan London: Great Plague Peak, September 12–19, 1665

METROPOLITAN LONDON
GREAT PLAGUE PEAK
SEPTEMBER 12–19, 1665

PARISH BURIALS
(ALL CAUSES)

- 601–800
- 401–600
- 201–400
- 140–200
- <140

SELECT PARISH BURIALS
(ALL CAUSES)

1 St Olave Southwark (Allin)   427
2 St Margaret Westminster (Albemarle)   411
3 St Gregory by the cathedral (Turner)   32
4 St Paul Covent Garden (Patrick)   30
5 St Olave Hart Street (Pepys)   20

How did Saint Margaret's only clerk feel as he registered those twenty-three nameless fatalities on that fateful day? The parish toll peaked in mid-August with 269 fatalities recorded of all causes, ten times the normal weekly number. The clerk struggled on but gave up the attempt to record nameless burials. Perhaps their numbers made the gesture too much for him to bear. Or maybe these anonymous dead were being picked up by a bearer and taken to a plague pit before a searcher could view their bodies and notify the clerk of the cause of death.

These searchers were experiencing their own difficulties and the conflicting emotions that accompanied them. Numbed by climbing the stairs of crowded tenements to view body after body during the terrible months of August and September, some of them began to report every fatality as plague. Who could blame them for not looking closely for buboes or tokens? It was unlikely that any neighbors came out to answer an inquisitive searcher's questions about the illness. Grieving family members might have been too overcome to be of any help.

Other searchers, wearied by the constant sight of diseased bodies, undoubtedly sympathized with the inability of the survivors in yet another infected dwelling to admit that plague was in their home. Even worse for a family at the height of this contagion was the humiliation of seeing a loved one strapped down and taken away on a board, sling, or barrow. This was not the parting from life to which a culture steeped in religious symbols and rituals was accustomed. Searchers could be forgiven in September as they had been in June for the simple courtesy of identifying a warm corpse with something other than the common sickness.

Were these women searchers driven by neglect, indifference, and greed, as Dr. Hodges believed? He did the best he could for the poor people he saw on behalf of the Guildhall. Hodges thought that searchers who would pocket a shilling to lie were almost as bad as the "wicked" nurses he said were known to strangle their patients for their money and tell the searcher they had died of distemper in the throat. One man, Hodges declared, was stripped of his clothes and money and left to die, only to recover after the nurse fled.[4]

Whatever the motivations of London's searchers, who had no way to speak in self-defense, they reported a total of 309 deaths in Greater London as "feaver" for the most fateful week of the year, September 12–19. Another 101 deaths were attributed to "spotted fever." Early childhood deaths, frequent in any year, soared that week, with "teeth" accounting for 121 fatalities. That tabulation undoubtedly was closer to the real number of childhood fatalities than were the figures for these other diseases; many young children succumbed either from the plague or from a breakdown of life-giving support in their stricken family. Curiously, "grief" carried away only three persons.

Everyone had to come to terms with the epidemic. Poets and artists found a ready audience, just as Italian painters had in the wake of the Black Death three centuries before.[5] Doggerel verses were more serious now than in the previous winter, when the poetic friend of Thomas Rugge had made light of the comets. The grim processions and gyrating skeletons printed from wood-cuts during past great visitations now reappeared in broadsheets that kept coming off the presses. They flooded the town despite the heavy mortality among printers. New printings of *Londons Lord Have Mercy Upon Us* enumer-ated plague burials and total burials down to the current week. In bold italic type the typesetter added a "cheap medicine": two cloves of garlic cut very small in a pint of new milk. The optimistic advice—"drink it mornings fasting and preserveth from infection"—may have been undercut by the tract's illus-trations of dead-carts and coffins. A doggerel verse ended stoically:

> Oh where's the vows we to our God have made!
> When death & sickness come with axe and spade,
> And hurl'd our Brethren up in heaps apace,
> Even forty thousand in a little space:
> The plague among us is not yet removed,
> Because that sin of us is still beloved.
> Each spectacle of Death and Funerall,
> Puts thee and I in mind: We must die all.

What were Londoners thinking as they mulled over these gloomy reflec-tions? Making his way up the river between the public fires on the sixth of September, determined to keep an appointment with Albemarle, Samuel Pepys could scarcely believe the scene. "Fires on each side of the Thames," he observed, "and strange to see in broad daylight two or three Burialls upon the Bankside, one at the very heels of another—doubtless all of the plague— and yet at least 40 or 50 people going along with them."[6] It must have seemed like Dante's inferno. In September the public began ignoring the magistrates' ban on funeral processions. People cried out for their rituals— even if it meant spreading the plague among the mourners.

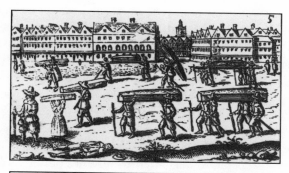

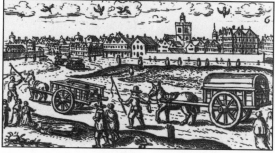

Fig. 11. Plague coffins and dead-carts in 1665. The first frame shows men with coffins on their shoulders and a woman bearing the small coffin of her child past the body of a fallen plague victim. The second frame features bearers with their identifying wands leading horses drawing an open dead-cart with coffins and a covered cart possibly holding uncoffined bodies. Courtesy of the Museum of London

Knells and Bells

Ye bells never cease to putt us in mind of our own mortality.
—JOHN TILLISON to Dean Sancroft, September 14, 1665

Day and night the church bells of London tolled their requiem message. Hodges said they were hoarse from continual use. The bell ringing might stop in a parish when the ropes broke or the bell ringer had so many deaths to ring for that he gave up ringing altogether. But nearby the bells sounded out the passing of yet another citizen.

Even in moments of silence, an unmistakable scent of death hung in the air. Down at Woolwich, Elizabeth Pepys couldn't find out whether her parents in Saint Sepulchre were alive or dead. Samuel had never stepped inside their door, and the messenger he sent to inquire had not come back. On his own travels back to London, Pepys was struck by the terror etched on people's faces: "How few people I see, and those walking like people that had taken leave of the world." On another day he was unnerved by their talk: "But Lord, how everybody's looks and discourse in the streets is of death and nothing else." He was obsessed by his own inability to think of other things. The death of his doctor, so long after his servant's passing, had made him forget what he wanted to do about his bookkeeping. And the plague pits preyed on his mind in a strange way. He walked toward Moorfields, knowing the dead were being buried en masse. "God forgive my presumption," he murmured. He had been curious "whether I could see any dead Corps going to the grave, but as God would have it, did not."[7]

Dean Sancroft had been away from Saint Paul's for two months. In that time the Destroying Angel's arrows struck so widely in the cathedral area that in some places the dead were piled in heaps on the ground before the buriers eventually took them away. Houses were locked up next to the court where the dean had lived before going for a rest cure at Tunbridge Wells and moving on to his brother's place in Cambridgeshire. The sacristan's wife had died of the common disease, and he had fled. John Tillison faithfully smoked Dean Sancroft's residence every Tuesday and Thursday, hopeful that eventually this plague would end and the dean would return.[8]

Samuel Pepys tried unsuccessfully to block out the sound. "Little noise heard day nor night but tolling of bells," he informed Lady Carteret. Alderman Turner was too occupied with public business at the Guildhall to pay attention to the bells of Saint Gregory's or, if he was conscious of the noise, he did not say. Across London Bridge, John Allin stared from the window of his rented rooms. Neither he nor the family with whom he boarded had come down sick, but the sights and sounds were unnerving. "I am, through mercy," he wrote, "yet well in the middest of death. And that, too approaching neerer and neerer, not many doores of[f], and the pitt open dayly within view of my chamber window. The Lord fitt me and all of us for our last end."[9]

Reverend Patrick was only too aware of the rising mounds in his churchyard, and his mood was mournful. The only topics of conversation, he wrote Mrs. Gauden, were the plague and death. "I can reflect on nothing so sadly as to be separate from my friends, and not so much as bid them farewell if I dye." The church bells at Saint Paul Covent Garden had pealed their sad message thirty times in seven days, all but one for plague victims. He had just come back from burying five parishioners that evening. The neighboring parish of Saint Martin in the Fields, which had six times the number of households and shared their common pesthouse, rang its bells for 286 burials that same week. Where were all these bodies going? Covent Garden's overseer of the poor, Thomas Rugge, knew the answer: many poor persons from these two parishes and others nearby were carted off to the pesthouse plague pit.[10]

For many, a church bell sounded the only acknowledgment of their departure. The rhythmic, pulsating sound broke the silence of empty shops in Cheapside and the abandoned navy office on Seething Lane. Samuel Pepys listened in spite of himself, knowing it might indicate how many persons in Saint Olave Hart Street had died that day. But he soon gave up the counting, thinking that the poor were too great in number to be accounted for. Nor could anyone measure the toll among the Quakers and other dissenters, "that will not have any bell ring for them." Pepys estimated that the full bill for the last week in August must be a quarter more than reported.[11]

At a rare meeting of the vestry of Saint Giles Cripplegate in September, the few members who gathered agreed it was God's punishment on the sins of the nation "and in a special manner this our parish."[12] How else to account for the second highest parish mortality in this Great Plague? In two decades, the parish had laid 28,000 bodies to rest; 8,069 of these interments came in 1665. Cripplegate's toll was greater than in any previous epidemic, in part because of the recent surge in population (see table 6).

Table 6. Saint Giles Cripplegate Burials
in Plague Years, 1603–1665

Year	Total Burials
1603	2,879
1625	3,570
1636	2,491
1641	1,650
1665	8,069

Funeral fees formed a large part of the year's poor relief budget at Saint Giles Cripplegate. Families that could afford it paid generously for their burials: A total of £282 14s. 4d. was received for "mortuaries," and £13 5s. 6d. was donated for "hearse cloaths." The parish took in £710 19s. 10d. from the poor tax and gifts, and spent £663 1s. 7.5d. The surplus was largely on paper; a parishioner had loaned £200 at 6 percent interest and had to be repaid.

The constant bell ringing placed a heavy burden on parish funds. Cripplegate had six large and mid-sized bells. Their repairs absorbed 22 percent of the operating budget:[13]

Expended to the carters when the bell went to be raised £100
Paid for raising the said bells, to Mr. Hudson £27
To James Allen for taking downe and hanging the great bell £5
Paid more for taking down the Treble and mending it £4
For bell clappers and ropes and mending the clock £8

On the gentle slope of Cornhill lay Samuel and Elizabeth Pepys' parish church. An observant passerby today may notice a mound in the churchyard. The ground was opened in 1891 for construction and then closed on the sight of uncoffined remains.[14] Entering the churchyard archway, one can look upward and reflect on the relief of skulls and crossbones, a grisly reminder of the toll in Hart Street and Seething Lane. When the plague finally withdrew from the parish, Samuel would look back on this time with a shudder. "It frightened me to see so many graves lie so high upon the Churchyard where people have been buried of the plague." He hoped the churchyard would be covered over with lime as required by the Guildhall as a health precaution.[15]

Roger L'Estrange's biweekly newssheets kept up a holier-than-thou drumbeat. In July they claimed that poverty and sluttishness caused half the plague deaths in the metropolis; in August, they saw little appearance of the infection in the main streets. The greatest mortality, L'Estrange asserted, was in "the sluttish parts of those parishes where the poor are crowded up together and in multitudes infect one another."[16]

Saint Olave Hart Street's death scene revealed a more complex and unsettling reality. Plague deaths had mounted from three in July to seventeen in August, climbed to sixty-four in September, and held at fifty-one in October. These bare statistics fail to reveal the reality that entire families were extinguished. John Hayward lost three daughters and a son to the infection in five days in September. A lodger, Edmund Poole, saw four sons and a daughter succumb between September 10 and 21; then he joined them in the churchyard. The Greenops, a poor family, lost five members.

Nor were the poor alone in this wholesale destruction of life. Saint Olave's well-to-do churchwardens and their families joined the dead. The upper churchwarden, Simon Giles, followed his son and wife to a fresh grave. His colleague George Green expired along with his son. A third churchwarden, William Poole, saw life slip from his wife and daughter; they were placed in a single coffin and lowered into the family vault. The parish clerk took pity on the surviving churchwarden: no *p* was placed beside the names of the two Elizabeth Pooles in the church register.[17]

The clerk, Mr. Hadley, survived the loss of two churchwardens but was overburdened with the official counts that he had earlier tried to hide in the published bills. When it was over, Saint Olave Hart Street's official count for the year in the Bills of Mortality stood at 160 plague burials and 234 total interments. Hadley's parish register included many more: 362 deaths from all causes that year. He had kept up his count for the parish's register, even when he didn't report accurately for the printed bill. Only 162 of the fatalities in the register were listed as interred in Saint Olave Hart Street's two churchyard areas, leaving two hundred others buried somewhere else. The parish bearers must have picked up scores of bodies in the streets, back ways, and abandoned houses and taken them to a nearby communal grave, keeping only a rough running count of the numbers. Among the dead were probably many lodgers and servants and some nurses. At the height of Saint Olave's epidemic in September and October, a bearer appeared with a dead-cart and hauled away a body from a terrified household, with little said on either side and no viewing by a searcher. This was part of the breakdown of the municipal order to shut up every infected house.

The total of 362 fatalities at Saint Olave Hart Street was stunning for a parish of only 274 households. If all the householders had stayed to wait out the plague, the mortality would have been the equivalent of more than one per family. But many substantial householders and their families were out of town. The true mortality rate may have been 40 percent or more of those who remained. And this was in a relatively wealthy parish, with a mean hearth number of 5.1. How might L'Estrange explain that deviation from his rosy picture of London's better neighborhoods escaping the infection?[18]

Trying to describe the increased tempo of the pestilence and the reality of an epidemic threatening to break down basic social norms, Nathaniel Hodges pictured family inheritances passing to three or four heirs in as many days.[19] Too many dwellings were infected to be taken care of by nurses and watchers. Little wonder that Mayor Lawrence spread the word for healthy citizens to stay indoors after dark so that shut-up families could come out for air and exercise. Pepys began to suspect strangers he passed on the street of having plague sores on them. The mayor, who prided himself on greeting petitioners at his door, addressed them from his balcony instead. The Guildhall was all but abandoned, the court of aldermen rarely meeting. The city's chamberlain juggled accounts so he could divert money to the parishes that had run out of relief funds and pay for new burial grounds and the brick wall closing them off from nearby dwellings.[20]

A Journey into Eternity

That the Burial of the dead . . . be at most convenient hours, always either before Sunrising, or after Sun-setting, with the privity of the churchwardens or constables, and not otherwise.

—*Orders Conceived and Published by the Lord Mayor and Aldermen*
of the City of London concerning the infection of the Plague, 1665

The Guildhall called them "tumultuary burials." Londoners knew them as "pitts." Whatever the name, they marked a rupture in the human civility to which surviving Londoners clung in their grief. Rugge referred to "a great hole" next to the Covent Garden–Saint Martin pesthouse; the other four pesthouses had similar pits for their dead, and Rugge again recorded the use of buriers from neighboring parishes. How many other cavernous holes were there around London? Rugge heard of pits "at every end of town" set aside for the numerous parishes whose churchyards were filled.[21]

Daniel Defoe remembered the legend of a "dreadful gulph" east of the wall, estimating its dimensions as forty feet long by fifteen feet wide. At twenty feet into the ground, the diggers struck water. If his sources and memory can be trusted, the pit was filled within two weeks in September, holding 1,114 bodies. To this day, Anglican rectors and vicars mention oral traditions of pits outside their churches, as at a circle in front of Saint John's Wood. With great assurance London taxi drivers show the curious where the Great Plague's pits were located. No two drivers report the same location. Open fields near the new pesthouse sheds on the periphery of the capital had plenty of vacant land to receive mass burials in 1665.

Plague pits in Finsbury Field within Cripplegate parish are thought to have held twenty-two hundred plague corpses. Communal graves have been found as far to the east as Chadwell and Wapping. Southwark's open fields were used when the churchyards could hold no more, causing people to re-name the land "Deadman's Place." It is unlikely that the stopgap burial place had been sanctified, for the bishop of London insisted that sanctified ground must remain so in perpetuity. The marshes at Gravesend became a mass grave for religious dissenters who had held services illegally and died on the *Black Eagle* prison ship before it could take them to exile in Jamaica.[22]

At Saint Bride's the vestry acted quickly as plague deaths mounted. The parish's regular bearer, Adam Baldwin, was joined by Edward Jennings and Henry Meades, who eagerly accepted the twelve shillings a week (soon raised to fifteen) offered by the vestry "for carrying the corps that shall dye of the plague." Their pay was to come from the customary fees for that service on "all persons visited that are able to pay." To lodge the new bearers at a safe distance from the public, the parish beadle cleared out the halberds and other arms stored at a shed inside the walls of the churchyard.[23]

Finding space for single graves became a problem. Saint Bride's grave-maker was initially instructed to make no graves without supervision by the churchwarden. Within two weeks the vestry added that he "digg the graves deepe" and asked the churchwarden "to give him something extraordinary for his paines as he shall thinke fitt." The neighboring parishes of Saint Dunstan in the West and Saint Martin Ludgate were charged heavily for burying their dead in the same grounds. These extra burials came to well over one thousand in addition to the twenty-two hundred residents of Saint Bride's who died during the year.

A week after his raise in pay, Henry Meades was dead. Two new bearers took his place. The upper churchyard was closed to all but families of the congregation who had held offices. All others were to be buried in the re-cently acquired lower churchyard, which contained more room and (more conveniently) no graves of past parish notables to be disturbed. The grounds quickly became an eyesore. To make it safer for the rector and his clerk to come there for burials, the bearers were forbidden to roam about in the churchyard or hang their clothes on the grounds. Saint Giles Cripplegate faced a similar problem, forcing neighboring houses backing onto the churchyard to lock their back doors and prohibiting the drying of clothes and collecting of rainwater from their roofs.[24]

By mid-August Saint Bride's was burying more than twenty bodies every night. The number reached the forties as September began. Laborers were hired at 2s. 6d. a day "for the digging of the pitts." Neighboring women were paid to serve breakfasts to the men, and food and drink were added as they labored. They were given new shovels and pickaxes as the old ones broke. By

September 19, the daily death count dropped to nineteen as the plague passed on to new territory; the pits had served their purpose.[25]

Death played no favorites, but final resting places were less egalitarian. In Covent Garden Reverend Patrick saw to it that his faithful parish clerk's wife and children had their own plots and prayers. When a noble lady's coachman and the churchwarden succumbed, their bodies were coffined up and placed in individual graves. For the poor, a single coffin was often used over and over again to transport bodies to the burial ground, where many were interred in a simple shroud. How much worse might the accoutrements of death have been for someone sent off to die in a pesthouse? Covent Garden's register bears no trace of where the Widow Page and the daughter of Widow Thorn were placed after they expired in the nearby pesthouse.[26]

Inside London's wall, cries of desperation from churchwardens reached the Guildhall. Ground was not available in any churchyards and space was lacking in the large burying ground next to the Bethlehem mental hospital. The city purchased vacant land in Finsbury Field north of the wall and put the keeper of Bethlehem's grounds under orders to "smother and suppress the stenches" from its mass grave and bury the bones and burn the coffin boards that had been dug up to make new room. In a time of critical need for burying space, the court of aldermen insisted that Bethlehem's keeper revert to single graves—a totally unrealistic command that he surely ignored.[27] Strangely, no mention had been made at the Guildhall after June of expanding the city pesthouse, including its burial ground.

Pesthouses

Sheds to be erected round the [city] pesthouse ground . . . in case the sicknesse continue to increase within the city and liberties.
—Order of the Lord Mayor of London, June 17, 1665

Pesthouse facilities had been on the minds of the king's councilors since April, but they put off action for six weeks, until the plague's spread from Saint Giles in the Fields to Saint Martin in the Fields threatened the courtier quarters of Westminster. The sole suburban pesthouse at the far end of Saint Margaret's was a long way from the site of the infection in the outlying parishes of Saint Giles and Saint Martin. To avoid having sick persons pass by the Piazza and Whitehall to that facility, the royal council ordered the two infected parishes to build their own plague facilities with a special levy on their householders.

Saint Giles in the Fields located a sizable plot north of the parish at Mutton Fields in the village of Marylebone. To placate villagers, the council had Saint Giles construct a separate path, ditch, and bridge for the entry of infected persons. A wall was built around the facility, and a well was dug for the inmates. A final proviso stipulated that all structures were to be torn down after the plague left.[28]

Saint Martin in the Fields agreed to share the erection of a pesthouse with neighboring Covent Garden, whose first plague deaths had been kept secret. The two parishes chose Clay Field, a five-acre plot in Soho Field. Its pesthouse became the largest plague hospital in the metropolitan area, accommodating up to ninety patients. Later, when the contagion took an enormous toll east of the city wall, a small facility was built in Stepney for the working-class eastern suburbs and infected prisoners and soldiers from the Tower of London.[29] The densely packed laboring suburbs across the Thames River in Southwark, where John Allin saw bodies entering the plague pit day after day, never had any pesthouse facility.

London's original pesthouse, constructed in Elizabeth I's time in Saint Giles Cripplegate next to Allen's Almshouses on Old Street, quickly proved inadequate for the sick poor within the walls and in the northern suburbs. Its makeshift burial ground was more accommodating, doubling as an adjunct to Cripplegate's overcrowded churchyard area. In June the mayor of London ordered new "shedds" to be added to the Cripplegate facility "with all convenient speed for the reception and accommodation of such persons as shall be sent thither from infected houses." The burden of death on the parish and pesthouse was such that the next year Cripplegate closed its overcrowded and odiferous churchyard for seven years.[30]

The old Westminster pesthouse at the Tothill Fields end of Saint Margaret parish was inadequate even for that parish's needs. The parish refitted the existing sheds and added ten "rooms" as the number of inmates soared. Two carpenters and a bricklayer, blacksmith, and ditch digger went to work for pay ranging from two to thirty-seven pounds for the completed job. Still, the expanded quarters were far too small for the cots and trundle beds crammed inside. In September eighty patients each week occupied the pesthouse. Westminster's Gatehouse prison took the overflow. A French physician, Dr. Grant, took charge of patients, dying in service.[31]

A veil of secrecy hung over London's five pesthouses. The three new facilities were not listed in the Bills of Mortality, and the weekly death counts

192 · THE ABYSS

from the two original facilities were far too low to be credible. For the entire year, the bills listed 156 plague deaths at the city pesthouses in Cripplegate, plus 3 from other causes. Curiously, the Tothill facility also reported 156 plague deaths. Undoubtedly, many in these cramped quarters expired without a statistical trace, while a few fortunate individuals survived their stay. What help were they given from the physician or surgeon in charge? How did expectant mothers go through the ordeals of childbirth? Records show that seven midwives went to deliver babies on six different occasions in Westminster's pesthouse, and a priest was listed as baptizing them. What courage these caregiving and religious acts demonstrated.

Although no account of life and death inside one of these pesthouses has yet been discovered, the churchwardens of Saint Margaret parish offer some clues in their weekly list of the inmates of Tothill Fields. A comparison of these counts with the same weeks' death counts reported in the Bills of Mortality yields an implausibly high survival rate that, at the peak of the epidemic, was far above the usual ratio of 10–40 percent for this disease. Such a deviation from the norm in a cramped facility where death was more likely than in many infected households defies all reason. The greatest likelihood was a breakdown in running the facility and counting the dying and dead.

When the occupancy of Saint Margaret's sheds jumped from four to fifteen in June, only four burials were recorded in the parish register for that month. In July the occupants doubled to thirty; again only four burials were recorded for each of the next two weeks. Then, as deaths in Saint Margaret's parish shot up from 200 to 350, with all but 12 listed as plague fatalities in the Bill of Mortality, the death count at the pesthouse was only 7. Yet the churchwardens counted 80 inmates that same week in this facility, making the survival rate a totally implausible 91 percent. Nor could the 39 pesthouse dwellers the churchwarden listed during the first week of August have been the same as the 39 persons reported buried there in the weekly bill, since 7 on the churchwardens' list were still there the next week!

Undoubtedly, the pesthouse keeper and his small medical staff were so overcome with caring for the sick that they lost track of who came in, who died, and who was discharged after recovering. Their confusion, however, was compounded by the habit of Saint Margaret's bearers of dropping some of their dead at the pesthouse pit instead of the churchyard. That would explain how the burial count for the first week of August reached thirty-nine despite the survival of seven inmates into the following week. A different tragedy awaited the people called Quakers, who kept excellent records of their fallen members.

For Whom the Bells Didn't Toll

I had not the freedom, satisfaction or peace to leave the city or Friends in and about London, in that time of such great calamity.

—George Whitehead, *The Christian Progress*

When George Whitehead left his home in Watling Street to attend a Friends meeting, he carried his nightcap in case soldiers burst in and took the worshipers to Newgate jail or the Gatehouse. The Quakers were a brave and nervy lot. They confronted Anglican priests on the street and in services about Christian orthodoxy. They met in secret, raising suspicions of planned insurrection in the minds of Captain General Albemarle at the Cockpit and the lieutenant of the Tower of London, Sir John Robinson. The diaries and newsletters of the plaguetime mention several roundups of dissenters; the Quakers were the most frequent targets, landing in infected jails.

The Friends' dedication to their sick and dying members was truly extraordinary. They were strong on fellowship and leery of ostentatious rituals. Their own burial grounds lacked even the simplest markers over the graves, yet nothing stopped them from visiting their sick or imprisoned.

Quakers lived throughout the metropolitan area, from Cripplegate to Southwark and from Stepney and other east-end suburbs to Westminster. Their beliefs forbade them to be interred in a consecrated Anglican churchyard. At the beginning of the visitation, they had a single large burying ground north of the wall by Checkers Alley in Bunhill Fields, which they made available to other dissenting groups. Able-bodied Friends went in teams with a barrow or other conveyance to the deceased's residence and took the body past the authorities to a quiet interment without ceremony in a single grave. When the numbers threatened the capacity of the Bunhill Fields ground in September, a second burial ground was opened in Southwark—convenient to the many Friends who lived south of the river and also to the local jail, where plague vied with jail fever among the diverse prison population.

Before the epidemic the Friends had about ten burials each month. According to legend their initial plague fatality was the wife of a charismatic Quaker preacher, Solomon Eccles.[32] The ensuing march of death left few tracks in any parish register, but the Friends' private register recorded everything from the complete name and parish of the fallen Friends to the cause of their deaths and sometimes the prison or deportation ship where they had breathed their last. In July 1665 the total number of fatalities rose to 35. During August, 254 of their dead were taken from homes and prisons across town for burial. September witnessed 478 Friends falling from the sickness. In addition to deaths in the prisons, 27 men and women died on the *Black Eagle* prison ship that September. George Whitehead found them crowded together on their deathbeds and dispirited but lifted up by his visit. The total number of Friends who died in this terrible "visitation" came to 1,117, a heavy burden for this widely scattered community of a few thousand.[33]

How many other religious dissenters fell during the Great Plague is unknown.[34] A Quaker in the city informed a country Friend at the peak of the epidemic, "Thousands more died than are in the bills."[35] He could not have been thinking only of their own congregations. Pepys alluded to others who would not have the bell rung for them. Presbyterians, Congregationalists, and Baptists were the main nonconformist communities of faith whose members vanished without a trace that summer. Some were buried in the parish ground near their homes, and a few in the Quaker burial grounds. The communal graves accepted anyone regardless of religious preference. The Dutch congregation of Austin Friars, including Mayor Lawrence, had mostly assimilated to the Anglican communion and the corridors of power. Some members took it upon themselves to stay and help; others followed English neighbors to the country.[36]

Virtually nothing is known about the fate of the Jewish community of London, which numbered a few hundred persons. They were not scapegoats, as Jews had been during the Black Death. They worshiped quietly at their Sephardic Synagogue in Creechurch Lane. On at least one occasion, Pepys attended a service there. The Jewish Historical Society has records of seven plague victims at their burial ground east of Aldgate and Mile End, but the sharply reduced attendance at synagogues after the epidemic suggests a much heavier mortality.[37]

The Last Reckoning

Many are sick and few escape. [Plague] raigned most heretofore in alleys, etc; now it dominates in ye open streets.
—John Tillison to Dean Sancroft, September 14, 1665

According to the Bills of Mortality, the epidemic in London reached its peak in mid-September. Yet death continued to stalk the city and suburbs, giving little comfort to persecuted dissenters and beleaguered churchwardens in the following weeks. As vaults in the church of Saint Olave Hart Street began to fill with plague-scarred bodies of well-to-do residents, Samuel Pepys wrote with a mixture of pride and anxiety to Navy Commissioner Sir William Coventry, "You, sir, take your turn at the sword [in naval engagement]. I must not therefore grudge to take mine at the pestilence." At Saint Paul's cathedral, John Tillison was awestruck by the wide path of death through streets and homes and shops that had previously been passed over.[38] The deadliness of the disease seemed greater now as the pool of healthy citizens was reduced.

We will never know the fates of most who fled, but a sampling of London's General Bill of Mortality for 1665 reveals that poor persons in crowded housing outside the walls suffered the greatest losses among those who stayed on. As summer ended, the infection swept into the eastern suburbs and south of the Thames. It also burrowed far into the countryside, spreading northward through the earl of Bridgewater's Hertfordshire. It turned eastward past Henry Foe's saddler's shop into Essex and narrowly missed Elizabeth Gauden's country haven outside Brentwood. The contagion appeared at the mouth of the Thames beyond Deptford, where John and Mary Evelyn lived. The archbishop of Canterbury issued a license to bury Greenwich's victims in a newly purchased site adjoining the pesthouse in Black Heath.[39]

The desire for dignity in death led increasing numbers of mourners to throw caution to the winds to give their friends a decent farewell. At Cripplegate, some wealthier congregants took up the tiles in the sanctuary to bury the dead. In Greenwich, Pepys witnessed "the madness of the town" following a corpse all the way to the grave, in flagrant defiance of the law. The innate desire for ceremony and finality was not to be set aside. Pepys and his navy colleagues tried to stop the practice, using their authority as ex officio magistrates of the dockyard town.[40]

Grim humor reflected both the troubled time and the spirit of endurance it evoked. A legend arose about a piper who collapsed on a London street in a drunken stupor. The bearers placed him on a dead-cart and piled on other bodies. As dawn approached the man regained consciousness and started to play his bagpipes. The eerie sounds terrified the bearers, who thought they were in the presence of the devil and fled, leaving the piper confused but very much alive. Many versions of this story exist; it was a natural tale for *A Journal of a Plague Year*. An elfin statue of this legendary piper, sculpted by Caius Gabriel Cibber, a Restoration artist, stands today in the Victoria and Albert museum.[41]

Table 7. Total Burials in Representative London Parishes,
December 20, 1664–December 19, 1665

Suburban Parishes outside the Walls	Total Burials	City Parishes inside the Walls	Total Burials
Stepney (northeast; highest metropolitan mortality)	8,598	Christ Church (by Newgate exit; highest city mortality)	653
St. Giles Cripplegate (north; second highest mortality)	8,069	St. Stephen Coleman Street (bordering the northern wall)	560
St. Olave Southwark (south; John Allin's parish)	4,793	All Hallows Barking (bordering the Thames River)	514
St. Mary Whitechapel (east)	4,766	St. Gregory by the cathedral (Alderman Turner's shop)	376
St. Margaret Westminster (southwest)	4,710	St. Olave Hart Street (Samuel Pepys' parish)	237
St. Giles in the Fields (west; William Boghurst's parish)	4,457	St. Helen (Mayor Lawrence's parish)	108
St. Bride (west of the Fleet River)	2,111	St. Mary Woolchurch (first city plague burial)	65
St. Paul Covent Garden (west; Rev. Patrick's parish)	408	St. Stephen Walbrook (Dr. Hodges' parish)	34
All 33 suburban parishes	82,099	All 97 city parishes	15,207

SOURCE: *A General Bill for this present year, ending the 19 of December 1665.*

Three centuries later, Albert Camus tried to make sense of plague's challenge to the human spirit in a novel set in twentieth-century North Africa. Setting the scene of unspeakable destruction, he pictured the charnel house of ancient Athens "reeking to heaven," putrefying pallets stuck in the mud floor of a converted Turkish leper house, and "the carnival of masked doctors at the Black Death." Not least of all he told of the "cartloads of dead bodies rumbling through London's ghoul-haunted darkness." The protagonist of Camus's 1947 novel, *The Plague,* is Dr. Rieux, a worthy fictional successor to the Great Plague's Boghurst and Hodges. As the bodies pile up around his city of Oran, Dr. Rieux hearkens back to the Athenians who had brought their dead to the water's edge after nightfall to give them a dignified burial in funeral pyres. There was not enough room for the dead, and so the living fought each other with torches rather than abandon their dead to a watery grave. Dr. Rieux feels strangely comforted by this contested scene: "The red glow of the pyres mirrored on a wine-dark, slumberous sea, battling torches . . . whirling sparks across the darkness, and thick, fetid smoke rising toward the watchful sky." Could future Algerians experience this anguishing brush with destiny? "Yes," he muses, "it was not beyond the bound of possibility."[42]

In Pepys' London as in Thucydides' Athens and Camus's Algeria, some people responded to this fright—this night of the mind—by shaping simple rituals to deny the victory of death. The urge for communal survival was evident among the ascendant Anglicans, the persecuted Quakers, and the other outlawed religious sects of the day. Young and old, poor and rich, male and female were affected by this spirit, including some who suffered the most and others who were waiting out the capital's visitation in the country.

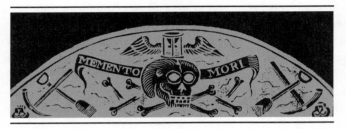

Contagion in the Countryside

I leave to your consideration whether it will be safe to stay a night in your house [in Clapham] till the plague be more abated. It is the last place I lay in after my owne lodgings, save that night only when I left you before you went away.
—SYMON PATRICK to Elizabeth Gauden, December 16, 1665

Safe Havens?

In early summer, the city's broadsheets called it a "Great Plague of London." By September, when astrologers were preparing their almanacs for the next year, it was a great plague of the nation. William Lilly's wistful prediction that Londoners would soon lose their fear of plague and return to trade masked a cruel truth he knew full well. The recent spread of contagion beyond the capital was hampering London's recovery as much as the lingering of infection in the city and suburbs.[1] "God's Angel hath drawn his sword," John Tanner wrote with a dramatic flourish, "and with a great stroke hath smote the Nation with the plague." His fellow astrologer Thomas Trigge predicted that the devouring enemy of humankind would strike more fiercely at the countryside than it had the capital.[2]

The Great Plague had stopped trade from London to the interior and marooned ships that normally took London's manufactured goods to provincial ports. Now the reverse flow halted because of contagion in the countryside. New cloth was no longer coming in from Colchester and the other cloth-making towns of Essex. Ships from Europe that had stopped as usual at a provincial port to unload some of their prized wine, brandy, oil, and raisins before going on to London were quarantined by the local infection.[3]

At the city and country ends of this new trauma, tensions mounted. Daniel Defoe captured the time with a tale of three London craftsmen fleeing through Essex. Armed with their practical sense and little else, they join forces with a band of refugees from Cripplegate. But as they approached Brentwood on the Roman road to Colchester, they encountered frightened villagers and the infection they thought they had eluded.[4]

Here fiction met fact. Elizabeth Gauden was staying just outside Brentwood during this terrible summer, awaiting the birth of another child. While Denis moved back and forth procuring naval supplies, Elizabeth settled into Hutton Hall, the spacious residence of her sister-in-law, widow of Bishop John Gauden (Denis's brother). A mile off the beaten path of the Roman road and away from Brentwood's dwellings, the house seemed a perfect haven from London's great visitation. It was. The town was eighteen and a half miles from London Bridge. Elizabeth could relax in the company of her sister-in-law, whose life as a bishop's wife had made her an excellent host and an entertaining companion. Elizabeth whiled away the hours with friendly neighbors, but the highlight of each week was the arrival at the nearby postal office of a letter from her faithful correspondent Symon Patrick in Covent Garden.

Elizabeth's pregnancy included some trying bouts of illness. Symon shared her joy in the safe birth of another boy and relief that she had escaped the terrible childbed mortality of the plague season. Symon passed on news he thought would divert Elizabeth with the caution, "You must not expect particulars from me."[5] But she did want particulars. Reluctantly he told her about the contagion's frightful toll on numerous clergy friends in the city and others who had fled to the country only to be cut down by the distemper. She related her postpartum ups and downs, the latest on her delicate baby's health, and her strong attachment for him.

Whatever the precise nature of this bond between a married woman and a bachelor minister (who could have married without breaking his priestly vows), they called it love. It was the perfect antidote for her flagging spirits out at Hutton Hall. Elizabeth dropped hints that they might be reunited despite this plague. Couldn't he come out to see her, she asked? The priest refused, at first gently and then more firmly. But the more he demurred the more she pressed. His life, she implored, was too valuable to risk his staying at Covent Garden. He replied as well as the theologian in him knew, "I am in the hands of the same God that delivered you." He was writing twice a week now. "What is the matter," he objected, "that you make such a long apology in your last letter about my not coming: It is enough that I am well, and to heare that you are so . . . I pray God preserve you and bring you and all your relations together againe."

Next she suggested he consider crossing the river to Surrey during the week and returning for Sunday services. "But if I should go," he replied, "why would you have mee to be at Clapham, when my brother is so neare [at Battersea] and you are not there?" Brushing aside her argument that his life was special, he shot back almost indignantly, "Am I better than another?" He would stay with his flock except for rare day-visits to his brother's place.[6]

Elizabeth watched in dismay as the weekly toll in the metropolis approached ten thousand. The infection had spread along the south bank of the Thames around the archbishop of Canterbury's palace at Lambeth, threatening Clapham and Battersea. She knew it was less safe than ever for her to return home, and she felt remorse for playing on Symon's heartstrings with talk of his escaping his parish's poisoned air.

By October the danger was more immediate. Brentwood's fashionable inns and other conveniences on the Roman road had attracted more than the usual traffic of Londoners, and plague had come with them. Before the year's end the infection would carry away 70 persons in Brentwood and 110 at nearby Romford.

The epidemic swept on through Essex, devastating its thriving cloth-making communities. A few miles from Brentwood in Bishop Gauden's first parish at Bocking, the church bell tolled for a hundred burials or more week after week until the epidemic finally ended in December 1666. A faded memorial in the adjacent town of Braintree remains to this day a mute witness to a similar tragedy: only 63 of the town's 284 households escaped the Destroying Angel. In these twin communities, more than one thousand women, men, and children perished of an estimated population of three thousand. The mortality rate was close to two times that of London.[7]

The two Mrs. Gaudens were captive residents as the raging distemper closed in on Brentwood. The local authorities hastily threw up a makeshift pesthouse near an inn that served as the postal office. A fatality in the pesthouse and the spread of the sickness into several parts of the town put a sudden halt to Elizabeth's correspondence with Symon; she dared not endanger a servant's life by sending him to the posting place until the area was clear of the infection.

Patience had never been one of Elizabeth's strong points. It seemed an eternity since she had been with old friends in Clapham. She prayed for the cool October air to banish the miasmas that hung over Greater London and make it possible to go home. Symon knew Elizabeth's temperament only too well, and that worried her also. He would be imagining the worst as the time since her last letter grew longer and longer.[8]

The View from the Country

That one parish of St. Giles [in the Fields] hath done us all this mischiefe.

—SIR THOMAS PEYNTON to the royal court at Salisbury, August 7, 1665

Thirty miles beyond Brentwood, Ralph Josselin's anxiety mounted. He had begun August conducting the Fast Day service and collection at Earls Colne for "distressed London." A week later his diary entries grew ominous: the weather had turned violent with a sad, strong wind; Saint Giles Cripplegate's latest toll was 690; and the Colne valley's market center at Colchester had become infected.[9] In the farther reaches of East Anglia, plague spread from Yarmouth to the interior of Norfolk and closed down the colleges of Cambridge. Elsewhere in the land scarcely a county remained unaffected. The Great Plague in England continued through the cold winter and all the next year, adding 100,000 victims in the provinces to the same number in Greater London in 1665 and several thousand additional fatalities in the capital in 1666.

When the pestilence moved northward through the Midlands, it marooned the countess of Huntingdon's son-in-law and grandchildren in Northamptonshire. The parish authorities in Hertfordshire, where the earl of Bridgewater had fled from Cripplegate, erected a pesthouse in the heart of the county. The distemper was approaching the cathedral city of Durham and the coal towns of Newcastle and Sunderland in the far northeast of England. Panicked rumors of contagion circulated in Dorset and Devon in the southwest. On the west coast, the major port of Bristol remained on alert for plague-bearing ships and infected inland travelers alike.

The coastal trade sped the contagion's spread. Sick sailors and Dutch prisoners brought the plague into Evelyn's hospitals in Middlesex and Kent and his colleague Sir William Doyly's makeshift facilities in Essex and Suffolk. From the Cockpit in Westminster, Captain General Albemarle gave orders to Pepys and Evelyn to double their efforts to supply and succor their charges, but there was no more room to house the sick and wounded, and

residents refused to put them up. The navy office's temporary home in
Greenwich was unsafe because of infection in the dockworkers' living and
working quarters. By the year's end 231 died of plague in the port town, and
many more followed in 1666.

Pepys was anxious at the Greenwich office, but Evelyn was nearly desperate. Unless the king outfitted an empty ship at anchor between Woolwich
and Deptford as a hospital vessel, he pleaded, the whole fleet could become
infected from sick sailors in port. To add to his worries, thirty houses had
been shut up near his own home. Fear went through his household when a
servant became sick "of a swelling." Mary Evelyn, who was expecting their
seventh child, objected strongly to leaving with the children, but she finally
relented at John's insistence. She took the children to her brother-in-law's
home in Surrey, while John remained at their Sayes Court estate, "a living
monument of God Almighty's protection," he said.[10]

Country people were as afraid as ever of catching the plague from London, as new arrivals from the city came their way every week. The harvesting
season brought a new threat from migrant farm workers. At Paddington,
then a village west of London, the vicar believed that the contagion had
come in with a crowd hired for pea picking who had been housed in a
farmer's barn. From rural Kent, word reached the peripatetic king that harvesting made it virtually impossible "to keep people in good order." "That
one parish of St. Giles at London," the informant added bitterly, "hath done
us all this mischiefe."[11]

Reverend Josselin found some comfort in his farm's bountiful harvest as he
pondered the empty pews of his church. The approaching plague was drawing
huge crowds to itinerant preachers calling on everyone to repent before it was
too late. The beleaguered pastor's diary jottings had become a jumble: "God in
mercy stop infection." "The weather sad, but this day cooling." "Died in London: plague 4237; all 5568." Saddest and most frightening of all was the danger
at hand: "Colchester [people] seeke into the country for dwellings."[12]

It was only six weeks since Josselin had first taken note of the massive
flight from London. Now wealthy merchants, professional people, and employers of the Dutch cloth workers in Colchester, a great provincial center of
10,000 to 12,000 inhabitants, began fleeing from their town's plague. God's
Destroying Angel had visited the town heavily in 1579, 1603, 1626, 1631, and
most recently during the Civil War in 1644. Colchester's current Bills of
Mortality recalled this unhappy history (see table 8).

During the first seven weeks of the current visitation in Colchester, the
parish searchers had viewed 787 plague corpses; 894 townspeople had died

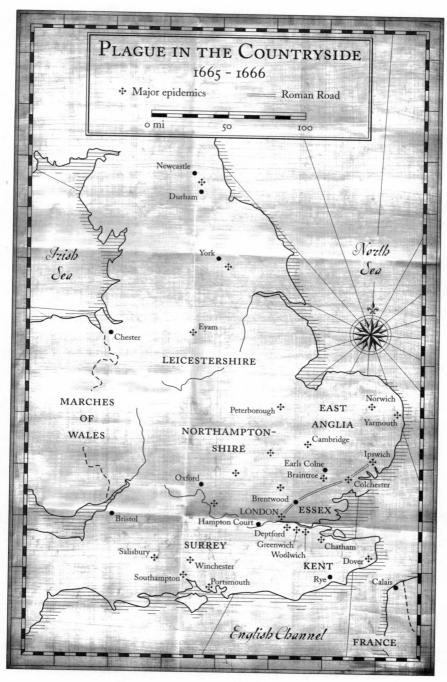

Map 5. Plague in the Countryside, 1665–1666

Table 8. Colchester Bills of Mortality,
August 14–October 6, 1665

Week	Plague Burials	Other Burials
August 14–21	26	2
August 21–28	66	2
September 1–8	122	4
September 8–15	153	22
September 15–22	159	25
September 22–29	100	26
September 29–October 6	161	27

from all causes. The next four weeks saw 334 burials, of which 276 were identified as due to plague. Confounding folk wisdom, the distemper continued through the winter. In December the gravediggers, greatly augmented in numbers, buried 200 bodies, 180 listed as plague deaths.[13] As in London, these official figures told only part of the grim truth. John Allin learned through his contacts with the English and Dutch dissenter communities in Southwark and Colchester that the toll among the town's cloth workers was much higher than was being reported. "God accept us and spare us for his mercy sake," Josselin wrote on October 4 as he sent his congregation's Fast Day collection to Colchester.[14]

The Greatest Plague

They bury'd upwards of 5,259 People in the Plague year, even more in Proportion than any of its neighbours, or than the Citty of London.
—DANIEL DEFOE, *A Tour Thro' the Whole Island of Great Britain*

Five hours' ride on horseback from London lay Colchester, atop a hill with long streets descending to weavers' cottages and water mills on the Colne River. The town's Norman castle dominated the north Essex landscape the way Saint Paul's cathedral did that of Middlesex and Surrey. England's country towns were all vastly inferior to London in population, commerce, and industry, but Colchester, the first capital of Roman Britain, was at the top of the second tier of provincial centers, exceeded in population only by Bristol, Exeter, Newcastle, Norwich, and York.[15]

Three times a week Colchester's markets beckoned to villagers with produce, livestock, and grain. A cluster of inns outside the town's six gates and on High Street catered to affluent visitors. Poorer country folk and urban laborers frequented the cheaper alehouses dotting the parishes just outside the town center. Shoppers crowded High Street, seeking fabrics and draperies made by the large Dutch and Flemish immigrant community and household stuffs and luxury items that arrived from London via the Roman road or via merchant vessels to the small port at the Hythe. The town's trade with European ports across the North Sea was brisk and lucrative. In two years, however, Colchester lost half its population, a catastrophe that a prominent local historian judges to be "the most destructive outbreak experienced by any large town in early modern England."[16]

Ralph Josselin knew the town's economic vibrancy from his many visits for goods and services, and he probably also sensed its major economic vulnerability: dependence on the volatile cloth-making industry. But it was plague that brought the town to its knees in August 1665. The locals could only guess whether the infection came in by sea or land, on infected goods and persons from Yarmouth to the north, or from London to the south. The mouth of the Colne River loomed as a highly likely flash point after a Colchester distiller helped a boatload of refugees from London slip past a suspicious constable.[17] Or the sickness might have accompanied the two thousand Dutch sailors captured during the battle of Lowestoft and brought to the castle jail by Evelyn's fellow commissioner, Sir William Doyly. A few escaped, and Doyly let it be known that, if any more got loose, the entire area was likely to be infected. The local Dutch population had their own contacts with families and friends in infected Amsterdam as well as London. One of them could easily have brought in the sickness with imported goods, especially cloth and clothing.[18]

The plague may have slipped in at several entry points. Cloth making in the Dutch quarter collapsed as workers died in huge numbers and their masters fled up the Colne valley.[19] A modern historian describes the downturn in the starkest of terms: "Manufacturing, trade, local government, and formal religious worship virtually ceased while the plague was at its height." Doyly wrote in panic to Evelyn: "The sickness is broken out most fiercely.

The present mayor hath noe authority to rule this numerous people." Like Albemarle at the Cockpit, Doyly at Colchester castle feared that the dissenting population, English and Dutch alike, would try to rise up under cover of the chaos created by the plague.[20]

Many of Colchester's forty-eight council members fled to neighboring villages, and the few attempts to call the town assembly into session at the Moothall on High Street were pitiful affairs. But perhaps town deliberations were not really necessary to set up the controls that the townspeople knew from previous experiences with plague. Despite Doyly's fears and the mayor's precipitous flight, in one key respect the assembly members were in a better position to fight this invader than were Albemarle and Lawrence in London. They had authority over the entire municipality, including its suburban liberties and adjacent semirural parishes.

Three men remained at the Moothall on High Street day in and day out, week after week, month upon month. The signatures of Deputy Mayor Moore and Aldermen Lamb and Tenneth appear throughout the pages of the thick assembly book beneath the columns of money they handed to the churchwardens and overseers of the poor from Colchester's sixteen parishes. As the crisis deepened, they took direct charge of many functions that in London were handled by the parish officers. A hurried scribe squeezed a list of their acts onto the bottom of the folio pages in a hand that became more and more crabbed and tiny until it was scarcely decipherable. They disbursed plague-relief taxes collected from an ever-widening arc of the surrounding countryside directly to needy persons who could still walk to the town center for their weekly handout. They hired masons and carpenters and glaziers and roofers to build two pesthouses. They paid doctors, apothecaries, and surgeons for physick and lancing of buboes.

No one seemed beyond the reach of these three men, who worked as hard and long as Alderman Turner and Dr. Hodges inside London's wall. When not gathering in and handing out money, they put on their judicial robes as justices of the peace and sentenced the few men and women brought before them by the town constables for breaches of the peace and defiance of plague regulations. In the Dutch quarter of town, lusty singing and carousing in taverns went on long after the nighttime curfew. Some individuals defied the constables to their face, and one called the justices foul names when hauled before their improvised court. The unraveling of mayoral authority that the outsider commissioner Doyly had predicted never occurred, however.

Colchester was famous for the Peasants Revolt after the Black Death, pre-

Reformation Lollards, and the summary execution of two arch-royalists at the castle wall by angry Puritans during the Civil War. Yet the town remained peaceful throughout the plague. For one thing the town government had by now assimilated prominent merchants and tradesmen from Dutch and other immigrant sects, making their dissenting rank and file less likely to cause trouble than in the past. Also, the heavily populated Dutch part of town suffered the greatest fatalities among the inhabitants; sickness and grief left little energy to resist plague controls.

Survivors of the terrible mortality in the pestered Dutch quarters by the river pooled their resources with all the vigor of wealthier citizens around High Street. Quakers and Baptists took care of their own. The Dutch Congregation (the town's only legal dissenter body) succored its sick and poor members. The sixteen Anglican churches of Colchester became the headquarters of official plague relief for their parishes, just like the 130 churches in Greater London. Warders, searchers, nurses, and buriers took up their parochial tasks. Overseers of the poor went to the Moothall and out into the country to collect money for the "visited poor" of their parish. Churchwardens kept their accounts. Every relief unit was badly shrunken by deaths and desertions, but some eighty courageous souls took up the slack, keeping order, burying the dead, and offering comfort to the living. When parishes ran out of poor-tax money and a plague-tax supplement, levies on the surrounding area and gifts from Josselin's and other churches saw them through the worst period of the epidemic. The total relief income for this hard-hit provincial center came to twenty-seven hundred pounds, a prodigious sum.[21]

The small graveyard of Saint Peter's parish could not hold all the parish's 691 plague victims. Even the ingenuity of the gravediggers at Saint Bride's in London would have been insufficient for the task. The bodies must have been taken somewhere out of town. Townspeople today speak of a plague pit off the Mersey road, where there is a suspicious-looking mound.[22] There are many likely spots. Possibly, there were common burial grounds adjacent to Colchester's two pesthouses, one in rural Mile End parish and the other closer in at Saint Mary at the Wall. (The location is better remembered for the royal cannon "Humpty Dumpty" that fell from the church wall during a Civil War siege, inspiring the nursery rhyme.) In 1665 and 1666, the loss of 40–50 percent of the town's population (estimated at five thousand persons) doubled the attrition ratio in metropolitan London. Colchester held the unhappy distinction also of having the longest visitation in the entire country, officially from mid-August 1665 to the first week of December 1666.

The continuous visitation with no interruption and far greater mortality in the second year than the first put a burden on the townspeople's material and emotional resources beyond anything Londoners experienced. The cloth-making industry, more central to Colchester's economy than in Cripplegate, experienced total collapse. The town suffered as nearly total an economic shutdown as occurred anywhere in England, except perhaps for Braintree and Bocking, which had virtually no middle-class tax base. The twenty-seven hundred pounds Colchester spent on relief for its poor almost doubled the sum that London's Saint Margaret Westminster paid out to keep its densely packed population in food, clothing, and medicaments during its plague ordeal.[23]

One isolated country parish suffered an even higher fatality rate. Eyam, nestled in a remote valley in northern Derbyshire, all but disappeared. The vicar, Reverend Mompesson, persuaded his flock to remain rather than flee and infect the countryside. This spared the surrounding area, while in the village 76 families were visited and 259 lives lost. Among the deceased was Mompesson's wife. When the plague siege that had begun in September 1665 finally ended in October 1666, he said in relief: "Now, blessed be to God, all our fears are over." The village lost between 50 percent and 80 percent of its residents, depending on how one interprets the evidence.[24]

The King's Service

I know none amongst our court greate-ones who do naturally care for our state. For all seek theire owne.

—John Evelyn to Lord Corniberry, September 9, 1665

The Destroying Angel was no respecter of persons; not even the sacred monarch could be sure of fending off her arrows. The royal escape route up the Thames River, Dr. Hodges affirmed, was a conduit for "tainted goods," and the royal court's hurried departure to the interior from the water's edge at Hampton Court had its own risks. The duke and duchess of York traveled northward to maintain order with their presence and an armed guard amid rumors of uprisings against church and state. The king headed southward, eager for the pleasure of inspecting the shipyard at Portsmouth and sailing in the Channel. On the first of August, he entered Salisbury with pomp and ceremony. His wife, mistress, ministers, and court followed at a more leisurely pace, bringing along the king's two nieces. The plague was not quite as far away as Charles would have wished, however. Before he left Portsmouth he ordered the town to build a pesthouse.[25]

At Salisbury, Charles and Catherine hunted stags, visited Stonehenge, and inspected a nearby noble estate in case they needed a new haven. Charles resumed the hallowed royal tradition of touching scrofulous subjects, perhaps to show he did not fear the plague. An attendant carefully inspected those who approached the sacred monarch for his magical cure before they knelt; the king healed scrofula, not the plague!

An ill wind blowing into the temporary royal capital soon claimed its first plague victim, the wife of a groom in the queen's stables. Charles's entourage swiftly banished to the open countryside everyone not on a list of courtiers and town residents.[26] Angry citizens murmured at paying doubly for this royal visit: first with a special tax to welcome their monarch and second with the infection that a "horde of harpies" had brought in their baggage. The royal court countered that the infection came from a poor, pestered suburb of Salisbury and ordered several of its cottages shut up.

Charles stood above the fray, providing a royal coach for the Spanish ambassador after discreetly closing his infected carriage quarters. When a royal farrier developed a swelling in his armpit that looked too serious to be explained by a kick from a horse (the initial story), the inn where he stayed was shut up. The king happened to pass by the inn and asked from a safe distance if they were all well. They politely replied that they were, and the obliging monarch assured them they would want for nothing and he would take care of the losses they sustained from their unfortunate confinement.[27]

After roaming the safest areas around Salisbury while an advance party prepared his next home, Charles galloped into Oxford, with its superb living quarters in the colleges, on September 27. His brother the duke of York joined him after a successful tour of the north, and the court was fuller than it had been since the infection entered Saint Giles in the Fields and Covent Garden.

In Oxford, the king summoned Parliament for its first session in six months, and peers and commoners swelled the throng. Tales of court hedonism and ribald verses on the pregnant condition of the king's favorite mistress reached London at an awkward time for the court: the capital was reeling from the worst weeks of the infection, and the war at sea was not going well. "The fleet came home with shame to require a great deal of money, which is not to be had," Pepys groaned. Either the sailors would come ashore and catch the plague, or they would remain on their ships at a greater charge to the Treasury. "As things look at present, the whole state must come to Ruine," he wrote in his secret diary.[28]

John Evelyn complained to a noble friend that no one at court cared about the state's needs.[29] Evelyn and his fellow commissioners were falling deeper and deeper into debt trying to cover housing and medical expenses. Nothing short of two thousand pounds a week would save them from utter collapse. Salary charges for physicians, surgeons, and officers, as well as quarters and medicaments, were eating up all reserves. The plague ships and makeshift hospitals and prisons were hopelessly overcrowded.

In desperation, Evelyn traveled to Westminster to plead his case to Albemarle at the Cockpit. Albemarle suggested stopgap solutions and wrote to the king for approval. But even this intrepid statesman had no solution to the overcrowding, and his mind was on public order. Some of Evelyn's prisoners had escaped to the countryside, he admonished him. Evelyn and his subordinates must tighten security at the hospital-prisons and be satisfied with the facilities they had.[30]

Pepys was managing to hold off his victualers with promises of money. But Evelyn and Doyly faced hundreds of new charges coming off the English and Dutch ships every week, most of them maimed or sick. Albemarle got £5,000 to Evelyn from the sale of booty from captured Dutch treasure ships and another £2,000 from a goldsmith in London. The commissioners placed their needs at £60,000![31] No personal remuneration, Evelyn said, could induce him to continue. His servants and officers, and Doyly's also, had fallen to the plague. "We have nothing more left us to expose but our persons," he informed a royal councilor. "We are every moment at the mercy of a raging pestilence by our daily conversations and an unreasonable multitude [of maimed and sick sailors] who dye like doggs in the streets unreguarded." Only faith and duty kept Evelyn at his post.[32]

Parliament's three-year supply of £2,500,000 for the Dutch war was all but gone after twelve months. Without blinking, the Lords and Commons voted a Royal Aid of £1,250,000. But how could this tax be collected? Pepys was skeptical. The king owed the city of London money, houses were vacant, and trade was in the doldrums. A desperate privy council ordered tax collectors to break open empty houses in London and sell what they found.[33] Evelyn and Pepys would see little of this money, if any.

The king and Parliament faced an even more daunting challenge from the plague, which they had been sidestepping so long. The subcommittee of the council assigned at the beginning of the epidemic to suggest new measures had disbanded with the flight of the court with little to show for its discussions. Now the greatest fear among the king's advisors was that dissenters might attempt some bold new attack on church and state. A new law plugged the one gap in the Restoration's suppression of activities by religious dissenters. The Five Mile Act prohibited ejected dissenting ministers from living within five miles of any incorporated community. That ruled out London, dissenter centers such as Colchester, and even remote places like Rye on the southern coast.

Almost as an afterthought, the two houses debated changes in the nation's Plague Orders. The Commons insisted on closing the loopholes that had kept pesthouses and home quarantines located away from courtiers' doors. The Lords insisted that there would be no shutting up of the homes of peers nor a pesthouse or burial place near the mansion of any gentlemen.[34] They were at an impasse. With relief, the two houses joined in a rousing vote of thanks to the king for "his great care in preservation of his people and the honour of the nation" against the Dutch.[35] On that happy October note, the Oxford Parliament ended; the revamping of the Plague Orders was left to another day, as it had been under the king's father after the last major visitation of the sickness.

Hutton Hall and Covent Garden

I am afraid you are troubled that I have not wrote this last post because I was so ill when I wrote last. But the reason I did omit it was because there was one dead of the sicknesse out of the pest house, and I thought it not safe to send [a messenger to Brentwood].

—ELIZABETH GAUDEN to Symon Patrick, October 5, 1665

Symon had just sent a frantic letter to Hutton Hall, wondering why he had not heard from Elizabeth. It was a relief to know from her October 5 letter that she was still alive. Her words bore another happy prospect. "The plague is in divers places in the towne," Elizabeth fretted, "but now the pest house is removed to another place in the towne more safe." Their correspondence could resume its normal rhythm.[36]

But new interruptions in the postal deliveries from Hutton Hall followed. Again Symon was beside himself: "What shall I think? Are you alive or do I write to another world? Is it possible that the post should be so unfaithful as to lose all the letters of the last week?" His questions continued to tumble out: "Are you ill that you dare not tell me how ill you are?" Symon's anxiety about Elizabeth's danger was heightened by the sight of recovered neighbors terrifying passersby with their embraces. The authorities in Westminster were no longer shutting up infected houses in some streets, despite the vigilance of Albemarle and Craven. Newly infected parishioners—the "vulgar, poorer sort," he confided in an uncharacteristic slur—were going everywhere.[37] Three days after writing that anxious note, Symon was in a happier mood on receiving a letter from Elizabeth. "My very deare friend, it was a singular joy to me when I did but see your hand last night."

Elizabeth, in turn, was delighted to hear of his improved mood and the pronounced dip in fatalities in the metropolis. Her spirits were buoyed by thoughts of heading homeward. Perhaps, Symon thought, this prospect would get Elizabeth over her headaches and ill spells. But he was concerned by her mood swings and tendency to become excited and impatient. She might still catch the infection. Clapham was not yet safe, nor were the routes around London to get there. Hutton Hall was her best haven, despite the encircling epidemic in Essex. She should remember her brother's advice: "Go far, stay long, return late." For her part Elizabeth persisted in urging Symon to take care of himself.

As the death toll in Greater London finally began to drop, Reverend Patrick seized on the chance to move to better quarters. "You must send your next to James Street, whither I am going the beginning of the week. I have an handsome study, a furnished room to lye in." Happily, he had hung it with Colchester "bay" cloth, "which I had of a safe hand, not thinking it fit to venture to enquire after anything better." Elizabeth was relieved at the knowledge he was taking better care of his needs, even to keeping his rooms warm with coverings on windows. But she worried that the move might delay delivery of his next letters. It was imperative not to lose touch, for the last part of his letter brought disturbing news. "My poore clerk," Symon admitted, "found his house infected, and acquainted me with it. I was so pity-full as to bid him come out of the house himself, and attend his business, and I should not be afraid of him."

She kept an anxious eye on London's Bills of Mortality as the temperature fell. One week the overall toll was lower; the next week it increased again in some inner and outer parishes. The plague was heavy at Wandsworth near the Battersea house of Symon's brother in Surrey, and right next door to him a girl had died, "not without strong suspicion of the plague." Elizabeth would know it was time to return when her brother reopened his London home and her husband found Clapham safe. The prospects looked good. The overall metropolitan bill had dropped for four weeks running: from 4,929 to 4,327, then to 2,665, and in this week's bill down to only 1,421 burials. Symon had buried more than a dozen persons, however, during each of those weeks. It was just as well that Elizabeth remain at Hutton Hall.[38]

Happier events greeted others in the country. "This morninge," John Evelyn's father-in-law, Sir Richard Browne, wrote to him at Sayes Court, "at half an hour past four I was awakened with the happy newes of the safe delivery of [your] daughter. The goodiest childe that ever your eyes beheld, and the mother (God be praised) in as good a state of health, strength and temper as can be desired . . . with the assistance of our Country midwife." That evening the father received the news by express mail. John Evelyn was overjoyed, and the timing of his daughter's arrival at his brother's place in Wotton could not have been better. It was the first of October, contagion had lessened in London, and Sayes Court remained miraculously uninfected. His servant's illness had been nothing but surfeit. John could travel to Wotton without worrying about carrying the infection.

Unfortunately, the sickness at Deptford kept his family from going home. After a joyous reunion John Evelyn took the road back to Sayes Court and his navy duties. Mary Evelyn broke the news to her father, who had recently come down from Oxford. "I find by Mr. Evelyn wee cannot with safety think of Deptford yet a while, the sicknesse being more dispersed than ever in towne." Mary carried on gamely at her brother-in-law's house: "The separation of friends is not the least misfortune I am sensible of in this sad time."[39]

From his windows overlooking the plague pit of Southwark, a middle-aged widower contemplated a different move. In August, John Allin had rejected the pleas of his friends in Rye to return to his old country parish. God had called him to give medical and spiritual help to poor dissenters in Saint Olave Southwark. Then plague broke out as fiercely at Rye as in Southwark, making it all the more imperative for his closest friends in the Sussex town, Jeake and Fryth, to keep watching over his three young children in his absence. Parliament's Five Mile Act made him change his plans again. As a dissenting minister Allin was now banned from all incorporated communities, London as well as Rye. He thought of moving to rural Sussex, he wrote Fryth, "but where I doe not know. If you can learne some place for me, somewhat about five miles from you, with honest people, you may doe well to let me know of it, where I may practice physicke."[40]

The Evelyn brothers, wives, and children celebrated Christmas and New Year's together at Wotton. Then John returned in the snow to Sayes Court and the king's service once again. Weeks went by without a chance to take a break from work and see his wife and their new baby. He waited impatiently to bring them home. The plague would continue in Deptford until the end of 1666.[41]

At Earls Colne, the shadow of contagion was just a hamlet away. One entry in Josselin's diary listed seven suspicious deaths and three plaguelike sores at Colneford Hill. When the annual Bill of Mortality came in from London in January 1666, the vicar took down the particulars: males dead, 48,569; females, 48,737; christenings, 9,967; increase in burials this year, 79,009. This was, he wrote, "the greatest plague in England since that in Edward the thirds time," the time of the Black Death. "And yet it continues very fierce in many places of England." By the coming spring, fever and plague would infect several families in his parish. The parish register, listing five plague burials, seems to have missed several other fatalities from the infection. Josselin's diary jottings on the effects of this Great Plague suggested a personal emotional toll that would not easily be forgotten.[42]

PART IV

Surviving

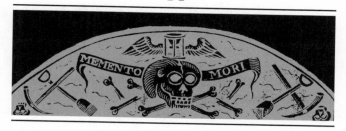

The Web of Authority

> Every six houses on each side of the way are to joyn together to provide one great
> fire before the dore of the middlemost inhabitant; and one or two more persons to
> be appointed to keep the fires constantly burning.
> —Proclamation of Sir John Lawrence, Lord Mayor of London, September 5, 1665

London Fires

At the peak of this terrible season, London's suffering citizens could scarcely
imagine how their great capital avoided plunging into utter disorder. For
weeks on end the mayor and aldermen held no meetings at the Guildhall.
The merchant guilds stopped meeting for the duration. The College of Physicians was abandoned, and thieves absconded with its treasure. The heads of
church and state were far distant—Dean Sancroft long since gone, King
Charles far away in body and spirit. In the parishes, center of most basic relief work, there were barely enough persons to carry on. Only top officials,
like Captain General Albemarle and Mayor Lawrence, and a handful of strategically placed persons, like Turner and Pepys, could see an overall structure
of containment behind the loose patchwork of visible civic relief efforts.

The most ambitious public act of the epidemic was the lighting of street
fires throughout the capital for three days and nights in September. Samuel
Pepys had just returned from the temporary navy office in Greenwich to finish packing at Seething Lane. The extreme heat of the day and the blazing
fires made the scene apocalyptic as Pepys' waterman rowed upstream to
Westminster on September 6. Samuel disembarked and went to Albemarle's
residence to discuss navy supplies, his mind still on the blazes. They had
been lit the previous day and were going continually. "A gloomy time," a

newsletter account said, reflecting on the death toll along with the darkened sky.[1]

John Evelyn saw the fires on the third day. He had come to Westminster to press Albemarle for a pest-ship for his infected sailors. Nearly ten thousand poor creatures were perishing every week in the metropolis, he recorded. Forlorn survivors crouched on their doorsteps as he passed the watermen's shabby quarters in Southwark, crossed over deserted London Bridge, and sped along Fleet Street and the Strand to Charing Cross, arriving at last at Saint James Palace near the Cockpit. Evelyn did not mention the coalfires; he was taken aback by "the coffins exposed in the streets, now thin of people; the shops shut, and all in mournful silence, not knowing whose turn it might be next."[2] How could the officials manage this crisis and keep law and order?

As Evelyn watched, a torrential downpour came from nowhere and within a short time extinguished the neighborhood fires. Skeptics knew the fires could do no good, and now God was confirming their judgment. Didn't the latest Bill of Mortality, published on the day of the storm, show an increase in plague deaths from 6,102 to 6,988? Then, after a short dip, the plague count reached the highest point yet, 7,165; only four parishes in the entire metropolis were plague-free, confirming the views of the fire naysayers.[3]

Had the continuous blazes of September been accidental, one would have thought hell had been let loose on earth. But King Charles himself had approved this action from Salisbury, hoping to "correct and purify the air" in his capital. Mayor Lawrence had promptly sent an order from the Guildhall to all the neighborhoods of the city and its liberties. Captain General Albemarle dispatched similar orders to the rest of the metropolis. By eight o'clock on the night of September 5, the fires were lit.[4]

Dr. Hodges was dismayed by this public health undertaking. He had heard too much talk about the smoke from street fires acting as a giant prophylactic against a possible weekly death count of ten thousand. The doctor supported the fumigation of homes to contain the contagion, but he was convinced these smoke-producing fires in the streets would only prove costly, useless, and harmful to the public's health. Later, Hodges claimed that the fires had precipitated the most fatal twenty-four hours of the entire Great Plague of London. Suffocated and enervated by the heat and smoke, four thousand Londoners expired in a single day![5]

Religious dissenters were likewise appalled by the fires and were scandalized that secular powers would attempt to usurp the role of God. Why had not the officials of church and state insisted that the citizens purge their sins rather than the air? These dissenters, although a minority, were angry and had to be taken seriously. Yet Albemarle brushed aside their protests and stepped up the arrests of those doing privately what others did at public services—imploring God to stay the hand of the Destroying Angel. Unfortunately, there was no sign of repenting, only an increase in persecutions.

The public fires were nonetheless an administrative triumph that also boosted public morale. Out in Earls Colne, Reverend Josselin believed that high temperatures and lightning dispelled plague. If nature could purge the air, he reasoned, why not help it along? The Covent Garden diarist Thomas Rugge recalled the use in previous epidemics of coalfires to change the quality of the air, and he hoped for the best.[6]

The sight of citizens setting those September blazes and steering gaping passersby around them was something to behold. Fire tenders were stationed by the Guildhall, at the western end of Saint Paul's cathedral, at Bridewell Gate, and at the Royal Exchange. Tenders built bonfires before the Three Cranes tavern, where Poultry linked Cheapside, and at Cornhill near the Stocks market. They set another below Thames Street by Queenhithe wharf. Fires burned at the Custom House near the ramshackle waterfront warehouses that housed smugglers' goods and homeless workers. Plague was rife there; the royal council later demolished the buildings.

The Guildhall had made certain that a fire was lit in front of Sir John Lawrence's house in Saint Helen's parish north of Cornhill and Leadenhall Streets. It was a fitting site, a handsome four-story house with an ornate façade bearing the arms of the family and city. Citizens had become accustomed to standing before the mayor's door. He might not be at the Guildhall every day, but Sir John still went through his daily ritual of greeting his fellow citizens. One certainly couldn't fault him for doing it now from the balcony above the front door; he was close enough to hear their petitions for help against the plague, ready with compassionate words that the city would help them in their time of need. It was reassuring to see a fire burning at his doorstep.

The duke of Albemarle and his aides designated where the blazes would be most effective in the Westminster area. In the huge outparishes where the plague had swept away the highest percentage of the local populace, the fires were more scattered. Messengers spread out with orders from the local justices, carrying printed instructions for each parish. Civic officials took special aim at areas that were known to breed disease. The flames that Pepys and

Evelyn saw all along the north and south banks of the Thames were designed to fumigate refuse that was constantly piling up there and routed river rats and other vermin from their burrows.[7]

The cost of these fires ranged from a few shillings in the smallest city parishes, to five pounds in moderate-sized Westminster parochial units, to still more in the largest outparishes. Seacoals were at a high price in September because of the slowdown of shipping from the north. The expense was borne by London's householders, who were charged eighteen to twenty pence apiece on top of their poor rate and a special plague-relief levy. In some streets other combustible materials were used, such as faggots of wood, lumber, scraps, and barrels of tar.[8]

The people who ordered the fires, lit them, kept them going, and eventually paid for them were demonstrating the same will to survive that they had shown for four long months. The web of authority was woven through every level of activity, from the proclamation of the Plague Orders at the start of the visitation to the relief of suffering and burial of the dead ever since. Men and women had been at work in every parish, ward, and quarter of the city and suburbs, expanding and improvising on preplague institutions and regulations.

But how had these officials at every level managed to maintain order amid the chaos? At the time of the fires, there were perhaps a quarter-million persons still alive in Greater London, most of them struggling.

Carrying On

I do not find this visitation to have taken away in or about the city any person of prime authority or command.

—ROGER L'ESTRANGE, *Newes*, October 21, 1665

After the mass exodus at the end of June, only a few city councilmen stayed on in their wards. The legislative council of two hundred members virtually ceased to exist. The record of the smaller executive court of aldermen was marginally better. Attendance fluctuated between fifteen and twenty during the first weeks of the epidemic and then fell to twelve after plague entered the city. The number rose again as the mayor and aldermen put the city's plague regulations into operation, before dropping a second time after the king and court left Westminster. Several aldermen sequestered themselves in their homes, sending servants out for necessaries. Others defied Charles II's orders to stay at their posts and followed his example, fleeing to the country-side.

Mayor Lawrence had convened the aldermen seven times in July, his voice becoming ever more strident as one emergency decree after another failed to stem the plague's progress. While he still talked of "cureing the infected" and staying the further spread of plague "by the blessing of God," his primary fo-cus shifted dramatically to easing the suffering. It was hoped that the city chamberlain could distribute the special plague levy to sustain parishes in the greatest need of money.[9]

After a two-week lapse, the mayor chanced another meeting in mid-Au-gust, encouraged by the attendance of several aldermen at a special service in the cathedral.[10] Thirteen members joined him in making final appointments to the public medical staff. Turner felt satisfied that his committee had found the best surgeons, apothecaries, and doctors of physick that the city budget could support. Parish collections of the special plague-relief tax were slow to come in, however, and Lawrence's threat to report delinquent officials to the king and his council in distant Salisbury was unenforceable. What to do? The Guildhall chamberlain dipped into the city's cash fund to meet the most crucial needs of individual parishes and citywide services.

Food and water had to be supplied to the infected jails. Bedding and other accommodations at the Cripplegate pesthouse had to be taken care of, as the supply ran short of the demand. The keeper of the pesthouse, Mr. Upton, was ordered to take in all poor visited persons recommended by the cham-berlain and to charge householders who sent their servants the top rate for inmates of two pounds. The Guildhall would cover the rest, hoping that its funds would outlast the visitation.[11]

Almost a month went by before Mayor Lawrence called another meeting of the court of aldermen. Meanwhile, out of sight of the public, the city gov-ernment was doing what it had to, although the infrequency of aldermanic sessions and new mayoral proclamations gave a false impression that nothing was happening at the Guildhall.

The mayor counted on individual aldermen to work with officials in wards and parishes to enforce regulations. The parish, after all, was the center for plaguetime action, collecting the special plague levy from taxable household-ers, relieving the sick, burying the dead, and paying the nurses, watchmen, searchers, and bearers. As for law enforcement, now that the law courts were no longer holding quarter sessions and jail delivery, the mayor had to rely on parish constables to enforce most plague controls. A few miscreants could be

sent to the justices of the peace for summary judgment and, if necessary, confinement to a jail or workhouse. At the Tower, a garrison commanded by Sir
John Robinson watched out for greater threats to public order, breaking up
conventicles of Quakers and other dissenters and keeping a watch for suspicious activity by old revolutionaries.

At times it seemed that anarchy reigned in the streets. Symon Patrick and
Samuel Pepys knew that some parishes in the suburbs and the old merchant

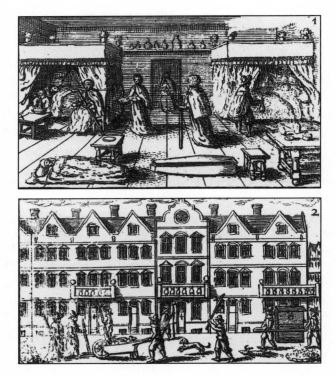

Fig. 12. Medical care in an infected household and outdoor plague controls in 1665.
In the first frame a nurse approaches a sick bed on the left and a doctor attends a sick
bed on the right. Nearby on the floor lie a body and coffin, while other members of
the household (infirm or recuperating from the plague?) support themselves with
canes. The second frame features red crosses on two doors and watchmen posted outside, two women searchers with their identifying wands, a parish raker carrying away
dead dogs in his wheelbarrow, the dog killer attacking a fleeing animal, and two men
bearing a plague victim in a sedan chair to the pesthouse. The two fires in the middle
of the street, positioned four doors apart, suggest the public fires ordered by the authorities on September 5. Courtesy of the Museum of London

center were unable to identify all the houses that were becoming infected. People were coming in and out of them at will. Certainly that was true of the Friends, who insisted on visiting their sick members whether their homes were shut up or not.

Only eight aldermen answered Lawrence's call early in the morning on September 5 for the lighting of the fires. Alderman Turner was one of them. Glaringly absent were the sheriffs-elect, mayor-elect Thomas Bludworth, and Sir William Peake, Turner's colleague on the medical advisory committee.[12]

Sir John Lawrence was nearing the end of his mayoral year. Almost a year had passed since Evelyn had watched from the high table as the new mayor raised his golden goblet and drank to the king's health. Sir John had grown in office as the city struggled through the coldest winter in a decade and faced the greatest plague epidemic of his generation. In the coming Age of Enlightenment, Lawrence would be eulogized by the poet Alexander Pope and Erasmus Darwin, the eminent scientist-physician and grandfather of his more famous namesake. Walter George Bell, who has little good to say about the king's flight in his classic on the Great Plague, heaps praise on the mayor as "a fearless, independent man."[13]

The journalist L'Estrange saw Lawrence as an embattled leader fighting against the odds: "Throughout this dreadful visitation he has, in spite of all hazards and mistakes, persisted in his duty." Among the hazards was the ultimate fear of the time. Sir John lived with his wife Abigail and their nine daughters; a son had died in infancy. In November, the *Newes* carried a somber item: "His own family was infected and the whole neighborhood utterly overspread with the Sickness."[14]

Sir John miraculously survived, but no records reveal whether his family recovered or succumbed. Other civic servants were less fortunate. The replacement of fallen officials was critical, and at the aldermen's last meetings in July they wisely authorized the mayor to fill vacancies on his own; formal aldermanic approval could come at their next meeting, whenever that might occur.[15]

Roger L'Estrange may have been correct in saying that no one in "prime authority" was lost in the visitation, for many among the ruling elite had fled and none of those who stayed fell. The distemper did carry off key civic persons, however. Early on, one alderman died of suspicious symptoms. Graveyards swallowed up several parish clerks and churchwardens along with several overseers and collectors of the poor. The grave beckoned the city's official remembrancer and its coroner, the master of Newgate jail, and three sergeants attending Sheriff Doe. A new jail keeper, Walter Cowdery, was immediately installed at Newgate jail after the keeper died. No one wanted that position to go unfilled; Cowdery was formally sworn in at the next aldermanic session.[16]

Sir John Robinson, commander of the Tower guard and an alderman, served in several capacities. He found new burial grounds outside the walls to take the overflow from city churchyards. He negotiated the acquisition of extra land around the Cripplegate pesthouse. He also had a hand in the erection of the Stepney pesthouse and became involved in its finances after some of his soldiers at the Tower became sick and were sent there. The pesthouse budget was already strained to the limit before these extra charges came in. Robinson's handling of this situation is uncertain, for he had the reputation of exaggerating his deeds. The pesthouse doctor later lodged a printed complaint of going into debt to feed, clothe, and provide medical care, without reimbursement from Robinson and the city.[17]

How much time and energy Robinson, his fellow aldermen, and Mayor Lawrence devoted to their emergency duties can only be guessed. Sir William Turner let his partners in Paris know he had "no time" to go over their joint finances in detail—a clear hint of pressing duties at the Guildhall. At first it was the Plague Orders and their enforcement. Then came the imposition of the plague tax; the appointment of the public doctors, apothecaries, and surgeons; and the replacement of fallen officials. In retrospect, the hurried early orders seemed far less crucial than had been believed at the time. The Guildhall had labored over keeping the conduits open for street cleaning. As mortality soared, there were complaints of far more alarming problems, including the stench and danger from overcrowded churchyards with uncovered graves. This situation demanded immediate attention, and the mayor ordered quicklime and piles of earth to be heaped on the graves. There was plenty to do in the public arena. The more the city emptied, the more there was to be done.

Four weeks after the public fires, Alderman Turner was relieved to see the mortality finally dropping. The weekly plague toll within the city wall remained above one thousand, however. The abruptness of his correspondence with the Pocquelins in Paris suggested a man still weighed down by civic burdens and the prolonged stoppage of trade: "Herewith I send you the accompt current. I had no tyme to looke them over but I presume you will find them right." He continued his sad refrain as autumn took hold and the sickness persisted despite cooler weather. Writing in French, the consummate English entrepreneur advised his partners: "The sickness increased during the past week, which increased the fears of those who were already wary of returning to the city." Between the lines the message was clear: the city's financial health and his personal spirits were at a very low ebb. Alderman Turner and his colleagues must find new sources of money to shoulder the burden of the parishes and put off paying some of the city's outstanding bills.[18]

At the Cockpit

Spoke with my Lord [Albemarle] in the parke, where I perceive he spends much of his time, having no wither else to go. And here I hear spoke of some presbyter-people that he caused to be apprehended yesterday at a private meeting in Covent Garden.
—SAMUEL PEPYS, *Diary*, August 21, 1665

In Westminster, the absent monarch had left Albemarle with a vast array of duties beyond fighting the contagion. He was captain general of the king's armies, master of the horse, admiral of the fleet in charge of all the navy's personnel and procurement needs, and commander of the garrison camped out at Hyde Park and a small guard at Whitehall Palace. Little wonder that Pepys found him snatching a few hours of rest and reflection at a nearby park whose high walls kept out intruders and presumably the infection.

With the help of his assistant, Lord Craven, and the justices of the peace in Westminster, Middlesex, and Surrey, Albemarle did what he could to keep order. Craven and Albemarle were powerful symbols of government at work, and yet their responsibilities in the capital's affairs were not clearly defined, in contrast to the duties of Mayor Lawrence inside the wall. Perhaps it was because these appointees of the king did not have the institutional base of the mayor: no court of aldermen, no remembrancer, no chamberlain, and therefore no records.

In the first weeks of flight, the earl of Craven could be found signing plague passes for the wealthy on their way out of town. As the weeks passed his concerns took him in a different direction. He found relief money in places others overlooked. He structured distribution of medicines and food, paying for much of this from his own purse. He roamed far from his Drury Lane neighborhood to see at first hand how the epidemic was affecting the poor. "Many good offices he did to the poor afflicted," Rugge wrote. Craven also came down hard on those who abused their office at the expense of private citizens. A foul-mouthed bearer named Buckingham had terrified the poor of Covent Garden and Saint Martin in the Fields by exposing bodies to the public and offering them as firewood with a mock "London cry": "Faggots, faggots, five for sixpence!" Word reached Craven; he called together the Westminster justices of the peace and had the offender taken to the pesthouse, whipped in front of the inmates, flogged through the fields, and then imprisoned for a year with a life prohibition from public service of any kind.[19]

Craven had something beyond the strong will and independent disposition of Albemarle and Lawrence. Nearing sixty, he was already distinguished by military service in Europe's Thirty Years' War and as a trusted advisor of great nobles and royalty at home and abroad. What distinguished him most, however, was his ability to look beyond himself; at a stage of his career when others would have been content to be effective managers of the status quo, he wanted change. The Great Plague made him restless and impatient to alter the way his superiors looked at England's perpetual cycle of public health crises. Here was a person of great talent, dedication, and influence, eager to rethink a national and metropolitan response to disaster that had been hobbled by hidebound beliefs, habits, and interests.

Traveling through the neighborhoods of Westminster, Craven saw the folly of shutting up the healthy with the sick. Families were living in undocumented hovels, hiding the sickness and escaping to the countryside when they could. Perhaps the current notions of miasmas and contagion needed to be rethought or adjusted to reality. He kept notes on the undocumented poor, shabby housing, and woefully limited pesthouse quarters, waiting for the chance to make a change. Once this nightmare was over, he promised himself, he would push for an overhaul of the outmoded plague regulations.[20]

A shroud of secrecy obscured the role of Craven's superior, Albemarle. The captain general remained what he had always been—a military man of decisive acts and few words. His greatest victory had been bullying the nation's wavering politicians into restoring the monarchy in 1660 by massing his troops in the capital. The erratic turns of this epidemic proved a far more elusive adversary. Albemarle's antiplague strategy, if he ever articulated it, remains buried in the archives. For all his authority as the king's leading representative in the capital, his name rarely appeared in public health measures against the pestilential invader. When plague swept through the suburbs in June and July, he dutifully ordered the distribution of sheets of Galenic plague cures to each parish for their residents' use. He collaborated with Mayor Lawrence in the great fumigation experiment of September. His most prominent plaguetime acts in the capital, however, centered on maintaining public order. The plague had kept alive the Puritan era's millenarian hopes of a Second Coming of Jesus and the end of the world as it was known; God's Destroying Angel was a new sign of a divine plan for the earth. However demoralized by defeat and repression these dissenters were in reality, Restoration officials, led by Albemarle, continued to fear the specter of old revolutionaries turning the world upside down right through this visitation and beyond.[21]

"Monstrous spirits" were demonstrating outside Saint Paul's cathedral, Stephen Bing reported to the absent dean. Canon Bing could hardly contain himself as he wrote. These mad dissenters blamed the clergy and magistrates for spreading this disease. "Down with them that would down with governors and government," Bing thundered. Sancroft's physician, Peter Barwick, was equally incensed at the subversive tracts hawked on the streets, "printed noe body knows for whom nor by what." Whoever the tract writers were, they seemed bent on pulling down the pillars of authority, starting with absent doctors and priests.[22]

Foremost in Albemarle's mind was the resurfacing of one of the Crown's most wanted men. Colonel Danvers, a former revolutionary soldier and fervent millenarian, had voted for Charles I's death as a member of the high court created by Cromwell to try the defeated monarch. "A Grand Contriver of the late conspiracies and long sought after," a newsletter reported. A warrant was out for his arrest, with execution likely to follow. Royal revenge ran deep: Cromwell's body had been removed from its Westminster Abbey crypt at the Restoration, ceremonially hanged, and reburied in ground set aside for common criminals; several of his surviving regicidal comrades were hunted down and executed, their bodies drawn and quartered. Danvers had an uncanny ability to slip through the net thrown over his hideouts. A lucky break led royal forces to his capture in a hideaway in Moorfields. On the way to the Tower, an obliging guard let him stop at a tavern to quench his thirst. His brother was nearby with a band of dissenters, and they whisked the colonel away before the alarm could be sounded.

Pepys got wind of this "great ryott" two days later. News of the daring escape reached the ears of Charles II at Salisbury. His privy council called on reinforcements for keeping the peace, doubling the royal forces at Hyde Park, Whitehall, and the Tower. At the Cockpit, Albemarle had to settle for embarrassing excuses. The hapless captain who had allowed the escape was sent to the Gatehouse jail in Westminster, sharing quarters with Quakers and jail fever.[23] The event was devastating for Albemarle. Bell calls him "a

benevolent dictator, a somewhat awesome mysterious figure, wielding un-
limited powers." Pepys was less flattering, characterizing him as a "block-
head" in meetings he dominated without any give and take. Evelyn kept his
opinions to himself.[24]

At the highest levels within Greater London, the thin web of authority
was holding, if imperfectly, against the triple threats of disease, dissenters,
and Dutch prisoners. The great testing ground of London's ability to survive
this crisis, however, remained the local parishes.

Men and Women at Work

The city chamberlain from time to time, until further order, [is] to issue and pay
out such money as the Lord Mayor shall direct towards releife of the poore visited
with the sicknesse.
—London Court of Aldermen, September 21, 1665

In the spread-out metropolis, action at the highest levels of authority could
only fill the cracks of neighborhood functions—supplying the all-important
communal burial grounds, for example, and supplementing needy parish
budgets with a vital transfusion of extra money. The most immediate and
crucial needs were at the level of the individual parishes. Parish leaders appointed the emergency personnel who kept London from collapsing into
utter chaos as they went out on their rounds.

The miracle was that the line of service in the parishes held firm. To be
sure, someone usually volunteered to take the place of a fallen workman or
woman, for any job was better than none. But the smooth changeover was
due to more than workers desperate for a job. Churchwardens and overseers
of the poor chose carefully among the applicants, arrived quickly at a pay
scale, and swore them in without any further ado. At Saint Bride's, common
laborers offered to serve if any gravedigger or bearer should fall victim to the
infection. Saint Margaret's pesthouse called in a midwife four times in one
week to deliver babies. The same parish paid two women on several occasions for their "extraordinary pains" in performing unspecified labors (probably as caregivers in their own homes for parentless children and other survivors of plague tragedies).

Nurses were in great demand. Young women who had lost their spouses
(and bread winners) to plague swelled the ranks of the normal nursing pool

of longtime widows on parish relief.[25] Searchers kept on searching and reporting to their parish clerks week after week right through the terrible days of September.

The indispensable parish clerk was in the front ranks of the vulnerable. Thomas Beard paused while writing in the register of Saint Martin Orgar, a long finger of a parish leading down to the Thames near London Bridge. Next to his handwriting was a smudge; the rest of the entry was completed by a different hand, that of the churchwarden. Beard died that evening and was buried the following day, August 6. Immediately John Robins was appointed to fill his place. Robins died on August 28, and by September 9 his wife had buried their three sons and a daughter.[26]

A fallen clerk's trained hand could be replaced by that of a churchwarden or minister.[27] The loss of a parish's two churchwardens, however, was nearly a catastrophe. They were the only ones who knew its finances, recording the income and outlays, paying out sums directly, and often taking over other duties when no one was immediately available. Yet each parish that lost a churchwarden managed to carry on somehow.

The crisis at Saint Bride's by the Fleet River was extraordinary. The junior churchwarden had vanished into the countryside at the first sign of plague. The vestry sent him a letter requesting his endorsement of a plague-relief loan offered by a parishioner. On arriving at the forwarding address, the postal messenger learned that the elusive official had gone farther away and could not be located. Henry Clarke served gamely alone as senior warden into September, juggling accounts, getting loan money without his colleague's warrantee, and procuring coals for the parish fires. Then on September 23, with the plague at its peak, Henry fell ill.

Mrs. Clarke turned her dying husband's books over immediately to his brother. The parish was fortunate: William Clarke had been one of the auditors of the parish accounts. Unluckily, William lasted only two weeks before he became sick. On October 8, the vestry met in emergency session, and this time made certain the parish had two churchwardens for the rest of the year. Together they managed accounts and delayed paying bills that could be put off. They continued supervising the digging of pits. And they sought out women to nurse orphan girls and boys who became ill. It was hands-on work of the sort that may have caused the deaths of their predecessors. Fortunately, for both themselves and the financial health of the parish, the new churchwardens closed out the fiscal year at Easter 1666 in good health. Their books showed expenditures twice those of other years, yet they ended with a surplus of over a hundred pounds.[28]

Part of their success was creative financing. Wealthy parishioners helped by loaning one hundred pounds without the guarantee of the absent churchwarden. In the end it was not needed, but it had given the churchwardens a cushion of financial and emotional security. The other source of their solvency was the chamberlain sitting in the Guildhall week after week juggling the city's accounts. Sir Thomas Player kept dipping into the city's cash reserves, sometimes on his own, at other times at the direction of Mayor Lawrence. City bills that could be deferred were left unpaid. Dr. Hodges would not receive the last of his salary until 1667, a delay that unfortunately contributed to a slide into bankruptcy as his health deteriorated and his practice suffered. Other emergency bills mounted for labor and bricks to build a wall around a new common burial ground and various laborers' fees for the pesthouse buildings. Most crucial of all were the needs of the poorest and most plague-stricken parishes in the city and its liberties. In July, Mayor Lawrence had warned of the "extremity of ye people" in the liberties and the "great disorder and danger" for the city if their needs were not met. In September the needs were spiraling out of the churchwardens' control.[29]

Fortunately for the city and its parishes, the chamberlain had not fled with his knowledge and skills like the elusive Saint Bride's churchwarden. And Sir Thomas Player had the good fortune to receive large donations from all over England for the infected poor of the capital at the time of the greatest need. Some towns sent in more than a hundred pounds. The sums went directly to the most desperate parishes inside the walls and adjacent outparishes.

The citizens who benefited never witnessed the weekly treks across town by their churchwarden or overseer of the poor to the chamberlain waiting inside the Guildhall. He stretched the Elizabethan Poor Law in a way that its creators could never have imagined. The parish officer came with his outstanding bills and the week's receipts from the plague-tax levy on resident householders. The chamberlain calculated where the need was greatest and transferred the excess plus the gift money from the countryside to these parishes. The lists remain in a city plague account book, cross-referenced with churchwardens' account books. Saint Giles Cripplegate and Saint Olave Southwark received the most. Saint Bride's was at the middle level of support; the ten to fifty pounds it received each week in July through September carried the ill-fated Clarke brothers through the worst of their parish's epidemic.[30] By then its weekly toll had dipped below one hundred, but it and other parishes were still suffering greatly as October began.

That month the financial fortunes of the city and its parishes sank to their lowest level. The cash fund was extremely low, the city's credit strained, the outside gift money almost gone. Six members of the court of aldermen showed up on the twenty-fourth of the month to confront the grim situation. One of the six was the ever reliable Sir William Turner. These city fathers decided to gamble by imposing a second year's plague-tax levy on the parishes within the metropolis under their jurisdiction. The money was collected slowly, with some of the parishes meeting their quota two years after the plague disappeared from the city. The chamberlain saw the year 1665 through by taking what he had, gathering in the sums as they came in, and allocating them to the parishes most in need.[31]

These are the bare outlines of the web of authority that helped the city and citizens of London through the darkest weeks of the visitation. The entire story is beyond telling, as only portions of the total city bill were recorded. Each street and parish had its own battle with the plague. The state church reached citizens in ways that the Guildhall could not. Preachers read proclamations from the pulpit. The bishop of London exhorted congregations to give generously and worked tirelessly to replace deceased or absent clergy with substitutes where possible. Clergy, like Symon Patrick at Covent Garden and Richard Pearson at Saint Bride's, and the dean's assistants, Stephen Bing and John Tillison at Saint Paul's cathedral, carried on with parish clerks and churchwardens who were religious as well as civic officials. Dissenters formed their own parallel networks, using their conventicles as centers of self-help. John Allin served in Southwark. The Danvers brothers and their fellow conventiclers in Cheapside performed good works despite the suspicions of the authorities. Presbyterians in the heart of Covent Garden took care of their own. The Quakers were everywhere. The merchant guilds also kept coming to the rescue of the city at its request, diverting money to plague relief from funds collected for their canceled annual banquet, supplying their allotments of grain and seacoals for the poor, and adding "ready cash" periodically as the mayor requested it. Their meeting halls were closed, but someone rounded up the money and supplies.[32]

These public servants and private citizens who had defied the odds by remaining in London, when many could have left, demonstrated a will to persevere through the darkest days of this visitation. Part of their determination, no doubt, came from material resources and professional skills. The ill-fated Henry Clarke, for example, was a successful merchant tailor whose understanding of the marketplace caused the parish to elect him their chief financial officer. The actions that led to his demise, however, showed an enormous faith in the triumph of life over death that is unlikely to have been only secular in inspiration. Chances were that Henry Clarke's faith tapped religious convictions as deep as the wisdom he had acquired in the market-place. Whatever he may have called it, this powerful resource had carried him through his daily tasks, just as it was sustaining the rector of Covent Garden, the commissioner of sick and wounded sailors and Dutch captives, and many others who lived to see the end of London's greatest plague.

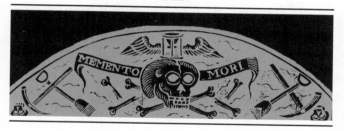

Not by Bread Alone

> In 1665 the yeare of the Great Plague my two brothers were sent to Board within
> a little way of Eppin and my two sisters to Sudbury neare Harrow on the Hill . . .
> Once in every weeke I went to see my brothers as also my sisters.
>
> —GEORGE BODDINGTON's Family Commonplace Book

George Boddington Jr. was no ordinary eighteen-year-old. A quick learner
with Latin and Greek at school and accounting at home, this oldest child of
George and Hannah Boddington had been writing letters and keeping the
books of their packing trade since his thirteenth birthday. Like Sir William
Turner, George senior had prospered with hard work through the ups and
downs of the marketplace, passing on his business ethic to his son by example. Hannah, a more religious person, "instilled good principles of religion
and morals" in her five surviving children, George junior later recalled, and
bore the loss of the other six with the same trust in God's unfathomable
goodness that the countess of Huntingdon and many others of their generation shared.[1] Between the two parents, George Boddington Jr. imbibed a
typical Puritan work ethic: people of faith used their talents to the full and
trusted God to bless their journey through life, whatever its end might be.

Hannah and George Boddington had taught young George more than
they had bargained for. When the plague came into London, they decided to
send George and his four younger siblings out of harm's way, while they
watched over the family business and George senior served as overseer of the
poor at Saint Margaret Lothbury, a well-to-do parish of a hundred households. George junior balked.

Looking back in prosperous old age on that early testing time, George recalled his experiences as vividly as if they had just occurred.[2] The country
house George senior had purchased for his parents and single sisters could
not accommodate the five Boddington children, but they could be boarded at
a safe distance beyond the Cripplegate exit. From his bookkeeping George
junior knew that family savings would pay for the children's lodgings and
keep his parents in food and drink at their city home for the duration of the
epidemic, even if their trade completely collapsed. Material considerations
were not alone in the parents' decision to remain in London, however, and
young George Boddington knew it. He turned their trust in God to his own
purposes.

George used two arguments. First, he had been attending a secret conventicle, and the minister's message of God's abounding grace had him on the
verge of a formal commitment to his Savior. Surely his parents could not object to him trusting in the Lord in the plague-ridden city. If that was not argument enough, George added a second: the neighborhood's pulpits, deserted by their Anglican rectors, were filling with dissenter preachers, and he
begged to stay on to hear their inspirational sermons.

Hannah and George senior resisted, but in the end his faith overcame their
reservations about the vulnerability to plague of someone so young. And so
the three of them remained in the handsome converted inn that had become
the family home on the north side of Lothbury Street, near the Guildhall. In
October, mother, father, and son celebrated their survival and his nineteenth
birthday. He occupied himself by running errands and keeping accounts current as if there were no plague at all. The Lord's Day was special. Every Sunday George went to hear at least one sermon. The first Wednesday of the
month found him devoting almost the whole day to the long services in
nearby churches, where he received "abounding consolations."

George got through most of the plague without his faith being fully
tested. Perhaps his youthful self-confidence and middle-class clothes were
enough to disarm wary country guards during his weekly visits to his sisters
and brothers in Middlesex. On his return through infected Saint Giles Cripplegate, he claimed not to have been afraid, even when he saw sixty corpses
being carried from the roadway to a common grave. He passed by "without
any amazement" about his own danger, he recalled, for he saw the plague as
"the Arrow of the Almighty and directed by Him."

George's crisis of faith came unexpectedly. He had gone out as usual on a
Friday to see his younger siblings. On the way to Harrow-on-the-Hill, he
met friends returning. They had been prevented by wary country people

from visiting their daughter at the boarding home she shared with George's sisters. George pressed on and was relieved to be let in for supper with his sisters. The next Wednesday being a Fast Day, George went to Saint Katharine Creechurch, where the most electrifying preacher of the plague, Thomas Vincent, was conducting the service. The gentleman he had met on the road on Friday entered the pew in deep mourning, sitting close to George. Inquiring about the couple's health, George was startled to learn that his wife had died since their last meeting and had been buried the night before.

George was at first "somewhat affrited" and about to flee. "But I remembered my selfe, and attended all day during the service (to my great comfort)." Years later Boddington remembered the four ministers who had officiated and marveled at his escape from the infection despite his staying on through the long service. God had cast him down, he declared, and then raised him up. With similar words the Baptist preacher and future author of *The Pilgrim's Progress*, John Bunyan, marveled at God preserving him while in an infected country jail: "He woundeth and his hands made whole."[3]

Faith and Fear

The Lord doth not afflict and torment them that abide in his Counsell with the fear and terror of these things, as the unfaithful and unbelieving are tormented and afflicted.

—WILLIAM CATON to English Quakers, September 8, 1665

No doubt George Boddington's faith carried him through the plague, just as he claimed. He had followed the rule that God had set down for the ancient Israelites during their forty years in the desert and that Jesus had repeated when tempted by the devil during his forty-day fast in the wilderness: "Man doth not live by bread only, but by every word that proceedeth out of the mouth of the Lord doth man live."[4] Still, Boddington's trust in God was surely made easier by his family's material security. His father's office holding in the neighborhood parish, too, helped assuage any fear he might have harbored of being jailed as a secret nonconformist. Many poor dissenters, especially Quakers, faced greater tests of their faith than this privileged young man ever did.

A Quaker leader in Holland, William Caton, heard of these London Friends' travails. "I know these things are not joyous, but rather grievous," he acknowledged, "and therefore would many be freed from them." Yet they should know also that neither persecution nor plague had visited them without the Lord's permission. This was not a judgment but a test of their faith: "spurs of Gods mercy and love to provoke you to watchfulness, to obedience and to faithfulness to the Almighty." Let them even see this pestilence as a God-given opportunity to reach out materially and spiritually to the ungodly who were without the hope of the Friends and ripe for conversion in their suffering.[5] This was strong spiritual medicine, not easily swallowed. Could these English men and women really hold to their faith and pass it on to nonbelievers with pestilence and prison a constant threat? Caton believed they could, exhorting them with the example of the Dutch Friends, who en-

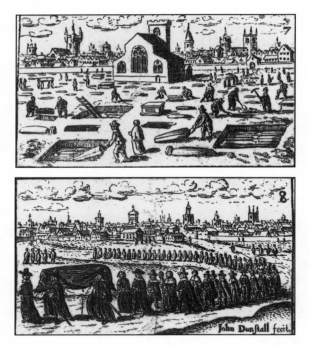

Fig. 13. Plague pits and a funeral procession outside London's wall in 1665. The first frame features plague pits in a large churchyard outside London's wall, with gravediggers, bearers, coffins, and shrouded bodies. In the second frame a very long procession of persons in mourning clothes escorts a black-draped coffin despite the prohibition of this public ritual. Courtesy of the Museum of London

tered infected dwellings to care for the sick. London's Quakers followed the Dutch example. Their severest critics acknowledged them to be among the bravest souls of the visitation.

George Boddington's favorite preacher, Thomas Vincent, sought to calm the fears of other dissenters. Baptists, Presbyterians, a few leftover Seekers and Ranters from revolutionary days, and probably more than a few Anglicans thirsting for spiritual help filled the city churches to overflowing when he preached. Their anxieties would be lessened, Vincent assured them, by reflection on the far greater torment of unbelieving and unrepentant sinners: "What dreadful fears do there possess the spirits, especially of those whose consciences are full of guilt and have not made their peace with God!" How different, Vincent declared, was the inspiring deathbed scene of true believers. "Let not the father or the mother weep to be in sadness," he recalled saying to the anguished parents of a dying son. The boy was only seventeen, yet he had told Vincent that the Lord had enabled him to look beyond this world: "When he was drawing neer to his end [he] boldly enquired whether the tokens did yet appear, saying that he was ready for them." He wanted to console those left behind, praying that his friends not feel guilty for failing to persuade him to flee to the country; it had been his choice. As his spiritual leader looked on, the boy told him where he wished to be buried, asking Vincent to preach on Psalm 16: "In thy presence is fullness and joy, and at thy right hand there are pleasures for evermore."[6]

Many persons must have left Vincent's services resolved to offer up their fate to God, only to feel fear well up again, often accompanied with grief. Reverend Patrick told his congregation that searchers were reporting people dying of grief. "Every day we hear of some or other that are ready to faint by reason of the anguish of their spirits," he acknowledged. Patrick composed one of his most moving sermons and had it printed for parishioners shut up in their houses; *A Consolatory Discourse persuading to a cheerful Trust in God in these times of Trouble and Danger* was remembered two centuries later, appearing in a collection of sermons entitled *Christmas Classics.* To families shut up with the plague and worried worshipers in his pews, he held out the same hope: God does not give us more than we can bear; He will dispose of us as He wishes, according to his plans.[7]

The Shadow of Death

I am environ'd with danger, and have nothing to trust to but your prayers to Almighty God, that (if it be his will) I may escape. If not, that my service [to the king] may be acceptable; for noe money should hire me to this hazard which I see everyman to flee from that has asylum.

—JOHN EVELYN to Sir Richard Browne, September 22, 1665

With the exception of physicians or nurses, no one felt the presence of pestilence more consistently than did John Evelyn. Whether at home or tending his Dutch prisoners and sick and wounded English sailors, Evelyn lived constantly in the shadow of death. The first scare had come when a household servant became ill, forcing John's pregnant wife and their children to flee to his brother's home. From her refuge in Wotton, Mary wrote to him, "I pray God preserve our poor [friends at Greenwich and Deptford]. I can doe noe more but my prayers for your health where these [are] daily made." Back at Deptford, the expectant father set his mind on tending to the king's business, "trusting in the providence and goodness of God."[8]

John received a second scare after visiting Mary a fortnight before her due date. It had been a harrowing trip back to Sayes Court. His nag lost a shoe, slowing him down to a bare walk. Stopping off for dinner, he sensed an "aguish disposition" coming on and took a posset drink for colds and a little theriac to ease his pain. The theriac (with its key ingredients of sleep-inducing opium and viper's poison to draw out any pestilential poison from the body) may also have calmed his spirits. He went on from Deptford to Greenwich, where three thousand new prisoners from captured Dutch warships had just arrived.

A week later, overburdened with work and still not fully recovered, Evelyn had to do battle with Albemarle in "very serious debates" over dinner. Dover castle held only sixty prisoners, and the nearby jails were all infected. All but one of Evelyn's officers at Chelsea were dead from plague, and this assistant had accompanied Evelyn "with it upon him, ready to sinke downe before my door." Still Evelyn forged on, uncertain about the fate of his sick companion. Arriving at his Sayes Court home, the navy commissioner found the plague spread all around Deptford and carrying off his closest neighbors. Parents, children, maids, and boarders, as well as nearby brewers, all dead or dying, he informed his father-in-law Sir Richard Browne, the original owner of the

Evelyn property—naming them one by one. "All the houses about ye doctor swept away, and at least 50 more shut up," Evelyn added.

As John laid out the grim scene at Deptford to Sir Richard, his fears turned in Mary's direction. She was facing greater trauma than he, for the nurse she had hired was shut up with the plague. He dared not worry her with the true extent of the mortality around Sayes Court, nor admit to fearing his persistent dizzy spells might be the plague coming on. "The truth is I much suspect the ague to be infected," he confided to his father-in-law, asking for his prayers and imploring him not to breathe a word to Mary.

John Evelyn offered up his own prayers to God and tried to focus on the blessings of his life, from family to financial security. Yet no matter how he tried, his thoughts kept returning to the present perils at Sayes Court and Wotton. It seemed an eternity since he had begun this year praising God for his mercies, receiving the holy sacrament, and setting his affairs in order.[9]

A short time after sharing his fears with his wife's father, John sent an express letter to Mary offering to replace her nurse with someone from Deptford. Then he let down his guard and revealed his full concern over "faintings and dizziness in my head now and then." Having made that admission, he acknowledged another: the "infinite hazards" of arranging for his newest group of three thousand prisoners had brought him to the point of desperation.

It was mid-September. Londoners wondered whether they would live through the next week. Evelyn braved the contagion on his visits to Albemarle in Westminster and risked infection at the half-dozen ports where sick and dying sailors kept coming in. Trying to shake a premonition of his approaching end, he told his wife, "If God be so mercifull to me, I may hope yet to see you once more before Sir Richard goes off to Oxford." In the meantime, Mary had two sources of strength to aid her: "You have a Gracious God to trust in, and (if I live) a most indulgent and affectionate husband to provide for you and ours, as far as our poore faculties will reach."

The end of the letter resembled a last will and testament. Mary should guard John's unpublished manuscripts and keep to herself what was not for other eyes. (The rest was presumably to be published or shared with virtuoso friends.) A key to his trunk, which he thought had fifty pounds in cash, was enclosed. "You are my selfe, and I trust you with all," he confided. He had drunk some of her cider last evening, and it had done more for his melancholy infirmity than all the concoctions he had taken to cure it. "I have no more to say, but to beg of God that he will blesse you, and restore you once more to me; for I am with all faithfulness and intire affection, my dear wife, your most inviolable loving husband and servant."[10]

With thoughts more inclined toward material than spiritual matters, Samuel Pepys reflected on his own mortality. "Lords day; up betimes, and to my chamber," he wrote as he skipped Sunday service and packed his papers and books for removal to the temporary navy office at Greenwich. He wrote out instructions to the executors of his last will and testament, "thereby perfecting the whole business of my Will, to my very great joy." The ever worldly Samuel brought his thoughts as close to the afterlife as he could: "So that I shall be in much better state of soul, I hope, if it should please the Lord to call me away this sickly time."[11]

The Plight of Pastors

Buried: John, son of John and Margaret Swethland, killed by the plague. Hence it will be seen in how greater danger I was placed, who, in the house of the infected, baptized him with the sacred stream, held him in my arms, and signed him with the sign of the cross.

—REV. DAVID FOULIS, curate of Paddington village church

Personal beliefs could carry a Christian only so far in these endless weeks and months of death and suffering, even if one possessed the faith of Mary and John Evelyn. Corporate worship helped to nourish flagging souls, and here Anglicans had an advantage over even the mildest of dissenting groups. John Allin's private gatherings in Southwark invited arrest by Albemarle's forces. Even public services in city churches by ejected ministers like Thomas Vincent were fraught with anxiety, though the large size of the congregation probably saved the worshipers from interference by the captain general (better to leave them alone than to incite a mass riot).

It comforted worshipers at Covent Garden and Cripplegate and Saint Margaret Westminster to know that they were all reciting the same words at the same hour. "For Jesus' sake, who himself took our infirmities and bare our sicknesses," they prayed in unison, "have mercy upon us, and say to the Destroying Angel, 'It is enough.'" When a family had to stay at home, the head of the household could read aloud scriptural passages on prudential action in time of trouble. Genesis 12 and 27, Proverbs 22, 2 Samuel 24, and Ephesians 5 were favorites. The rest of the family might join in, reciting familiar verses on

God's providence from Ezekiel 9, 2 Kings 20, and 2 Chronicles 16.[12] Psalm 91, offering serenity in place of fear, became a staple of Reverend Patrick's sermons. "You would not expect to be free of robbers, war, suffering, or fever," he exhorted his listeners. "Why think you will be never without plague?"[13]

In June the bishop of London had drawn up the special services of propitiation with the dean of Saint Paul's. The prayer books, printed in old Gothic script, were distributed throughout the diocese early in July. They were used immediately in the 130 parishes of Greater London. By August, Reverend Josselin at Earls Colne and his fellow priests in Colchester and country parishes throughout the land were using them.[14]

The order of service reminded worshipers to forgive their enemies if death should approach and while they lived to give generously for the infected poor. Prayers of supplication called on Almighty God to protect his earthly creatures' bodies and souls from harm and evil. But worshipers were also warned by their pastors not to lapse into fatalistic resignation: faith should be combined with physick, for the counsel of physicians as well as that of priests came from God.[15]

These pastor-shepherds needed to listen to their own counsel, for they risked their lives by staying on to feed their flocks. The curate of Paddington village, Reverend Foulis, held a newborn infant in his arms to administer baptism, only to learn two days later that the infant was dead of the plague. Reverend Josselin had a scare when a parish boy came back from Colchester and died nearby of the infection.[16]

Reverend Patrick recounted to Elizabeth Gauden his own close encounter with death. The chaplain at Poultry Compter, a city prison, dropped by the home of Reverend Outram, rector of Saint Mary Woolnoth parish in the heart of the city, when Patrick was there. The conversation came around to the recent death from plague of a minor cleric and all his family. Chaplain Bastwick knew all the details. The evening wore on, and Reverend Patrick took his leave after wishing them all well; Bastwick stayed on until late. Five days later the chaplain was dead of the distemper. A badly shaken Dr. Outram broke the news to Patrick, saying that the man's countenance had changed later in the evening, but Bastwick had said nothing to him. Symon told the whole story to Elizabeth Gauden and concluded, "You see how much we are beholden to God in keeping us from dangers to which we are exposed."[17]

The dissenter John Allin's spiritual anguish ran much deeper during that terrible September in London. His old parish at Rye had been off-limits to him since the Restoration, and now the pestilence was in houses on either side of his rented quarters. Then his brother-in-law died of the sickness in the city, a devastating blow. Peter Smith had been a pillar of emotional and financial strength ever since the death of John's wife. Who would help him pay for his children's needs? And what would happen to them if John died? He had not seen Peter since a bubo appeared under his ear, and John's detailed knowledge of plague gave him to believe that he might have been infected before then. There was nowhere to go, he wrote in alarm to his friend Philip Fryth, "none in heaven nor earth to goe unto, but God onely." He dipped into the well of his spiritual support: "The Lord lodge mee in the bosome of his love, and then I shalbee safe whatever betides."[18]

But he could not remain calm. Allin slipped down the slope of doubt and despair. He became distracted and fatalistic, worrying about his three "dear babes." His anxieties brought on severe headaches, which again worried him. His letters read like a last will and testament, as he ticked off his valuables to be passed on to his children and his own writings on astrology, alchemy, and medicine (including plague) to be entrusted to his close friends Jeake and Fryth.[19]

Unexpectedly, a blessing occurred. Allin's friends in Rye collected money for his children and himself. The very persons who had so feared receiving his letters gave generously. Allin was overcome with emotion at this sign of God's grace. "To think that He should bee employing the vials of his wrath upon others, yet heaping coales of love upon my head!" He wondered whether he was worthy of his good fortune. In a convoluted spasm of tension, he wrote to his friend Samuel Jeake that this wonderful outpouring of love could all end in "bitterness." He must show true gratitude by thought, word, and deed to merit God's continued favor.[20]

Across the river in Covent Garden, Reverend Patrick spoke of God's saving grace in less stringent terms, for he dwelled on the peace of the next life. Elizabeth Gauden thought he might pay a little more attention to his material needs in the present life, but he scarcely listened. Symon had grappled with these transitory concerns in August as his father lay dying in the Midlands. After working through his grief from the loss of his father and thoughts on his own mortality, Symon informed Elizabeth that he was no longer worried about his time on earth. Then came a series of frights in rapid succession. His brother across the river had a troublesome, lingering illness, and Symon experienced a worrisome pain in his leg right after a servant caught the distemper. He confided little of these worries to Elizabeth, reserving them for his memoirs. This personal crisis could not have come at a worse time. In the metropolis, ten thousand persons had died the past week, and smoke from the public fires hung in the air.[21]

Symon continued to dwell on God's providence. Many times he had been short of cash for his poor parishioners, yet money appeared almost miraculously when he was most desperate, sometimes in a note of credit from a parishioner peer at court and occasionally "in some corner or another, where I could not remember that ever I had laid up any." This set him to thinking about his parishioners who had come out of their infected houses to talk to him. How did this happen? And what of his recalling in his memoirs that he had actually entered infected dwellings to pray with the household? If doctors of physick could do this, why not healers of the soul? "We are in the hands of God and not of men," Symon affirmed. He would do what he could for his parishioners, "who I think would not be so well if I was not here."[22]

Reverend Patrick told Mrs. Gauden of their many fallen clergy friends. John Allin remembered dissenters who fell.[23] At Saint Paul's cathedral, the remaining clergy kept Dean Sancroft current on vacancies in the city pulpits caused by deaths or flight. Other clergy recommended that he appoint to permanent posts priests who had filled in for absent rectors "in the midst of great danger and mortality." The pleas of these substitute pastors sometimes came from their own lips. Francis Lewys, after filling in at Saint Botolph Bishopsgate, where the mortality rose sevenfold to claim thirty-five hundred victims, sought a city parish of his own with words that revealed his need for a living and his anxiety in requesting it of someone far above his rank. "I shall not alledge any argument to prevaile with you," he wrote to Dean Sancroft. "I do no more then my duty. It is God preserving me (blessed be his name) in these more than dismal tymes of mortality, in the very valley of the shadow of death, to be a surviving miracle of his mercy."[24]

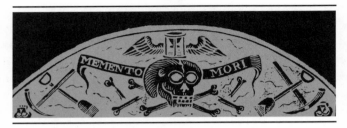

The Awakening

> Since my last on Tuesday night I have no newes to add to the inclosed [Bill of Mortality]; by which you will also perceive ye sickness is now againe increasing [at] divers fresh houses since the returne of fresh persons hither.
>
> —JOHN ALLIN to Philip Fryth, December 14, 1665

Coming Home

It began as a small line of people on foot returning in early November. The first snow had left a dusting that accented the large mounds in most churchyards. The sight of these graveyards and empty old haunts must have been a stark reminder of what they had escaped. Beggars and transients crouched in the cold on householders' doorsteps, all but ignored by the neighborhood constables.

The influx of Londoners returning from the country added to the urgency of the moment. Here was a new pool of potential plague victims, each lacking the emotional and physical immunity that survivors had gained. Dr. Thomson worried that an individual's archeus might be tricked into imagining the sickness, causing him or her to come down with the real thing. Dr. Cocke's *Rules for Returning Citizens* warned returnees to approach their homes with a calm spirit and extreme caution (perhaps a conflicting message). The infection might be on "cunning persons hiding their plague sores" or dogs that had been pawing at graves. Most important of all, people were warned not to enter a house before having it fumigated and disposing all of the old bed linen.[1]

The new lord mayor of London had been installed at the end of October without the festive mood of other years. The streets were all but deserted, the wharfs and Custom House devoid of activity. Few boats could be seen on the river. Scarcely any of Samuel Pepys' business associates stopped by the Royal Exchange; there was little news and less gossip to exchange. Londoners hardly noticed the transfer of civic authority from Sir John Lawrence to Sir Thomas Bludworth. The master of the vintners' guild and a member of Parliament for Southwark, Sir Thomas had to play out his greatest triumph on an empty stage. L'Estrange strove to put a good light on it in the next day's *Newes*, "the splendor and order of the Solemnity being somewhat interrupted by the present visitation."[2]

Recorded fatalities from all causes had dropped sharply for six consecutive weeks, from a high of 8,297 for September 12–19 to 1,388 during the week of October 24–31, a remarkable improvement. Yet the plague lingered, and without warning the death toll shot up again. The jangled nerves of the survivors made them receptive to the worst rumors. It was hoped that the cold weather would bring the plague toll down again, but one never knew what to expect from one week to the next.

At his shop by Saint Paul's, Sir William Turner hid his uneasiness as he wrote at the end of October, "We are much joyd here by the continued decrease of ye sickness." His credit still held, and perhaps he could soon cash letters of credit and bills of exchange "at sight" with the help of his goldsmiths. Unfortunately, Turner's customers were not returning in large numbers, and those who did return couldn't be cornered into paying bills for past services. In November he admitted to his associates across the Channel, "The merchants doe not yet come to towne so that I have not received one penny of our money." Still he reassured them, "You may be confident I watch all opportunities." Finally running short of patience, Sir William turned politely but with determination on his most objectionable debtor: "As long as civility or reason could require it, I have waited the pay of the sume due to mee . . . I am too well acquainted with all manner of delayes and excuses to be contented. Please to lett me know by [this carrier] where and when I may receive my money without referring me to your returne or anything else." Two weeks later, Sir William wrote triumphantly to his Paris partners, "Mr Wade hath payd mee £500. Mr Humphryes and others have promised me; and I entend this week to send my man to Oxford to solicit Smith and others there."[3]

That same month Samuel Pepys took stock of his own prospects as the comatose city started to stir. He couldn't help exulting in his good fortune at having an office with the Navy Board. "How little merit doth prevail in the world, but only favour. Chance without merit brought me in, and diligence only keeps me so." His diligence had garnered him new deals with suppliers in October even though the money supply from his goldsmiths and the Treasury had gone dry. To keep up his frantic pace required blinkers. He anesthetized himself against the appalling mortality and misery in the city and countryside. He couldn't even react to the sight of bodies lying by the roadside or left unattended in a coffin. This disease, he said, "[is] making us more cruel to one another than we are [to] dogs."[4]

Certainly, Pepys' wheeling and dealing sometimes left him out of sorts and impatient, in contrast to the polite and measured Turner. After hearing Albemarle, Craven, and Robinson ramble on about state finances and poor relief, Samuel simmered with frustration, "But Lord to hear the silly talk between these three great people." On reflection, he saw that he could tolerate inefficiency at the top because these "very great friends" opened doors for him. Happily, as November drew to an end, he found the business climate inside the wall dramatically different from a month before. "So to the Change, where busy with several people, and mightily glad to see the Change so full, and hopes of an abatement still [of the plague] the next week." A great frost, he exclaimed, "gives us hope for a perfect cure of the plague."[5] His eyes and everyone else's remained riveted on the weekly bills, anxious to see whether the downward trend would continue (table 9).

Table 9. Greater London Bills of Mortality,
October 31–December 19, 1665

| Week | Number of Burials | | Change from Previous Week | Number of Infected Parishes |
	Plague	Total		
October 31–November 7	1,414	1,787	+399	110
November 7–14	1,050	1,359	-428	99
November 14–21	652	905	-454	84
November 21–28	333	544	-361	60
November 28–December 5	210	428	-116	48
December 5–12	243	442	+14	57
December 12–19	281	525	+83	68

When the parish of Saint Olave Hart Street recorded only one death for the week, Elizabeth Pepys decisively orchestrated a return home. Her husband's erotic adventures were on the increase again, and yet he energetically took part in her move back to Seething Lane. On the second of December, she settled back in their London apartment. He returned to Greenwich, where much of his business was still centered, while planning to see her as often as possible. Two weeks later, after one of their reunions, Samuel triumphantly paid all his outstanding bills with the help of his goldsmiths and treasury officials. He had also steered thousands of pounds from the royal coffers to his victualing superior Denis Gauden and arranged for Denis's older sons (stepsons to Elizabeth Gauden) to join the navy victualer's staff. If Denis should fall to the plague, his wife would be protected, much to the relief of the Gaudens and their old friend Symon Patrick.[6]

Elizabeth Pepys busied herself redecorating her home with newly purchased draperies. From the Pepys homestead in Cambridgeshire, Samuel's father wrote that a wagon filled with passengers had departed for London. Samuel could now see up to twenty shops open in a handful of places, though few after dark. As Christmas approached, a worldly Pepys had much to be thankful for, despite new scares from plague at his Greenwich quarters and around Seething Lane.

At Hutton Hall in Essex, Elizabeth Gauden read the bills every week, asking Symon Patrick if it wasn't time to return to the Gaudens' Surrey mansion at Clapham. Symon demurred politely, saying her soul conflicted with a noncompliant body. Elizabeth's volatile emotions and headaches made her far too vulnerable to the distemper to risk moving yet. While he admitted that only one of his returning parishioners had succumbed to the distemper, he noted that most of those who had gone into the country were wisely delaying their return. Symon was certain that some of the early returnees had brought the infection with them, causing the fatalities to shoot up again. Perhaps in a month, if the sickness didn't increase, the city would fill, making it safe for Elizabeth to come home. It wasn't an encouraging letter. His mood was darkened by poor church attendance: "We had nothing so good a congregation yesterday as we used to have" at the height of the epidemic, he wrote sourly, "and therefore God may in mercy quicken us again to mind our duty and rouse up dull souls by this new alarm."[7]

Just when things seemed almost back to normal, plague deaths reported in the bill suddenly shot up again during the second week of December. A new fatality in Saint Gregory's by the cathedral churchyard caused Turner to inform his partners in Paris of the bad news for their trade. The highest toll was in the Hart Street parish; Pepys put off plans to move back in with his wife. Allin, Pepys, Turner, and Patrick all sprang into action before the sun set on December 14, when the increase in deaths was published.

In Southwark, John Allin had just finished drawing up astrological tables for 1666. A copy was in Samuel Jeake's hands, accompanied by a note of Allin's forebodings of "a very sickly if not a mortal day very neere approaching me." Then the bill came out on December 14. In haste, Allin penned a note heavy with apocalyptic meaning to Philip Fryth. The plague toll had risen once again, the increase being "wholly in the city." Allin linked it to people returning carelessly from the country.[8]

Samuel Pepys learned the bad news at the Exchange the day before. "We hope it is only the effects of the late close warm weather," he speculated, "and if the frosts continue the next week, [the count] may fall again." Yet he worried, "The town doth thicken so much with people" it would be surprising if the plague did not "grow again." Pepys rushed to Seething Lane to see his wife, "who is well (though my great trouble is that our poor little parish is the greatest number this week in all the city within the wall, having six (from one the last week)." Distracted and distraught, he started losing track of his assets again, "which doth trouble me mightily, fearing that I shall hardly ever come to understand them thoroughly again, as I used to do my accounts when I was at home." Samuel swore an oath not to drink until he made an accurate accounting, fearing that if he died, no one would be able to make any sense out of his reckoning. "I hope God will never suffer me to come to that disorder again."[9]

Sir William Turner's records were in perfect order. As always, he knew exactly where he stood financially. This latest increase in the death toll, however, set him aback. The Pocquelins in Paris heard from him immediately: "I doe all I cann to procure money," he wrote on the fourteenth, "but it is so scarce that wee must have patience perforce. Since the £500, I have only received £50 of Mr. Russell."[10]

Symon Patrick also paused on the fourteenth to take in the bad news. The Piazza remained largely deserted, with the peers and gentry holding back in the country until the king and queen made their move from Oxford. Patrick finished his letter to Mrs. Gauden, "God alters the weather as he pleases . . . If [the plague] does not leave us this winter, God knows when I shall see you." He dearly missed her company. The next week Symon reported the town filling up again, while noting the "great increase" in the sickness that had unsettled Pepys, Turner, and Allin in their own idiosyncratic ways. Symon was now writing almost every day to Elizabeth, perhaps because of an increase in his free time, perhaps because he felt conflicted by her impending move. He happily changed the subject to a trip to Denis's London office, where Denis handed him a letter from Elizabeth. The visit and letter quickened Symon's desire to see her.[11]

Elizabeth scribbled the beginning of her reply on the back of Symon's letter. "What shall I think? For I cannot speake enough of that laborious love of yours that digs so deepe to please and ease." She had grown more hopeful than he of their coming together soon; the overall lessening of the sickness and the coming cold season augured well. The bill for the next week and the week after showed significant drops in London's mortality figures. Elizabeth read the first of these two encouraging bills on her own. Without waiting to hear what Symon thought, she set her sights on leaving for Clapham. Two days after Christmas she broke the news that her lonely friend might not hear from her for some time as she journeyed homeward.[12]

Symon got the news after a quiet Christmas; he saved a goose and hare in case his brother visited him soon. After New Year's he learned of Elizabeth's arrival at the Gauden mansion across the river, a tonic for both of them. They were so close that they wrote of their signs of love reaching one another. Cautiously, he waited for a further drop in mortality around his parish before going to see her.[13]

One last scare came in January. "Blessed be God, wee are in a pretty good state of health at this end of the towne," Symon assured Elizabeth. The surge in fatalities, he said, was partly due to the carelessness of returning residents and of those who had stayed on and were throwing caution to the winds. He was far from alone in thinking this way. Dr. Hodges blamed people for sleeping in the beds of deceased persons before they were cold. Boghurst criticized returnees for exposing themselves needlessly to likely sources of the infection. A high official at the Exchequer exclaimed that people coming into London "tumble over the goods and household stuff in infected houses."[14] The vital statistics of the bills in part caused and in part reflected these concerns (table 10).[15]

For all the agonizing bill reading and deliberation by Londoners, there was comic relief in the flamboyant return from his country estate of Charles II's boon companion and navy commissioner Lord Brouncker, in the vanguard of returning peers. On January 5, 1666, he set out with his mistress and his fellow member of the Navy Board and the Royal Society, Samuel Pepys, for London Bridge. As they clattered through the slowly awakening city streets, the eyes of Londoners stared in disbelief. Such a scene of a great lord in his elegant coach had not been witnessed in the city for five or six months.

Table 10. Greater London Bills of Mortality,
December 19, 1665–January 30, 1666

Week	Number of Burials		Change from Previous Week	Number of Infected Parishes
	Plague	Total		
December 19–26	152	330	-192	46
December 26–January 2	70	253	-77	31
January 2–9	89	265	+18	35
January 9–16	158	375	+110	47
January 16–23	79	272	-103	30
January 23–30	56	227	-45	29

"Porters bow everywhere to us," Pepys exclaimed, "and such begging of beggars." From the porch of his church, Reverend Patrick could spot Brouncker in his twenty-hearth townhouse on the Piazza. It was a welcome sign, for the residents of Covent Garden and elsewhere in Westminster continued to be thin on the ground by comparison with the old city. Two days later Pepys returned for good to his Seething Lane home. On the twenty-second he joined returning friends from the Royal Society at the Crown tavern for the first informal meeting since plague had set in. Pepys and Brouncker had long anticipated this reunion.

At last Westminster sprang to life with the return of Charles II on February 1. Bonfires and bells greeted the joyous event throughout the metropolis. The return of His Sacred Majesty signaled the end of danger from plague, though in fact the disease was not yet spent. By mid-February only a few shops remained closed. People eagerly prayed for renewal, a way to forget and a way to heal. The plague death toll for the month was 222, down from 382 in January. In March only 107 died, most of them in poor areas.

At the Royal Society's tavern supper, Pepys pricked up his ears in anticipation as Dr. Goddard addressed his fellow virtuosi. Goddard had fled from the pestilential air and was defending his exodus and that of most of his colleagues in the College of Physicians. These society doctors had been "left at liberty" after their own patients left town, Goddard explained. Pepys was not at all convinced, recalling the death of his own doctor. And one of Samuel and Elizabeth's surgeons had risked death while continuing to serve the poor at Saint Bartholomew and Saint Thomas Hospitals.

Pepys was curious to know what the rector of Saint Olave Hart Street would say at his first service since returning. Snow had fallen the night before and mantled the churchyard's bloated contents like a great burial shroud, offering a mute reproach to a pastor who had left his flock to grieve and pray on their own. Samuel and Elizabeth gathered with others in the church to thank God and meditate on Reverend Milles's sermon. Samuel anticipated a "great excuse" from this man who had fled the parish before anyone else and had come back last. "He made a very poor and short excuse, and a bad sermon," Pepys recorded.[16]

There was much to be forgiven and many lessons to be drawn from this collective human tragedy. Another great plague would surely come, with or without the astrologers' doomsaying predictions. Twelve aldermen—twice the number of a few weeks before—now showed up at the Guildhall to reckon with unpaid plague bills and battle the lingering contagion. The king was back at Whitehall with reform of the Plague Orders on his agenda. The question was: Did these leaders of the capital and country have the will and the ability to act boldly?

Unfinished Business

The shutting up would breed a plague if there were none. Infection may have killed its thousands, but shutting up hath killed its ten thousands.

—*The Shutting up of Infected Houses, as it is Practiced in England, Soberly Debated* (1665)

In January 1666, Mayor Bludworth discharged the public physicians from further duty to the city, and the court of aldermen thanked them for their services. Monetary compensation for the surviving medical personnel and the widows dragged on. The delay in final payments of Great Plague expenses is puzzling. Perhaps the city cash fund was too depleted by the economic impact of plague, and then of the Great Fire of September 1666, to allow the Guildhall to pay all past and current bills, and nonplague items took priority. In February 1666, the city fathers asked Turner, Lawrence, and two colleagues to determine whether the bills of several apothecaries were valid. The last plague-related payment was sent to Edmond Higgs in July 1670 for a surgical bill of thirty pounds; it had been approved three years before. In Westminster the king presented handsomely inscribed silver plates to Westminster's small public medical corps for their treatment of sick householders and pesthouse patients. These official acts and a jumble of other accounts tell us something of the enormous monetary outlay for the Great Plague.

Guildhall accounts listed more than twelve thousand pounds spent on the city's medical team and supplies, pesthouse and burial-ground construction and maintenance, and subsidies to needy parishes. Another fifteen hundred pounds came in from the countryside to the Guildhall for distribution.[17] The merchant guilds contributed money, grain supplies, and other necessities for the poor. Expenses of the 130 parishes, ranging from a few hundred pounds in the smallest parish units to more than fifteen hundred pounds for large parishes like Saint Bride's and Saint Margaret's, added greatly to the expenditures. Assuming a modest average of two hundred pounds per parish for expenses on plague-related items not paid from city funds, the parishes' total would have been twenty-six thousand pounds. And, finally, there were the unknown sums that Albemarle and Craven, from his own resources, spent on the suburbs.

The grand total for the Greater London area was clearly much higher than the "few thousands of pounds" that historian Walter George Bell estimated went to public relief and interments during this great plague in London. The real bill came to forty thousand pounds, probably more.[18] For a metropolitan area whose economy had come to a standstill and whose population was reduced 20 percent by deaths plus perhaps 40 percent by flight, that financial outlay was impressive. To be sure, it fell considerably short of what must have been spent on rebuilding London after the Great Fire gutted the center of the metropolis a few months later, and it paled by comparison with the astronomical cost of the Dutch war, which, by Pepys' itemized accounting, came to more than one million pounds just for the six-month period of April to September 1665.[19] Restoring the capital materially from its smoldering ruins and combating the nation's greatest commercial rival on the sea counted far more with those in power than did fighting an unconquerable disease, which victimized mostly poor people. Given the Poor Law's goal of minimal maintenance of the "deserving poor," however, holding to that level of assistance amid the horrific mortality and loss of employment in the capital in 1665 constituted a considerable commitment of financial resources.[20]

It was true that Samuel Pepys kept virtually all of the more than three thousand pounds he made in 1665, with only a few pounds going to the poor.

Sir William Turner, being wealthier, more religious, and more civic minded, had undoubtedly contributed considerably more and still retained the several thousand pounds with which he had begun the year.[21] But common laborers or scullery maids, whose annual income could have fallen far short of two pounds each that year, might well have judged their material resources during the plague adequate. They had been kept in bread and beer with perhaps some vegetables and meat. If plague had entered their households, a nurse and medicaments might have been supplied. And if death had ensued, the parish's knells and bells fund covered burial expenses.

People of Turner's and Pepys' class may have considered these relief measures a credible response to the ravages of plague, given the public and private resources of the time.[22] But conquest of the disease lay beyond their power and knowledge. Only divine intervention and nature's cyclical return to autumn and winter seemed to have stayed the hand of the Destroying Angel. To be sure, the Plague Orders had some tangible results; witness the removal of some 40,000 dogs and 200,000 cats from London! Nothing had prevented the infection from reaching England's shores, however, or spreading through the capital after it broke through the initial watch surrounding Saint Giles in the Fields. As London awakened from its long nightmare, it was easier for the authorities to focus on tightening existing public health controls than to strike out with new theories and plans.

Mayor Bludworth ordered the city law courts back into session to speed up the enforcement of obvious measures. He forbade citizens to reenter an infected house until its contents were smoked and aired out.[23] Churchwardens were to see that graveyards had an extra foot of lime placed over the graves, which was not always possible because of lack of parish funds and the scarcity of lime after its continual use. Constables rounded up drifters and sent them packing to their original parish if it was known; London's lockup facilities at Bethlehem Hospital and Bridewell prison scarcely sufficed for the city's mentally and physically ill "deserving poor" and "able-bodied" beggars and prostitutes.[24] Alderman Turner made a mental note of this. When business returned to normal, he intended to tackle the problems in Bethlehem and Bridewell.

Bolder proposals germinated in tracts and private writings. The most far-reaching idea came from Sir William Petty, who calculated that the loss of workers during this epidemic was a tragic waste of human resources. When plague threatened again London should evacuate its healthy population en masse to existing and new housing within a thirty-five-mile radius of the capital. This might, he admitted, cost more than the Great Plague had in pounds (at an estimate of fifty thousand pounds for transporting and maintaining the evacuees), but it would save fifteen times that amount in human labor preserved.[25]

Other reformers turned their wrath on the double scandal of shut-up houses and inadequate pesthouse space. At the peak of the contagion, the five metropolitan pesthouses could have accommodated no more than 300 or 400, suggesting a total occupancy of 5,000 at most for the entire epidemic. The other 65,000 plague victims acknowledged by the Bills of Mortality, plus an estimated 10,000 unrecorded ones, succumbed either unattended or shut up with the rest of their household. While no estimate of the number of shut-up households was possible then or now, this massive confinement of the healthy with the infected failed to stop the spread of the plague and, at the height of the epidemic, proved unenforceable in parts of the city and suburbs.

Hodges fumed at the inhumanity of cutting off healthy persons from everyone except sick inmates, making them emotionally "easier prey to the devouring enemy." Boghurst talked of friends "growing melancholy" due to their separation and this sadness contributing to the spread of the disease through an entire family. The double standard of allowing de facto exemptions to privileged citizens rankled. Many peers had avoided finger pointing by leaving the capital. Mayor Lawrence eluded the stigma of the red cross on his infected household; neighbors who tried to shut up his house on their own were promptly arrested.[26]

In February 1666 the king and his council asked the earl of Craven to survey the enforcement of existing regulations with the two chief justices and thirty-three justices of the peace from the metropolitan area. The easiest solution appeared to be the elimination of pestered places. When Craven's investigators took a closer look, however, they met resistance from everyone: landlords who brandished their contractual agreements, tenants who faced eviction without other affordable housing, and employers who needed their cheap labor. The proposal to clear out cellars and restore multi-unit tenements to their original single-family state was abandoned.[27]

Undaunted, Craven set his sights on a radical shift in focus. Contagion, not miasmas, caused plague, he told the king. That being so, the royal government must embark on a major anticontagion project too expensive for local government to undertake on its own. Craven envisaged plague hospital facilities for England's capital on the grand scale that Charles I's French physician had envisaged and that Evelyn had seen in Italy. Craven's words fell on deaf ears.[28]

That was not the end of it. In spring the number of deaths rose again, "the plague, as we hear, increasing everywhere," Pepys shuddered. The king reconvened the privy council's emergency plague committee, which had put off major reforms at the beginning of the visitation. Albemarle had gone to sea to fight the Dutch; Craven replaced him. Once more Craven argued that plague was carried not through air but contagiously from person to person. There was only one viable solution: large pesthouse complexes were needed.[29]

The privy council objected to the cost of a general hospital, and medical theory was conflicted on its usefulness. If the disease were truly miasmatic, what good would it do to segregate the infected from the healthy? Hadn't external quarantining of ships, with their infected cargos and passengers, at major ports, including Colchester and London itself, been a dismal failure? So the king and his advisors decided to confirm the existing Plague Orders with very modest changes. The most significant innovation, requiring every town and city in the kingdom to maintain a permanent plague facility "in readiness in case any infection should break out," failed to dictate the size of the facilities or provide any funding for them. As for home incarceration, which by default was to be the lot of most poor households in a future visitation, the new orders simply tacked on to the quarantine period an additional twenty-day fumigation period, with a white cross replacing the dreaded red.[30]

Plague without End?

It had been a year of prodigies in this nation: plague, fire, rain, tempest and comet.
—John Evelyn, *Diary*, March 6, 1667

Mary Evelyn and her children came home in February. John felt some relief from his duties, and aunt Susan made up clothes for the family from country cloth, feeling it safer than apparel from London. For the next few weeks, the parish church at Deptford enjoyed a full congregation. "Blessed be God for his infinite mercy in preserving us," John wrote gratefully. Charles II and Albemarle thanked Evelyn in person for tending the sick and wounded sailors when "everybody fled their employments." Albemarle was in a repentant mood, telling Evelyn he would never have let the king appoint him commissioner had he known of the mortal danger he faced.[31]

Spring brought new setbacks. Admiral Albemarle suffered an ignominious defeat at sea. Evelyn and Pepys failed to get approval for a large infirmary at Chatham to house sick sailors. The plague count soared in Deptford. John and Mary Evelyn were forced to hold church services in their home, and the town appealed to the privy council for help.[32]

Deptford joined a queue of beleaguered towns in the countryside of southern and central England, each crying that this second year's toll exceeded the first. Reverend Josselin recorded an alarming rise in deaths at Colchester, Braintree, and Cambridge. As he wrote, one of his parishioners at Earls Colne was dying of the infection, and the man's wife would succumb a week later. But Colchester offered the saddest story. The acting mayor appealed to the royal council, "Within the space of seven months [the plague] hath taken way 3,500 inhabitants and brought the town to extreme poverty." Neither the town nor the county of Essex could carry the burden of relief any longer.[33]

London's response was immediate and substantial. The bishop of London exhorted his parishes to contribute weekly until further notice. Five huge sacks of money reached Colchester on the twenty-sixth of May. Colchester's acting mayor and chamberlain counted out £360, not a penny less than the amount entrusted to the carrier. The next installment came on June 2. Yet another arrived on June 9. The relief monies came up the Roman road through June and July, when Colchester reached a weekly peak of 175 deaths. When the Great Plague finally ended in Colchester in December 1666, the most reliable death count from all causes since August 1665 stood at 5,259.[34] The town received outside relief money in taxes and gifts of £2,700, of which £1,307 10s. had come from metropolitan London. The capital's generosity proved essential to Colchester's relief undertakings.[35]

Counting the Blessings

One gentleman would have carried me to the king, and acquainted him with my care of my flock. But I did not think it fit to accept of his kindness, having happiness enough in being preserved and assisted in the performance of my duty.

—SYMON PATRICK, *Brief Account of My Life*

Samuel Pepys delighted in the great and small harbingers of renewal that Symon Patrick and Sir William Turner failed to record. As the end of 1665 drew near, Pepys attended a church wedding at Greenwich "which I have not seen [in] many a day, and the young people so merry with another." At Christmastime, turkeys given to Samuel provided a feast for Elizabeth and her friends at Seething Lane, while he dined at the country house of the navy commissioner and engineer, Lord Brouncker, as they talked about reform of the navy administration and Samuel's musical compositions.

Celebrating New Year's at home with his wife, Samuel Pepys broke into self-congratulatory reflections. "Thus ends this year, to my great joy, in this manner," he recounted in his diary. "I have raised my estate from £1300 to £4400." More soberly he continued, "It is true we have gone through great melancholy because of the plague, and I put to great charges by it, by keeping my family long at Woolwich, and myself and another part of my family, my clerks, at my charge at Greenwich, and a maid in London."

How predictable was this navy entrepreneur and bon vivant! Though he could still be jarred by what he saw and felt, he continued to screen out unpleasantries from his mind and pen. He had lost track of a few of his financial successes and missed appointments, but not his dalliances, even for a week. Bathed in self-satisfaction, he wrote, "I have never lived so merrily (besides that I never got so much) as I have done this plague-time." The naval war had been good beyond measure to Samuel Pepys, while the sailors were desperately short of pay and services. He had been compelled to put down near-riots at the ports, he admitted. He ended with a lament: "Many of such as I know very well [are] dead . . . yet to our great joy, the town fills up apace and shops begin to open again."[36]

Pepys' diary entries left unrecorded a very different balance sheet of this Great Plague. The labor of London's working poor had made it possible for their city and its better-off citizens to keep functioning, even as these workers suffered enormous losses of life. The surviving workers, in turn, were kept afloat by the web of support from wealthier Londoners, which had maintained the semblance of a safety net when institutional structures weakened and the economy collapsed. The interdependency of the two "Londons"—one of the rich and the other of the poor—had cushioned the blow of the Great Plague.

Perhaps it had accomplished more. By keeping their city and its suburbs functioning at a minimal level through the entire period of this visitation, the poor and the rich, workers and entrepreneurs, the governed and their governors may have laid the foundations of the remarkable revival of the metropolis that Samuel Pepys and Nathaniel Hodges saw in the bustle of activity as Londoners returned and country people moved in to fill the jobs of those who had fallen.

Sir William Turner felt grateful to be alive. A religious man, he still marked his ledgers as he had before the Great Plague, "Praise to God." The row upon row of empty stalls and abandoned shops around Saint Paul's and the Guildhall testified mutely to the deaths of others. For a merchant guildsman like Turner, the bitterest pill to swallow was that he had had to survive without the absent master merchants and professional men who were major components of private commerce and public finances.

Reverend Patrick had much to be thankful for and expressed it fully. His returning parishioners were "wonderfully kind to me," he wrote. Symon accepted their thanks but did not want any special praise from court or king. As do many who survive a tragedy, Patrick wondered why God had spared him when others had fallen. It must have been for some purpose. Rededicating himself to a life of service, he urged his surviving parishioners to reflect on their own blessings. They should write down the vows and promises they had made in their time of trial and carry them out now that the shadow of death had been removed.[37]

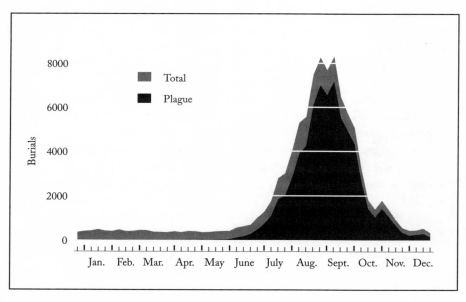

Fig. 14. Greater London Bills of Mortality: Total Burials and Plague Burials, December 27, 1664–December 26, 1665. *London's Dreadful Visitation; Or, a Collection of All the Bills of Mortality* (1665); GL, MS 3604/1/1 Parish Clerks Company Weekly Bills of Mortality, December 1664–October 1669

A second trial was in the offing. In three days in September 1666, the Great Fire razed central London. The medieval Guildhall and old Saint Paul's were reduced to shells, while Covent Garden's church and Whitehall Palace were spared the westward spread of the flames. Four-fifths of the housing within the wall vanished, leaving thousands of Londoners camped out in tents in empty land near the city pesthouse.

Money poured in from a countryside still reeling from its own Great Plague. Colchester was among the most generous towns, sending £103 8s. 9d. to the capital that had recently contributed so much to its relief. The town's inhabitants had responded from a deep gratitude for their deliverance.

As for the recent tragedy of London's Great Plague, the official tallying at the end of 1665 had counted 97,306 burials for the year, of which 68,596 were listed as plague (see appendix A). The actual toll from all causes was at least 110,000. Thousands of unidentified bodies lay in plague pits, and hundreds more were buried without official records, among them religious dissenters. In 1666, plague claimed 1,998 Londoners; again, the records were incomplete, this time partly because many churches within the wall had been destroyed and their records suspended. But life went on. Sir William Turner absorbed personal losses from trade and lived to profit once more. Parish life returned to normal, and the city government resumed functioning as it was supposed to. The five metropolitan pesthouses stood abandoned and in disrepair, as people struggled to forget. Much the same occurred in the countryside. In Colchester, citizens dismantled boards from the pesthouse at Mile End for their own needs, prompting the town assembly to sell what remained.[38]

The plague toll continued to decline in metropolitan London. In 1667, thirty-five persons were listed as dying of plague, twenty-three of them within the wall. In 1668 the figure was down to fourteen, and in 1669 a miniscule two. During the next decade only occasional outbreaks and rare plague deaths occurred in southern England.[39]

As the shadow of the distemper lifted, people's concerns turned to other diseases. "The smallpox [is] very much in London and other parts of England," Rugge lamented in January 1668. But there was a difference. Smallpox lacked the wildly escalating fury and indiscriminate destruction of life and livelihood that characterized plague and lived on in people's memories. Fear of the Destroying Angel's returning to English soil carried well into the future. The Royal Society's secretary, who had stayed in Westminster through the entire ordeal, was haunted by the mystery of this greatest of all diseases. He ascribed the survival of people who would otherwise have fallen to "the

A generall Bill for this present year,

ending the 19 of *December* 1665. according to
the Report made to the KINGS most Excellent Majesty.

By the Company of Parish Clerks of *London*, &c.

	Buried	Pla.		Buried	Pla.		Buried	Pla.		Buried	Pla.
Albans Woodstreet	200	121	St Clements Eastcheap	38	20	St Margaret Moses	38	25	St Michael Cornhil	104	52
Alhallowes Barking	514	330	St Dionis Back-church	78	27	St Margaret Newfishst	114	66	St Michael Crookedla	179	133
Alhallowes Breadst	35	16	St Dunstans East	265	150	St Margaret Pattons	49	24	St Michael Queenht	203	122
Alhallowes Great	455	426	St Edmunds Lumbard	70	36	St Mary Abchurch	99	54	St Michael Que ne	44	18
St Alhallowes Honila	10	5	St Ethelborough	105	106	St Mary Aldermanbury	181	109	St Michael Royall	152	116
St Alhallowes Lesse	239	175	St Faiths	104	70	St Mary Aldermary	105	75	St Michael Woodstreet	122	62
St Alhall. Lumbardst.	90	62	St Fosters	144	105	St Mary le Bow	64	36	St Mildred Breadstreet	59	26
St Alhallowes Staining	185	112	St Gabriel Fen-church	69	39	St Mary Bothaw	55	30	St Mildred Poultrey	68	46
St Alhallowes the Wall	500	356	St George Botolphlane	41	27	St Mary Colechurch	17	6	St Nicholas Acons	46	28
St Alphage	271	115	St Gregories by Pauls	376	232	St Mary Hill	94	64	St Nicholas Coleabby	125	91
St Andrew Hubbard	71	25	St Hellens	108	75	St Mary Mounthaw	56	37	St Nicholas Olaues	90	62
St Andrew Vndershaft	274	189	St James Dukes place	262	190	St Mary Summerset	342	262	St Olaues Hartstreet	237	160
St Andrew Wardrobe	476	308	St James Garlickhithe	189	118	St Mary Staynings	47	27	St Olaues Iewry	54	32
St Anne Aldersgate	282	197	St John Baptist	138	83	St Mary Woolchurch	65	33	St Olaues Siluerstreete	250	132
St Anne Blacke-Friers	652	467	St John Euangelist	9		St Mary Woolnoth	75	38	St Pancras Soperlane	30	15
St Antholins Parish	58	33	St John Zacharie	85	54	St Martins Iremonger	21	11	St Peters Cheape	61	35
St Austins Parish	43	30	St Katherine Coleman	299	213	St Martins Ludgate	196	128	St Peters Cornehil	136	76
St Barthol. Exchange	73	51	St Katherine Creechu.	335	231	St Martins Orgars	110	71	St Peters Pauls Wharfe	114	86
St Bennet Fynch	47	22	St Lawrence Iewry	94	48	St Martins Outwitch	60	34	St Peters Poore	79	47
St Benn. Grace-church	57	41	St Lawrence Pountney	214	140	St Martins Vintrey	417	349	St Stevens Colmanstr	560	391
St Bennet Pauls Wharf	355	172	St Leonard Eastcheap	42	27	St Matthew Fridaystr.	24	6	St Stevens Walbrooke	34	17
St Bennet Sherehog	11		St Leonard Fosterlane	335	255	St Maudlins Milkstreet	44	22	St Swithins	93	56
St Botolph Billingsgate	83	50	St Magnus Parish	103	60	St Maudlins Oldfishstr.	176	121	St Thomas Apostle	163	110
Christs Church	653	467	St Margaret Lothbury	100	66	St Michael Baffishaw	253	164	Trinitie Parish	115	79
St Christophers	60	47									

Buried in the 97 Parishes within the walls, 15207 *Whereof, of the Plague* 9887

	Buried	Pla.		Buried	Pla.		Buried	Pla.		Buried	Pla.
St Andrew Holborne	3958	3103	Bridewell Precinct	230	179	St Dunstans West	958	665	St Sauiours Southwark	4235	3446
St Bartholmew Great	493	344	St Botolph Aldersga.	997	755	St George Southwark	1613	1260	St Sepulchres Parish	4509	2746
St Bartholmew Lesse	193	139	St Botolph Algate	4926	4051	St Giles Cripplegate	8069	4838	St Thomas Southwark	475	371
St Bridget	2111	1427	St Botolph Bishopsg	3464	2500	St Olaues Southwark	4793	2785	Trinity Minories	168	123
									At the Pesthouse	159	156

Buried in the 16 Parishes without the Walls 41351 *Whereof, of the Plague* 28888

	Buried	Pla.		Buried	Pla.		Buried	Pla.		Buried	Pla.
St Giles in the Fields	4457	3216	St Katherines Tower	956	601	St Magdalen Bermon.	1943	1362	St Mary Whitechappel	4766	3855
Hackney Parish	232	132	Lambeth Parish	798	537	St Mary Newington	1272	1004	Redriffe Parish	304	210
St James Clarkenwel	1803	1377	St Leonard Shordicht	2669	1949	St Mary Islington	696	593	Stepney Parish	8598	6583

Buried in the 12 out-Parishes, in Middlesex and Surrey 28554 *Whereof, of the Plague* 21420

	Buried	Pla.		Buried	Pla.	
St Clement Danes	1969	1319	St Mary Sauoy	303	198	
St Paul Covent Garden	408	261	St Margaret Westminst.	4710	3742	*The Total of all the Christnings* 9967
St Martins in the Fields	4804	2883	hereof at the Pesthouse		156	*The Total of all the Burials this year* 97306

Buried in the 5 Parishes in the City and Liberties of Westminster 12194 *thereof, of the Plague* 8403 — *Whereof, of the Plague* 68596

The Diseases and Casualties this year.

Abortive and Stilborne	617	Executed — 21
Aged	1545	Flox and Small Pox — 655
Ague and Feaver	5257	Found dead in streets, fields, &c. — 20
Appoplex and Suddenly	116	French Pox — 86
Bedrid	10	Frighted — 23
Blasted	5	Gout and Sciatica — 27
Bleeding	16	Grief — 46
Bloody Flux, Scowring & Flux	185	Griping in the Guts — 1288
Burnt and Scalded	8	Hangd & made away themselves — 7
Calenture	3	Headmouldshot & Mouldfallen — 14
Cancer, Gangrene and Fistula	56	Jaundies — 110
Canker, and Thrush	111	Impostume — 227
Childbed	625	Kild by severall accidents — 46
Chrisomes and Infants	1258	Kings Evill — 86
Cold and Cough	68	Leprosie — 2
Collick and Winde	134	Lethargy — 14
Consumption and Tissick	4808	Livergrown — 20
Convulsion and Mother	2036	Meagrom and Headach — 12
Distracted	5	Measles — 7
Dropsie and Timpany	1478	Murthered and Shot — 9
Drowned	50	Overlaid & Starved — 45

Palsie — 30
Plague — 68596
Plannet — 6
Plurisie — 15
Poysoned — 1
Quinsie — 35
Rickets — 557
Rising of the Lights — 397
Rupture — 34
Scurvy — 105
Shingles and Swine pox — 2
Sores, Ulcers, broken and bruised Limbs — 82
Spleen — 14
Spotted Feaver and Purples — 1929
Stopping of the stomack — 332
Stone and Strangury — 98
Surfet — 1251
Teeth and Worms — 2614
Vomiting — 51
VVenn — 8

Christned	Males — 5114		Buried	Males — 48569		Of the Plague — 68596
	Females — 4853			Females — 48737		
	In all — 9967			In all — 97306		

Increased in the Burials in the 130 Parishes and at the Pest-house this year — 79009
Increased of the Plague in the 130 Parishes and at the Pest-house this year — 68590

immediate preservation of Almighty God."[40] A physician who read all of Albemarle's reports on the Great Plague could not free his mind from the thought of what might happen again: "In 1665 and 1666 there died about two hundred thousand men, women and children of the pestilence, which was a visitation beyond any formerly in this Nation; and I hope and pray that God will never send the like, and that we nor our Posterity after us may never feel such another judgment."[41]

Facing page

Fig. 15. The General Bill of Mortality for 1665, with a breakdown of burials by cause as well as the total for all causes and the increase in burials from the previous year. Note the suspiciously high number of fatalities attributed to ague and other fevers, consumption, convulsion, dropsy, and stomach disorders (gripping of the guts, stopping of the stomach, and surfeit) and the high mortality associated with childbirth and infancy (childbed, chrisoms and infants, and teething and worms), which were undoubtedly connected to the disease of plague and the disruption of living conditions that it caused. More difficult to understand are the low counts of persons found dead in the streets and fields and of deaths associated with emotional trauma (distracted, suicide, grief, and lethargy). The minimal fatalities attributed to "overlaid and starved" suggest that the searchers did not hear many stories of people starving to death from lack of provisions. Guildhall Library, Corporation of London

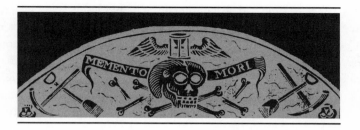

Epilogue

Of Once and Future Plagues

O let it be enough what Thou has done,
When spotted death ran arm'd through every street,
With poison'd darts, which not the good could shun,
The speedy could out-fly, or valiant meet.
—JOHN DRYDEN, *Annus Mirabilis* (1667)

Twenty Years After

"Men eat, and drink, and laugh as they used to." The words came easily from the pen of the greatest economic forecaster of the age. Twenty years had passed since the Great Plague, and Sir William Petty was as happy as anyone to focus on England's good fortune. "The Exchange seems as full of Merchants as formerly; no more Beggars in the Streets, nor executed for Thieves than heretofore," he joked. The number and splendor of coaches exceeded former times, the theaters were magnificent, and the king had a greater navy and stronger guards "than before our Calamities." Yet Petty's statistical mind told him that the calamity of pestilence returned to England every twenty years; this time, he calculated, it would kill 120,000 persons in the capital.[1] The public authorities also remained wary, keeping that special column for plague in the metropolitan Bills of Mortality until 1703—just in case. But no plague death was entered in that column after a single case in a remote downstream parish in 1679.

[263]

The passage of time had also dimmed the memories of London's citizens, blurring the twin calamities of plague and fire in 1665 and 1666 into a nightmarish sequence best forgotten. Or, better still, one could reflect on the city's quick recovery. The image to remember was that of the phoenix rising from the ashes, as the poet-playwright John Dryden had written so eloquently in his *Annus Mirabilis*. It was an apt metaphor, for London's citizens had rallied the capital against both the plague's terrible blows and the conflagration that destroyed the old city center.

After fire broke out at a bakery in Pudding Lane during the early hours of Sunday, September 2, 1666, Samuel Pepys brushed aside Mayor Bludworth's excuses for inaction. The risk-taking plague survivor dashed to Whitehall to alert his king, and Charles II was braver than he had been the year before. By the third day he was supervising the firefighting and relief for a hundred thousand displaced citizens. Carters from the countryside transported the homeless and their goods to tents north of the city pesthouse, where twelve months before thousands had been taken to nearby plague pits.

At the eastern wall Pepys buried valuable papers, coin, wine, and Parmesan cheese in a neighboring garden and huddled in his office wrapped in his assistant Will's quilt. Fearing the worst, he later moved his wife, servants, and £2,350 in gold to their plaguetime quarters at Woolwich. When he returned he found the nearby streets "all in dust," but to his joy their home was intact. Dynamiting operations had stopped the inferno short of the navy office, Tower, and bridge. John Evelyn led a similar operation to protect royal Whitehall and the hospitals housing his sick and wounded sailors.

Rev. Symon Patrick remained with his frightened parishioners, the poor not knowing what would happen to their livelihood, the richer sort wondering whether their mansions would be among those blown up by the king's orders to save the west end. Inside the wall Sir William Turner stood ready to serve as he had the year before, but it was beyond his powers to save the Guildhall. The crumbling medieval cathedral of Saint Paul's, which Evelyn and others had been planning to repair, also went up in flames, the molten lead of its roof flowing across the glowing stones of the churchyard past Turner's shop. A decade later, an unlettered workman fetched a flat stone from the churchyard rubble to mark the center of the dome on the floor of the new Saint Paul's. By pure chance he had unearthed a gravestone bearing a single decipherable word, "RESURGAM." As the new edifice arose over the ruins of the old, this same magical word, symbolizing London's rebirth, appeared on the south transept over a phoenix rising from the ashes.[2]

John Evelyn submitted a design for a new London featuring broad avenues and verdant squares. Robert Hooke, newly returned from the country, and Christopher Wren, back from travels in France during the year of the plague, had equally bold schemes. But these visions yielded to pressure from Londoners to rebuild their homes and shops on existing sites and return business to normal as quickly as possible. Sir William Turner became lord mayor in 1668–69, when construction and financing lagged for the largest public structures, and donated the four hundred pounds bestowed on bachelor mayors by the king and much of his own money and talents to completing the material restoration of the city.

Red brick and stone replaced combustible wood. Slate and tile roofing made residents safer from fire and vermin than had overhanging thatch. Drainage at the curbside improved on filthy ditches in the middle of streets. The trademark spires of Christopher Wren's churches, exemplified by the triumphant octagonal spheres at Saint Bride's, which inspired the design of multilayered wedding cakes, softened the city's grief for the thousands of plague victims buried below. Towering over the new cityscape was Wren's dome at the new cathedral, Protestant England's response to Catholic Rome's basilica of Saint Peter.

The restoration of central London, spectacular though it was, only camouflaged the chronic dangers to public health. A hundred narrow streets grew straight and wide, but back alleys remained. The Fleet stream became a canal but continued to receive its habitual household and industrial pollutants. Miles of new water pipes replaced the old but carried water of dubious purity. Old food markets inside the wall were combined and new ones opened in the suburbs, but sanitation around the animal slaughters remained a neighborhood responsibility. The tangle of tumbledown sheds and warehouses cramming the alleyways running down to the Thames River had been consumed along with their flammable contents of oil, pitch, and tallow. But even as the quays were opened up and warehouses moved back, their resident rats, which were the bane of London's householders and a boon to city rat-catchers, migrated upstream and downstream to the crowded suburban waterfront areas that had escaped the Great Fire. When all was said and done, the repairs to the central city left unchanged the suburban areas where plague and other diseases concentrated. Thus is disproved the myth, which persists to this day, that the Great Fire ended the danger of a new Great Plague.

People might not talk about "the sicknesse" anymore, but medical experts and ordinary citizens kept the frightening words *miasma* and *contagion* in their vocabulary. In the privacy of their medical casebooks, doctors and apothecaries kept their "diagnosticks" and "treatments" for the dreaded disease. A new outbreak of plague in Europe, they knew, would bring panic again to England's shores.

William Boghurst left his firsthand account of the Great Plague in manuscript form, while publishing a poem on the "Antiquities and Excellencyes of London." Boghurst died in obscurity at fifty-four in September 1685, twenty years to the month after the plague of 1665 had peaked. "He was an honest, just man," it was written, "skillful in his profession, and in the Greek and Latin Tongue, delighting in the study of Antiquity; and plaid exceeding well upon the lute." He had worked hard to provide comfortably for his survivors, "a sorrowful widow and six children." At the country churchyard where he was buried, a worn tombstone retains the following spare Latin verse: "Here lies the bodies of Anne, James, William and Henry Boghurst of singular piety and conspicuous honesty."[3] Boghurst's plague study finally reached the public two centuries later, when plague raged again in faraway, British-held Hong Kong.

Nathaniel Hodges, a year younger than Boghurst, outlived him by three years. His dangerous work in 1665 with the city's public health committee had been duly acknowledged and well, though belatedly, rewarded. He gained notoriety by defending Galenist orthodoxy against the chemical physician George Thomson, who had conducted the controversial plague autopsy. His account of the Great Plague, *Loimologia*, appeared in Latin in 1672, to the acclaim of the College of Physicians. An English translation for the general reading public was published posthumously as plague raged in Marseilles in 1720. At the height of his career, Hodges was given the honor of delivering the annual oration named for England's greatest medical discoverer of the century, William Harvey.

From this lofty position Hodges sank to an ignoble end. His medical practice fell off, perhaps because of the alcoholism that had been apparent during those death-defying rounds of 1665. He died a debtor in Ludgate jail. A plaque was placed in his parish's Wren-restored church of Saint Stephen Walbrook. "Here lies in his grave Nathaniel Hodges, Doctor of Medicine," it reads simply, "who while a child of Earth lived in hope of Heaven. He was formerly of Oxford, and survives by his writings on the plague."[4]

Samuel Pepys and John Evelyn enjoyed a more enduring public fortune. Their goal of a large naval hospital at Greenwich eventually came to fruition. Evelyn continued to publish erudite works on gardening and other exotic subjects, while Pepys headed the administration of the Royal Navy from 1683 to 1689. This adept moneymaker realized a small fortune. In the first five years after the plague, Pepys more than doubled his assets to ten thousand pounds, sported gold lace on his sleeves, and bought a coach with four horses, to his own immense satisfaction and that of his wife. Then he abruptly cut back on conspicuous consumption to avoid the jealousy of colleagues who felt he had overstepped the bounds of his social status. Just how wealthy he became is unknown. He turned secretive about his income, and his weakening eyesight put an end to his diary writing, with its monthly tallies of his wealth. He was perhaps worth twenty thousand pounds at his death, while the government still owed him close to thirty thousand pounds more![5]

Having survived plague and fire, Pepys channeled more of his energy into helping others than he had during the epidemic. His administrative ability helped to transform the Royal Navy, an achievement recognized to this day. Less well known is his imprint on a school for orphans and other poor children at Christchurch Hospital near his cousin Kate's inn. From the early 1670s to the end of the century, he fought for improvements at the school, eventually overcoming recalcitrant colleagues on the board of governors and hostility at the Guildhall. Enrollment soared to eight hundred, teaching and financing improved dramatically, and he realized his dream of establishing a mathematics program geared to public and commercial navigation. A sketch of a boy and girl at Christchurch Hospital can be seen in the Pepys Library, Magdalene College, Cambridge.[6]

Pepys' support of scientific projects drew distinguished visitors to his home, including a fellow plague survivor, Sir Isaac Newton. In the mid-1680s Pepys reached the pinnacle of scientific success for someone who was a mere observer of experimentation, presiding over the meetings of the Royal Society. His name adorned the title page of the most famous scientific work of the age, Newton's *Principia,* whose central concept of universal gravitation first came to the great scientist while he waited out Cambridge's plague in 1665–66 at his mother's country home.

The Pepys and Evelyn households continued much as they had before. Mary Evelyn gave birth to two more girls after the harrowing plaguetime arrival of their seventh child and first girl.[7] John was not untrue to Mary as was Samuel Pepys to his Elizabeth. The Evelyns' strong bond of affection sustained them through the sadness of losing most of their children by early adulthood. The couple lived into old age in the next century, John dying first.

Elizabeth and Samuel Pepys continued their tortuous relationship of the plague year into the aftermath of the fire. Pepys' promiscuity became more pronounced, in tandem with bad dreams of the fire, dreams that may have included the plague. A year later a fifteen-year-old girl entered Elizabeth's service. He avoided the temptation by a new round of liaisons outside the household. But in 1668, Elizabeth caught him in a sexual encounter with her maid. The crisis, combined with fears of losing his eyesight, made him far more considerate of his wife's physical and emotional needs. "I have lain with [her] as a husband more times since this falling-out [than] in I believe twelve months before," he wrote in one of the last entries in his diary. "And with more pleasure to her [than] I think in all the time of our marriage before."[8]

Elizabeth Pepys had never experienced robust health. The plague and fire had been unsettling, to say the least, and the threat of flames to her home and possessions may have contributed to the loss of her hair shortly after. In 1669 she came down with a severe fever. Elizabeth had just turned twenty-nine. The Hart Street rector, whom Samuel had criticized for fleeing from the plague, came to Elizabeth's bedside for a final communion. Her grieving husband placed her body in a vault high in the chancel of Saint Olave Hart Street. Samuel later eased some of the pain and loneliness by taking in a housekeeper whose lower social status and sharing of his quarters scandalized those close to him. He navigated the troubled religious waters of the later Restoration years by being loyal to the covertly Catholic Charles II and his openly Catholic brother James II. Briefly arrested on the spurious grounds of treason, Pepys retired from public life when the Glorious Revolution of 1688 replaced James with his Protestant son-in-law William III.

It had been more than twenty years since plague had swept through the capital, and many of Pepys' friends who had survived that nightmare were now dying. Among them was his longtime colleague in the navy victualing business, Denis Gauden. In perhaps Pepys' finest hour, he eased the financial burdens of his friend's last months by forcing the state to honor more of the procurement debts that had bankrupted him. The Gaudens' mansion at Clapham passed on to Samuel Pepys' old servant Will Hewer, and it was there that Samuel retired, dying in the house during his seventieth year in 1703. His body was placed in the family vault next to Elizabeth's in Saint Olave Hart Street church. His enormous range of papers, letters, and other writings are in four locations: the National Maritime Museum at Greenwich, the Bodleian Library in Oxford, the Public Record Office at Kew, and the Pepys Library at Magdalene College, Cambridge, where the diary can be seen with its shorthand entries, first decoded in 1825 and available since 1971 in the eleven-volume scholarly edition of Robert Latham and William Matthews.[9]

Two prominent Londoners continued to serve the common good in the unique ways they had shown during the Great Plague. The inveterate bachelor Sir William Turner remained a model civic magistrate with his Puritan-tinged probity, as noted in his account book headings, "Laus Deo," Praise to God. As trade revived after the plague and fire, his private wealth grew enormously, increasing his opportunities to shape the rich and poor citizenry of London in the image of his scrupulous work ethic. In addition to being lord mayor in 1668–69, he was elected master of his guild a second time and played a prominent role in the East India and Royal Africa Companies. The energy that he had thrown into maintaining public health in 1665 was now channeled into presiding over two civic institutions that housed members of marginal groups of society: the mentally disturbed at Bethlehem and "able bodied beggars" and prostitutes at Bridewell. He also founded a hospital and free school in his family's ancestral town of Kirkleatham, Yorkshire, where his body was interred at his death in 1693. He had lived for seventy-seven years and left more than forty thousand pounds in his will. A portion was bequeathed to his guild for annual grants to three poor cloth workers.

To the end of his life, Sir William displayed the moralizing rectitude that his customers and colleagues had witnessed during the Great Plague. He did not shrink from challenging James II's Catholicizing mission, and he reached the height of his moral and political authority after the Revolution of 1688 as Member of Parliament for London. A revealing epitaph took Turner's true measure:

Here lies interred, under this stone
A worthy magistrate, well known,
Lord Mayor of London in Sixty nine,
And one who led a life divine;

A true son of the English church,
Whose name to Harlots smells like Birch,
Who while he lived on this stage,
Made Bridewell their chiefest cage,
Then rest, dear ashes, in thy urn,
Until the earth consume and burn.[10]

Turner's ecclesiastical counterpart, Rev. Symon Patrick, continued faithfully at Saint Paul Covent Garden for two decades after the Great Plague. He spurned an offer to move to neighboring Saint Martin in the Fields, the most lucrative parish in all England. His parishioners, he said modestly, had been wonderful to him, and he would not leave them. The honor of serving as one of the king's chaplains was bestowed on this modest servant of the church, "whether he would or not." Later in life he married and found this alliance nurturing and satisfying. Elizabeth Gauden's letters to him have not been found, except for a few drafts on the back of his letters to her.

Twenty years after standing against the plague, Reverend Patrick was thrust into the center of national turmoil over James II's pro-Catholic campaign. He debated with leading Catholic apologists and joined a successful clergy boycott of the king's attempt to legalize worship for Catholics. After the Revolution of 1688, he was elevated to the bishopric of Chichester and soon after transferred to Ely, where he died in 1707 at age eighty.

Patrick was immortalized with a likeness above his gravesite inside Ely cathedral and by his publications on life's traumas. The dual themes of suffering and survival so prominent in his Great Plague sermons reappeared time after time. At a Fast Day Sermon in 1679, he reflected on sinners cut off in an instant and sent down to the pit. What will be your destiny, he asked his listeners "who still survive the war, the plague, and all the rest of God's judgments?" Let persons who think themselves blameless reflect, "Of those eighty or ninety thousand that fell by the plague, think you that they were sinners above all men that dwelt in London and Westminster?"[11]

Reverend Patrick outlived the other protagonists of our story who had grappled with the meaning of life and death in the midst of the plague. Elizabeth Gauden, who had wondered about Symon's certainty of the afterlife, was gone, along with Denis. After her death, Symon's letters were returned to him, which cushioned the loss of his dearest friend and confidant. The house at Clapham that he had visited so many times bore a triple loss: first Elizabeth, then Denis, and finally Denis's associate Samuel Pepys. Sir William Turner was also gone, leaving behind his account books and letters from the time of the pestilence. In the countryside, John Allin and Ralph Josselin had lived out the biblical three score years serving their communities as they had during the time of the Great Plague. Allin moved to Woolwich, where Elizabeth Pepys and her maids had waited out the epidemic, and obtained a local license to practice medicine openly. He continued his chemical experimentation and worked to free imprisoned dissenters. Reverend Josselin continued to serve his parishioners and farm at Earls Colne to the end of his days.

Two Hundred Years Later

Long after the *dramatis personae* of the Great Plague were gone, the disease continued to threaten Europe from the Ottoman Empire and Central Asia, which had become its apparently permanent base. Around 1680 it invaded

Vienna, Budapest, and Prague with massive mortality, causing grateful survivors to erect votive monuments and altars. In 1710 a deeper incursion struck the Baltic seaports, a major source of the English navy's building materials. "We are terribly afraid of the plague," wrote the great English satirist Jonathan Swift. Daniel Defoe reprinted the terrible Bill of Mortality of September 12–19, 1665, to remind Londoners of what might happen to them.[12] Then in 1720 plague struck the major French port of Marseilles on the Mediterranean, causing consternation on the Thames because the two cities were linked through continuous shipping. Nathaniel Hodges' *Loimologia* was translated from Latin to English. His companion piece, *A Letter to a Person of Quality*, joined other sources from 1665 in *A Collection of Very Valuable and Scarce Pieces Relating to the Last Plague*. One self-appointed authority tried to calm his readers by reminding them that in 1665 plague "did not reach those who smoak'd tobacco every day."[13]

Defoe's popular *Journal of the Plague Year* of 1722 kept popping up in London's bookstalls for decades with slight changes to title and text to look like a new work.[14] Every once in a while, a brand new tract on this ancient disease reached the booksellers of Saint Paul's churchyard.[15] There was obviously a market for the subject. While the disease stayed away from Western Europe after the Marseilles visitation, it struck repeatedly at southern Russia from Persia in the 1720s and 1730s. Then in 1770 plague slipped past a Russian imperial quarantine, killing 100,000 persons around Moscow. That epidemic lasted three years—the equivalent of the Great Plague of London—and defied the wisdom of the Russian medical profession.[16] The inhabitants of the British Isles and Western Europe had good reason to wonder whether they could rely on the *cordon sanitaire* of guards that the Austro-Hungarian Empire was now posting against the entry of infected goods and persons from the Turkish lands. Every outbreak in Europe and beyond caused the English authorities to quarantine ships from suspect sources, hoping this would keep the poison out.

The Industrial Revolution, which began around 1760 and continued for seventy years, contributed to unsanitary working and living conditions and gave new meaning to the old idea of "miasmas." Rapid modes of transport made communities all the more fearful of "contagious" goods and passengers. By 1846 the London presses made a point of publicizing the findings of the French Academy of Medicine on the difficulties of sealing Europe off from plague in Asia.[17] But quarantine was England's only obvious defense.

Meanwhile, a mysterious new infective disease entered the Russian Empire from India in 1829. Soon Asiatic cholera became the great killer-disease in the West, the *new* "plague." Old fears merged with new terror. In desperation, European states fell back on existing quarantine mechanisms in hopes of fending off the new invader. But Europe also searched for transnational ways to respond to a collective threat and found a vehicle in international sanitary conferences, beginning at Paris in 1851, the precursor of the World Health Organization of today.[18]

The officials and scientists meeting at Paris, Constantinople, and Vienna in the succeeding quarter-century took all infectious diseases as their domain, while focusing on cholera, "the classic epidemic disease of the nineteenth century."[19] Between the first and second conferences, an Italian microscopist and an English anesthetist published pathbreaking works on the new disease's mode of transmission. Filippo Pacini traced the illness to an "organic, living substance of a parasitic nature." John Snow connected the outbreak of cholera to drinking water; the clue was a London pump whose users had become sick. Public health authorities in Europe and the succeeding international conferences, however, failed to follow up these fresh clues to understanding infectious diseases. As is often the case with scientific riddles, new information on everything from cholera to plague was folded into the old views of Hodges and Boghurst rather than being gathered into a fresh theoretical or practical approach. Something was missing.[20]

Answers began to emerge on the fringes of the medical communities in Europe. In 1850, two obscure investigators, combining microscopic observation with an ability to draw new conclusions, isolated the anthrax bacillus in the blood of dying animals and achieved the startling feat of transmitting the disease to healthy members of the herd!

In the mid-1850s a French professor of chemistry, Louis Pasteur, responding to the plight of a brewer whose beer spoiled during fermentation, stumbled unwittingly into this new realm of bacteriology. From the spoilage of beer and wine, Pasteur's path led to disease-producing organisms in animals and humans, including anthrax, chicken cholera, and rabies. In 1885 he produced a preventive vaccine for rabies, and four years later the Pasteur Institute at Paris came into being.

Robert Koch, a German country doctor twenty years younger than Pasteur, set up a laboratory of sorts in a friend's garden. In 1876 his findings on the life cycle of the pathogenic anthrax bacillus were published. Plucked out of obscurity by medical benefactors, Koch refined the staining techniques then emerging for identifying bacilli with microscopes far more powerful than the ones Pepys had read about in 1665. By 1880 Koch was drawing eager young assistants from around the globe, succeeding in identifying the bacilli that caused tuberculosis and cholera.

Others began researching various diseases and their microbes with impressive results. By the last decade of the nineteenth century, "microbe hunters" had identified the pathogenic organisms for anthrax, cholera, diphtheria, leprosy, malaria, pneumonia, strep sore throat, tetanus, tuberculosis, and typhoid,[21] leading the way to new therapeutics and eventually to the wonder drugs of the twentieth century.

A major plague epidemic broke out in China as the curtain was falling on the nineteenth century. Fear and hope combined in a dramatic race to find the microbial source and natural habitat of this ancient scourge. On May 4, 1894, Dr. James Lowson, director of medical services at the British colony of Hong Kong, booked passage on a night boat to plague-ridden Canton. Lowson had heard rumors that the pestilence was spreading from China to Hong Kong. After stopping for a vigorous game of tennis, he accompanied a physician friend to the Canton city hospital to see the plague at first hand. Back in Hong Kong, the colonial authorities denied the presence of plague, but Chinese residents were dying at an alarming rate. The signs and symptoms would have been familiar to both Hodges and Boghurst.

By May 10 there were twenty cases of plague in Tung Wah hospital, the only facility in Hong Kong that made the Chinese population comfortable by employing Eastern as well as Western medical practices. Lowson, in charge of the colony's hospitals and the treatment of infectious diseases, was at the center of a crisis. He immediately turned the ship *Hygea* into a quarantine facility on the water, away from the population. On the night of the thirteenth, he wrote in his diary, "Hot sun. Cases pouring in. Outlook appalling." A Chinese medical worker along with twenty-four other persons died that day, and twelve sick persons entered the *Hygea* facility. On the following day twenty-two more corpses were reported, but a far different count appeared in the London *Times:* 100 fatalities a day, a total of 1,500. The *Times* also reported that 100,000 persons had fled Hong Kong, perhaps exaggerating the mass exodus from the city of 150,000 persons but not the panic causing it. Lowson sent forth an urgent plea for medical expertise in identifying and treating the disease.

Seven weeks after Lowson's visit to Canton, two expert microbiologists, one Japanese, one French, arrived in Hong Kong within three days of each other, after receiving urgent messages by telegram. Thus began a contest between rival nationalities and competing schools of medical analysis, each employing knowledge and tools that Dr. George Thomson had lacked in his controversial autopsy two centuries before.

The Japanese specialist, Shibasaburo Kitasato, had played a role in discovering the tubercle microbe and an antitoxin for anthrax at Koch's German laboratory. He came in with a team of Japanese specialists and impressive equipment: glass slides and stains, solid and liquid media for growing bacteria, inoculating needles and loops, the latest Zeiss microscopes, and the indispensable autoclave for preparing and sterilizing media, glassware, and disposed-of cultures. To the local Chinese physicians, this Japanese native's offer of help represented a double irony: he came as a native of a country about to wage war with China, bearing Western techniques alien to Chinese tradition.

The arrival of Swiss-born French expert Alexandre Yersin reflected different ironies. He had worked at the Pasteur Institute and had collaborated with Emile Roux on the discovery of diphtheria toxin. Growing restless with laboratory life, he had left the Pasteur Institute on a quixotic adventure. Colleagues were shocked when this young scientist abandoned a promising career and took passage as a ship's doctor on a vessel bound for French Indochina. The diminutive, almost reclusive figure quickly settled into an alien culture and language, teaching himself the skills of cartography and meteorology. Yersin mapped the coasts and explored the jungle, braving encounters with pirates, hostile tribesmen, a tiger, and debilitating bouts of malaria and diarrhea. Letters to his mother related the pleasure of treating the native people for smallpox, cholera, dysentery, and rabies and his relief at escaping the tedium of research in Paris. "My firm intention is to never return again to work at the Pasteur Institute," he informed a disappointed mother. "Life in a laboratory there would seem impossible to me after having tasted the freedom and life of the open air." Then a telegram arrived from his former friend and colleague Roux, forcing him back into the world of research: the Pasteur Institute wanted him to help the British fight the plague. He hastily departed for Hong Kong, hand-carrying the microbe hunter's barest essentials—his microscope and autoclave.[22]

When Kitasato and Yersin reached the stricken port city in mid-June, they found the streets almost deserted. The Chinese were in near panic, bewildered by Western medical techniques and resisting quarantine orders issued by foreigners. The colonial authorities tried in vain to isolate the sick members of the Chinese community; the infected Chinese simply fled to their ancestral villages to die among their own people, past and present, an ancient custom that treated death with dignity and communal support. The British residents were stranded and frightened as shipping companies stopped transporting passengers from Hong Kong. Two additional hospitals were reserved mainly for the British sick. The labor market was paralyzed, and revenues from the opium trade dwindled. But the most daunting problem was sanitation. There were hasty burials, as evidenced by shallow graves in wayside ditches. Official reports characterized the Chinese waterfront dwellings with four words: "unfit for human habitation."

Yersin had to make do with a makeshift hut as his laboratory and bribe British soldiers disposing of infected bodies to let him have some for testing of the victims' blood. By contrast, the Kennedy Town Hospital, manned by English doctors, provided Kitasato's team, which had arrived first with great publicity, with their up-to-date facilities and a constant supply of bodies. As often happens in medical research, however, the successful route among the rival paths to discovery was not the obvious one. Kitasato, brilliant, exacting, and superbly equipped as he was, stumbled.

The day after Kitasato's arrival, his assisting pathologist, Dr. Aoyamo, hastily performed a postmortem without a bed, blanket, or mosquito netting. A photograph from Aoyamo's research paper shows half-naked patients lying in a large warehouse, where numerous mosquitoes entered at night.[23] (Some mosquitoes were later found to be infected with plague but lacking the ability to transmit the organisms.) That first plague patient had experienced a temperature reaching 40° Celsius (104° Fahrenheit). Lymph nodes in the groin were swollen and of a red-bluish color. The connective tissue displayed small red spots. The spleen and other organs were enlarged. Other dissections followed, but Aoyamo and a coworker became infected and entered the isolation ship. Aoyamo survived; his colleague died, recalling the rumored deaths of Dr. Thomson's collaborators in 1665.

Kitasato pressed on with his work, sending illustrations of his findings to the British medical journal *Lancet*.[24] Under the microscope, small, rod-shaped bacteria were visible. The Koch-trained expert had stained his samples with a reliable enough gram stain, giving a purple color if the bacteria were gram positive or a red hue if gram negative. But Kitasato hesitated as he looked at his blood samples. They contained both gram-negative, nonmotile bacilli and motile, gram-positive diplococci, round bacteria associated with pneumonia. He inoculated live mice to try to verify whether he had found the plague bacilli. The small rodents showed signs of plague, but Kitasato remained unsure of the bacillus.[25] Probably his samples had been contaminated.

Three days after Kitasato's arrival with his team, Yersin had appeared unaccompanied. Five days later he wrote in his diary, "At first glance, I see a real mass of bacilli, all identical. They are very small rods, thick with rounded ends and lightly colored." He categorized them as gram negative and non-motile. Yersin sent specimens in test tubes to Paris for corroboration and confirmed his diagnosis when his plague bacilli produced the same signs in his animals as in infected humans. On August 18 his illustrated report reached the world through the Pasteur Institute's *Annales.* The bacterium, initially called *Pasteurella pestis* after Yersin's mentor Louis Pasteur, was later fittingly renamed *Yersinia pestis* after its discoverer.

Kitasato's and Yersin's dramatic search for the plague bacillus brought them to the next step of discovery: finding a reservoir where the bacteria flourished. Both men had observed a large number of dead rats and flies in Hong Kong. It did not take long to confirm their suspicions that the rats were involved in the plague epidemic. Drawing blood from dead rats, Yersin found it packed with plague bacilli. "The rats are certainly the great propagators of the epidemic," he concluded.[26] Yersin knew that the flies were also infected but questioned how they could pass on the microorganisms.

The discoverers pondered the route of the bacilli from rat to human, wondering how to break the chain of transmission. Kitasato posited three entry routes of the bacteria to human victims: an external wound, ingestion, and respiration. Yersin went further in his probing. Discounting ingestion and respiration, he suspected an insect to be a transmitting carrier. He located an inoculation site near an infected bubo but did not know the perpetrator. Epidemiology was just on the threshold of identifying parasitic "vectors" of communicable diseases.

Five short years after the epidemiological breakthrough at Hong Kong, Paul-Louis Simond of the Pasteur Institute demonstrated that the rat flea was a missing biological link in the world of the plague pathogen, with some fleas infecting rats and other fleas transferring plague from dead rats to human victims. So Yersin was right in looking for an insect vector contributing to bubonic plague. But Kitasato was also on the right track in suspecting respiration as the human contributor to pneumonic plague through the sneezing, exhalation, and inhalation of infected droplets.

Scientific sleuthing had now uncovered the bacillus that caused modern plague (and presumably its early modern precursor) and linked the four participants whose interaction resulted in the outbreak of plague in human communities, the famous *ménage à quatre* of the bacteria, flea, rat, and human.[27] The challenge now was how to defend the human population against future plague epidemics. Should the environment be cleaned up or humans protected more directly by vaccination?

Each of these modern approaches found backing in ancient medical tradition: on the one hand, cleaning up polluted waters and rubbish to banish airborne "miasmas"; on the other hand, arming oneself against the "contagion" of contact with sick persons by smoking or chewing tobacco and carrying herbs around one's neck or in the head of a cane. Plague waters mixed by apothecaries and concoctions that included viper's poison had their long history as common defenses. The Europeans had their Venice treacle, the Chinese their special herbs, the Muslim world a wide range of prophylactics.

Yersin and Kitasato saw merit in both the environmental-miasmatist and prophylactic-contagionist approaches, but each focused solely on one approach, trying to adapt it to their understanding of microbial infection. The Koch school, familiar to Kitasato, concentrated on sanitation-based control of an infectious disease, once the bacteria and their source were identified. The question was basic: What were the appropriate preventive measures? Their answers were in line with traditional thinking about miasmas and therefore intelligible to the public: general hygiene, good drainage, pure water supply, and cleanliness in dwelling houses and streets.[28] The Pasteur school's approach, while resembling the rival contagion theories of the past, was more daring and probably less intelligible to the general public: instead of the standby herbal and chemical prophylactics, it sought to derive antidotes from the disease itself.[29] By cultivating plague bacilli in various media, Yersin hoped to use them to trigger the body's immune response, thus giving protection against the invading organism.

The hygienic attack on plague at Hong Kong took place with little chance of success. Living conditions in the poorer parts of Hong Kong were so appalling that the logical solution was to burn down the Chinese town along the wharves. Budgetary considerations saved the Chinese from that sad fate. The sewer system was also an obstacle because of the smallness of pipes. The public health program that Lowson put into effect echoed the Plague Orders of 1665. The authorities relied on obligatory street cleaning, cleansing of the houses of the infected with carbolic acid and lime, burning or boiling the clothing of the dead, and burning bodies or burying them under three meters of soil.

Meanwhile, Yersin worked feverishly in total isolation to find a modern microbial solution. Skipping meals and sleep, he dissected buboes and made media right through the long hours of the night. "From a bubo of a patient who had recovered and had been convalescing for three weeks," he wrote wearily but with hope, "I was able to isolate a few colonies which completely lacked virulence in mice." He had found the long looked-for antidote! On a visit to the Pasteur Institute in Paris the next year, he cultivated attenuated bacilli and serum antibodies that became the source for future vaccines. He returned to Indochina, established a local Pasteur Institute, and remained there to the end of his life except for short trips to give lectures and accept awards. In the summer of 1896, his vaccine proved successful in countering a fresh outbreak of plague in Hong Kong.[30]

The race between these two great microbiologists in the climactic year of 1894 in Hong Kong had brought an outcome very different from the relief measures undertaken by London's plague fighters in 1665. Building on the foundational work of Koch and Pasteur and the achievements of Yersin and Kitasato, twentieth-century microbe hunters would go on to develop the long-sought wonder drugs that could cure plague. The end of an ancient scourge of humankind was at last clearly in sight.

Of Future Plagues

Plague will not be soon eradicated, despite the major advances made since the beginning of [the twentieth] century in the knowledge of the disease, in public health, and in therapy.

—Pasteur Institute, Paris, 1994

In 1995 Elisabeth Carniel and her colleagues at the Pasteur Institute in Paris wrote that la peste d'aujourd'hui could be considered a reemerging disease. Madagascar, one of the world's persistent plague centers, averaged 1,250 cases per year; in 2001 the figure rose to 2,000. In India a pulmonary epidemic in 1994 infected 876 humans.[31] Plague remains in our global village despite public health measures and vaccines and antibiotics. Endemic foci of the plague bacillus exist in Africa (Madagascar, Zimbabwe, Mozambique, Tanzania, Kenya, Zaire, Botswana, and Uganda); Asia (Vietnam, China, India, Mongolia, Kazakhstan, and Myanmar); South America (Bolivia, Brazil, and Peru); and North America (California, Arizona, New Mexico, Nevada, Colorado, Oregon, and Idaho).[32] A mortality rate of 25 percent is not uncommon in the western United States for unfortunate campers who pick up dead rodents or place their sleeping bag near burrows harboring infected animals.

The human symptoms of modern plague are easily recognizable to trained personnel with a checklist of signs, of which buboes are the most obvious. The primary hosts vary considerably, mainly consisting of wild rodents. Secondary hosts can be as disparate as rabbits, camels, and humans. The plague microbe *Yersinia pestis* has been able to adapt to a wide variety of mammals. The virtually inaccessible burrows of its wild rodent hosts are scattered throughout the globe. The host usually becomes infected by fleabites and in rare cases from contact with the soil. Fleas serve as vectors by feeding on infected rodents and transferring the bacteria to new hosts. This happens when uninfected rodents share nests or burrows with infected ones. Even if exterminators reached these remote areas and destroyed their occupants, the bacteria could survive for years in the den of the dead animals. The arrival of the next occupiers of the nests would trigger a new epizootic, potentially leading to a human epidemic.[33]

As the twenty-first century begins, we are on the threshold of a new relationship with this dread disease. The early microbe hunters, led by Pasteur and Koch and their protégés Alexandre Yersin and Shibasaburo Kitasato, laid the groundwork by identifying the microbe. The twentieth century followed with a detailed mapping of its cycle of transmission, the development of effective vaccines and antibiotics, and the sequencing of the DNA of *Yersinia pestis*.

But is it certain that this *Yersinia pestis* of the third plague pandemic also caused the two plague pandemics that preceded it? Some skeptics suggest an entirely different pathogen, such as the Ebola virus or anthrax, as the microbial source of early plague visitations.[34] Yet it seems impossible that Ebola could maintain itself during such large-scale epidemics. In Africa, Ebola attacks have wound down after an initial wave of cases. Similarly, anthrax is not able to create a sizable bubo and would probably not leave such large numbers dead in the streets as are described in seventeenth-century accounts. Anthrax bacteria can be found in the soil, and spores can exist on the hair or wool of animals (causing so-called "wool-sorters disease"), but the pathogen is most lethal in an airborne spore form. Human mortality from anthrax infection is not as great as with plague; furthermore, it cannot be passed from person to person.

Most microbiologists remain convinced that the causative plague organism, *Yersinia pestis*, has been the same in all pandemics. Testing this belief, Dr. Julian Parkhill and his colleagues at the Sanger Center in Cambridge have decoded the complete DNA sequence of *Yersinia pestis*. Genetically, this microbe has remained extremely constant through time.[35]

These scientific findings fit well with the repeated description, across centuries, of the same symptoms appearing on plague victims. The symptoms described by William Boghurst, Nathaniel Hodges, and Gideon Harvey in

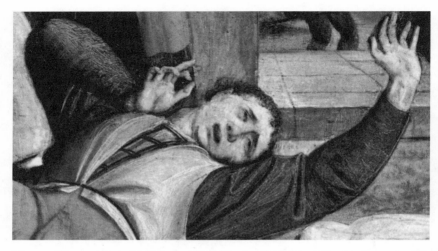

Fig. 16. Plague victim with bubo on the neck, detail of *Saint Sebastian Intercedes during the Plague*, Josse Lieferinxe, 1497–99. This fifteenth-century artistic rendition of a plague scene, featuring Saint Sebastian as a spiritual consoler and aid to the victims, displays on a victim's neck the bubo swelling of the lymph nodes that has been the most common identifying sign of plague since the Black Death. Other diseases can also cause this swelling but without the other common body signs and symptoms and high mortality rate characteristic of plague. The Walters Art Museum, Baltimore

1665 would fit a present-day diagnosis. Their external observations mirror with considerable precision what was happening internally. Their greatest contribution is letting us know that the disease's pathology has not fundamentally changed during a long history.

What has fluctuated over time is the plague bacillus's cohabiting relationship with vector fleas, primary host animals, and incidental human hosts. The result has been an ebbing and flowing of plague in the human population. This is partly explained by the plague genome's elasticity; it can integrate small snips of foreign or rogue DNA, called plasmids, which have infiltrated the bacterial DNA. Some added pieces of DNA increase the bacilli's virulence, and other plasmids give adaptability to insect vectors. These snips of DNA are so well integrated that researchers can't distinguish them from the rest of the *Yersinia pestis* genome.

The role of the black rat poses the most problematic link in the chain of human plague infection. Rats were virtually unmentioned in 1665, yet they were presumably the primary hosts of fleas searching for a warm bloodmeal.

A possible explanation is that rats have a habit of going back to their nests when they become ill. The Pasteur Institute's researchers, from Henri Mollaret to Elisabeth Carniel, have emphasized this characteristic. Dead rats in the alleys and cellars of London in 1665 may not have been present in sufficient number to capture people's attention. The ratcatcher, after all, was a regular feature of this society; rodents abounded, and some of them turned up dead. Charles I's French physician Theodore Mayerne voiced a rare suspicion of a connection between rat and pestilence. Most people pointed to live dogs and cats prowling the city streets as the most likely animal carriers of the disease.

Two British historians and an anthropologist from the United States argue that the Black Death spread too rapidly across Europe to have been dependent on rats for dispersal.[36] Perhaps they have not considered fleas on travelers' clothing as a likely medium for the plague's rapid advance. Medical observers in 1665 knew nothing of the etiology of plague. Yet they suspected that the disease entered a community frequently on cloth and clothing, especially light-colored material, which is particularly attractive to fleas. This not only fits with the role of fleas as a vector of the disease but helps to explain how plague could travel great distances and strike persons at places, like Eyam in Derbyshire, that were remote from the source of infection.

Some *Yersinia pestis* skeptics look to the temperature charts of the midseventeenth century and say that it was too cold for the rat flea, *Xenopsilla chopsis*, to be a key link in the chain causing a human plague epidemic.[37] In response, continental European researchers suggest that human fleas played a crucial role during this period. They argue that the human flea, *Pulex irritans*, could withstand the temperatures of early modern Europe's Little Ice Age. These fleas could have spread the disease from person to person and did not need rats as a source of the plague bacillus once it entered the human arena. Many researchers, however, point out that *P. irritans* is not a good vector.

At least at the beginning and through much of the Great Plague of 1665, it seems likely that an epizootic in rats caused by bites from infected rat fleas was needed for the human epidemic. Rats in the "pestered places" of London's poor attracted infected rat fleas, which may have come by a cargo ship from an infected port. The fleas could have survived in the warmth of the rat habitat. It follows logically that, when rat die-off began in the late winter and early spring of 1665, isolated cases of human plague followed. An occasional infected flea, ravenous after its proventriculus (the pouch of the esophagus leading to the midgut) became blocked with bacteria, searched for a warm-blooded meal. These fleas, in a feeding frenzy, abandoned dead rats and went looking for the closest warm body. Thus an epidemic began. When the rats started dying in large numbers, the plague mortality in humans shot up as the secondary human host alternated with the primary one.[38] This chronology fits the early stages of Great Plague mortality.

One last point about the causal organism concerns the multiple diseases reported at the time of the Great Plague.[39] Certainly, there were cases of smallpox at the beginning and perhaps other diseases as well. Since the mortality curves of all nonplague diseases reported in 1665 mirror the distinctive plague death curves, as shown by graphs, it seems obvious that the parish clerks and searchers frequently listed plague as other diseases. This side-stepped quarantine and masked the enormity of a crisis that left uncounted victims dead in the streets.

As medical science now understands it, plague in humans usually begins with infective fleas piercing the skin. Fleabites are known to regurgitate 25,000 to 100,000 bacilli into the victim's tissue.[40] With radarlike certainty these invading microbes attach to approaching white blood cells that have been alerted by chemicals released from the invaded tissue at the site of the injection. The people of 1665 could not have seen this first stage of a battle royal within the body, but they did see the resulting tokens that accounts described as resembling fleabites.

What happens next could be neither seen nor imagined by the humorally centered medicine of 1665, though Fracastoro's invading seedlets of disease and the body's sentinel-like archeus imagined by Thomson vaguely fit the two sides of the microscopically detected battle: the microbes and the body's defense system. Among the first white cells to arrive at the site of the invasion are large macrophages from the blood, lymph, or tissue. These baglike cells are phagocytic—that is, they engulf the bacteria and release killing enzymes. The plague bacillus, in turn, has two avoidance mechanisms: antiphagocytic surface molecules and a capsule that prevents destruction by cellular enzymes.[41] Protected by these two defenses, the plague bacteria proliferate and turn the macrophages into centers of multiplying *Yersinia pestis* organisms. Other white cells (T cells) carry the infected macrophages through blood vessels or tissue to the nearest lymph nodes, where more white cells try to destroy the organisms.

At this point in the battle within the human body, the physicians in 1665 picked up the external signs again. They could see the protruding buboes and observe the victim's excruciating pain as the parasitic bacteria and host blood cells proliferated rapidly there, causing the nodes to swell. The buboes are usually discernible in three days, matching the descriptions of Boghurst and others.

The bloodstream soon becomes infected with bacteria. The body's defense response produces a raging fever, which is the body's attempt to kill foreign microbes. It is the symptom that Gideon Harvey, Thomas Sydenham, and Thomas Willis used as a chief diagnostic indicator of plague. If the bacteria survive this counterattack, the vital organs of the liver, the spleen, and more rarely the lungs are next in line.[42] Finally, the heart is involved and heartbeats become erratic, as reported by the physicians of the Great Plague. Death ensues, usually brought on by toxic shock.

The battle between the response mechanisms of the human cells' immune system and the invading microorganism's stratagems has been termed a Microbial Dance of Death. Such a struggle might be seen as a game of chess for immortality, reminiscent of Ingmar Bergman's *The Seventh Seal*. (More highly evolved pathogens than the plague bacillus have a more accommodating relationship with their human host cells.) When the buboes begin to appear, the victim has a mortality probability of 60 percent or more if not treated. If the bacteria attack quickly through the bloodstream, as in septicemic plague, the body is completely overwhelmed with little immune response and no bubo formation. Death comes in two days in the vast majority of cases. If the plague victim develops a lung infection, the disease is even more deadly, approaching 100 percent mortality if untreated. A patient must be diagnosed quickly and treatment begun within twelve to fifteen hours of the fleabite.

An equally frightening aspect of this pneumonic plague is that a cough by the victim can pass the infection to other humans via droplets containing plague organisms. Although plague in the seventeenth century probably did not enter the pneumonic stage, folk memories had carried the visions forward from the Black Death, as seen in George Wither's descriptions in 1625 and 1665 of the spotted siren killing with her "noisome breath." This image blended with the medical opinion of the time that one could catch the disease from a sick person's exhalations. Pneumonic plague is short lived after the initial transfers, unless a reservoir of infected rats or fleas exists. Such an outbreak occurred in India in the late summer of 1994, terrifying but brief, with antibiotics helping to bring it to a quick end. A footnote on this outbreak provides yet another connection with the Great Plague of 1665. Although laboratory analysis was available in the 1994 outbreak, technicians lacked training in plague identification and diagnosis was delayed. Officials

handling plague patients detected the signs and symptoms used diagnosti-
cally by Hodges, Boghurst, and other 1665 caregivers and administered antibiotics immediately. Later diagnosis by laboratory results from the Pasteur
Institute confirmed the presence of *Yersinia pestis*.

Ecology and Evolution

Little genetic distance separates a rarely encountered mild food- and water-borne
zoonotic pathogen from one of the most feared pathogens of human history.
—B. JOSEPH HINNEBUSCH, "Bubonic Plague: A Molecular Genetic Case
History of the Emergence of an Infectious Disease" (1997), referring
to *Yersinia pseudotuberculosis and Yersinia pestis*

AIDS now appears to be the ultimate microbial challenge to contemporary
medical research. But the wily plague bacillus is not far behind with its speed
and stratagems. An obvious defense for persons in an endemic plague area is
vaccination. Several vaccines were used during the Vietnam War. Unfortunately, the vaccine's protection lasts only about six months, it offers no protection against pneumonic plague, and it carries potentially harmful side effects. Unless someone is traveling to an area where plague frequently infects
humans, the preferred strategy bypasses immunization, treating with antibiotics after a diagnosis of plague. Streptomycin has been the antibiotic of
choice. Alternative drugs (harder to find and more expensive) may be available if a patient has a resistant strain. The discovery in 1997 by Dr. Carniel
and her colleagues of plague strains in Madagascar resistant to multiple antibiotics, including streptomycin, chloramphenicol, and tetracycline, has
caused great concern.[43] In 2001 another strain resistant to streptomycin was
identified, again in Madagascar.

The slow pace of discovering new antibiotics is troubling. If drug-resistant
microbes should cause an epidemic, we might be returned to a pre-Pasteu-
rian world. This makes us wonder what could have caused the end of a cycle
of epidemics, as occurred in the late Roman Empire during the eighth century and again in the eighteenth century in Europe. If scientists can determine what caused the pandemic of the Black Death to end after four centuries in Europe without antibacterial intervention, perhaps this knowledge
may be adapted to our newest antimicrobial techniques.[44]

Historical hindsight suggests that something happened to the cohabiting relations among the four players: microbe, flea, rodent, and human. It is impossible to sort out all the possible changes in this *ménage à quatre,* as Dr. Henri Mollaret, emeritus expert on plague at the Pasteur Institute, has noted. Nevertheless, several intriguing hypotheses merit consideration.[45]

Improvements in sanitation, hygiene, and general living conditions have sharply reduced the threat of infectious disease over the past three centuries. Did they come early enough to help explain the disappearance of plague from Britain after the Great Plague of 1665 and from the rest of Western Europe a few decades later? A popular myth holds that the Great Fire of 1666 started the downward cycle of plague by clearing out the rat-infested dwellings of London. The myth dies hard: the fire actually took out the wealthy core of the city, leaving most pestered buildings in poor suburban areas intact as breeding grounds for black rats and their fleas. In the long run, such new behaviors as frequent changes of clothing and bedding cut down on the proximity of fleas to humans, and the elimination of thatched roofs and the building of brick houses kept the rats at bay.

A further deterrent was the disappearance in the eighteenth century of the urban-dwelling black rat. Its successor, the Norwegian brown rat, did not live close to humans and could not swim, making it a less likely source of plague transference to human communities.

Many historians of epidemics now favor the hypothesis that external quarantine sharply reduced the prospect of a plague outbreak in Europe during the eighteenth and nineteenth centuries.[46] European officials, suspecting that plague epidemics began with the importation of plague on people and goods from the East, posted guards at the Turkish border and quarantined ships at European ports. This may have placed a hold on suspected goods and people, but it stretches credulity to believe that this *cordon sanitaire* could have kept back all the infected rats and fleas. Some fleas on clothing and rats in grain sacks would have passed through, bearing the microbial agent. The infected fleas could have lived 230 to 396 days by varying modern calculations, long enough to take them across Europe.[47] At that point, environmental conditions favorable to wild rodents and fleas that remained in European communities would probably have been tinder for a new pestilential conflagration.

The search for causes of plague's disappearance and failure to return to Europe therefore leads inevitably to *Yersinia pestis* itself. We can assume that, if plague bacilli remained or were reimported, the wild rodent primary hosts settled into a coexistence with their bacterial tormenter. This theory states that the rats did not die, and the fleas had no need to leave this primary host

for a human.[48] A new plague epidemic would await either a bacterial mutation into a more virulent strain (fitting Boghurst's notion of endemic plague
in pestered places getting out of hand) or the importation of a new, deadly
plague strain (which fits Hodges' theory of plague coming from Turkey via
Holland).

The relationship of the human hosts to *Yersinia pestis* must also be considered. What of the persons who have been so prominent in our story: the
ever-daring Samuel Pepys, the caring physicians Nathaniel Hodges and
William Boghurst, and Symon Patrick, who visited stricken parishioners?
All of these men came close to infective rat fleas during their great plague.
Many nurses, midwives, searchers, and bearers ran even greater risk of being
bitten by infected fleas. Were these women and men blessed with natural immunity during the epidemic? What about immunity in populations in the
years following this last Great Plague?

Interesting evidence might shed light on this. One could have acquired
immunity by exposure to a relatively benign microbe that is genetically close
to the plague bacillus. In the eighteenth and nineteenth centuries, officials in
parts of the Middle East reported a chronic form of plague that caused dis-
tressing intestinal sickness and nothing more. Researchers have now identified a bacterial agent, *Yersinia pseudotuberculosis,* that closely resembles *Yersinia pestis* and produces mild intestinal disorders. Although it is transmitted
by contaminated food or water rather than an insect bite, it belongs to the
same genus as *Yersinia pestis,* with ribosomal RNA (from small structures
called *ribosomes* within the cell transcribed from original DNA) that is 97.8
percent identical with that of the plague bacillus. It is now believed that *Yersinia pseudotuberculosis* was the original form of *Yersinia pestis.*

In this near-clone of plague, researchers have found similar antigenic
molecules—proteins that cause the body to produce protective antibodies. If
this close cousin infects humans or rats, its antigenic molecules will protect
against plague. It abounds in many European ports and has been widely
identified in France, from which plague retreated after the epidemic at Marseilles in 1720–22. Testing of the sewer system of Paris in the last century
showed high levels of this organism.

The plague bacillus has remarkable homogeneity, with little discernible
change since it mutated from *Yersinia pseudotuberculosis* 1,500 to 20,000 years
ago, probably in the central Asian plateau. In a fascinating search backward
from what we know currently, Dr. Carniel and her co-investigators have
drawn on the ribosomal RNA of *Yersinia pestis,* a template of the original par-

ent DNA found on ribosomes within the cells of all organisms. From seventy specimens of plague in sixteen different places in the world, they distinguished three plague types, or biovars, whose territorial coverage appears to fit the spread of plague in its three historical pandemics. These types have been appropriately named *Antiqua, Medievalis,* and *Orientalis* (see appendix D).[49]

The *Antiqua* ribotype, O, is believed to have moved from an ancestral home in central Asia into the heart of Africa, then up to lower Egypt, and to Alexandria. From there it spread by ship to Emperor Justinian's capital at Constantinople and throughout the Late Roman imperial lands, where only O types are found today. The *Medievalis* group also has type O but is distinguished from *Antiqua* by its inability to reduce nitrates as part of its metabolism. Its geographic locations today fit the historical path of the second pandemic, originating in central Asia as well. It traveled along the silk route to the Crimea, migrated into the Mediterranean, and spread throughout Europe. The widespread locations of *Orientalis,* with its distinctive type B, span four continents plus the Pacific islands, mirroring the known travels of the third pandemic from its origins in China's Yunnan province to Hong Kong in 1894 and then by steamships, with infected rats and their fleas, around the globe.

A fundamental link in the evolution of *Yersinia pestis* is suggested by microbiological understanding of both B and O types. *Orientalis* type B lost its ability to ferment glycerol as part of its metabolism (both O types can) but is believed to have evolved from the first *Antiqua* strain, since they share the ability to reduce nitrates.

Definitive proof that *Yersinia pestis* caused the first two pandemics awaits evidence from the testing of dental pulp DNA in skeletal remains from the first and second pandemics. Samples of dental pulp from cadavers of the fourteenth, sixteenth, and eighteenth centuries, discovered in mass burial sites and charnel houses in southern France, have been analyzed. These samples tested positive for *Yersinia pestis,* on the basis of DNA testing. Some specialists conclude from this evidence that the Black Death and later visitations during the second pandemic were definitively bubonic plague similar to what we have today. Another group questioned the findings, suggesting the possibility of contamination; testing of large numbers of cadavers is needed for convincing proof.[50] Papers on this research were discussed at a world conference on plague in Marseilles in July 2001.[51]

Perils and Prospects

Perhaps, as we grow almost smug about influenza, that most quotidian of infections, a new plague is now gathering deadly force. Except this time we stand armed with a better understanding of the past to better survive the next pandemic.

—GINA KOLATA, *Flu: The Story of the Great Influenza Pandemic of 1918 and the Search for the Virus That Caused It*

The most dreaded disease ever to afflict humankind shares a crowded stage with infectious diseases that have not yet made their last curtain call. A wide variety of bacterial and viral pathogens have clung tenaciously to life for hundreds or thousands of years. In the seventeenth century, 30 percent of all reported deaths were associated with epidemics. Wave after wave of typhus, smallpox, dysentery, and influenza struck capital and countryside.[52] The threats continue. Benign microbes far removed from the *Yersinia* bacilli may suddenly pose a threat, propelled by "minor genetic changes that alter [their] route of transmission or extend [their] host range."[53] The recent history of malaria, tuberculosis, and AIDS reveals reasons for maintaining vigilance against all potential microbial killers.

Malaria, a protozoa-caused disease with a long history, is believed to have originated in tropical Africa. The parasite probably infected several primates besides humans. Hundreds of years later it radiated out to Mesopotamia and subsequently spread up the Nile River to the Mediterranean Sea, making a debilitating mark on the ancient Greek and Roman world.[54] Drs. Willis and Sydenham treated it with quinine in the seventeenth century, and today it carries away three thousand children daily. One in ten of the global population suffers its debilitating fevers and chills. A new, highly virulent form of malaria appeared at the end of the twentieth century, with vector mosquitoes resistant to chemical extermination. The situation remains critical in sub-Saharan Africa, where close to 90 percent of the fatalities are of children under the age of two. As of this writing the leading antimalarials have failed in 80 percent of cases. Responding to this crisis, the United Nations Development Program, in collaboration with the World Health Organization, UNICEF, and the World Bank, launched a campaign against the disease in 1998. Among the promising antidotes is a plant extract that has been used in China for two thousand years against fevers. The active ingredient in this plant seems to attack malaria at many stages in its life cycle, completely destroying the parasites.[55]

Among ancient bacterial diseases, tuberculosis *(Mycobacterium tuberculae)* continues to be a monumental threat to human health. The seventeenth century knew it as consumption; later it became known as "the white plague." One-third of the world's population today is infected with tubercle bacilli; eight million individuals a year develop tuberculosis from the infection. Only humans are susceptible to the bacillus. Sunlight and fresh air retard the infection rate; stress and crowded, unsanitary conditions accelerate it. The bacilli can pass through the air on droplets of moisture and can also be transmitted by contaminated milk or water. The breakdown of immune resistance in AIDS patients has greatly increased the incidence of tuberculosis. In New York City, the disease increased threefold between 1979 and 1989, when AIDS was just emerging as a known threat to human life. Forty percent of the cases were HIV-related, 82 percent of the patients were unemployed, and 68 percent were unsuitably housed or homeless. Streptomycin became a magic bullet for sufferers, but compliance in taking the drug is a serious problem, and some new strains are resistant to this antibiotic.[56]

Viruses pose a greater problem than bacterial pathogens, even their most deadly representative, *Yersinia pestis.* Antibiotics have no effect on viruses, and the raging fever employed by the human body's defense system to destroy microbial invaders utterly fails. Today's most dangerous viral pathogen is HIV—the acronym for human immunodeficiency virus, which causes acquired immune deficiency syndrome (AIDS). HIV carries a strand of RNA of around 250 bits, ten million times less than human cellular DNA—a formidable David to the human's Goliath-like gene structure. Its virulence is somewhat mitigated by its parasitic nature; it cannot replicate or organize itself without co-opting a living cell. But for humans who become infected, no adequate therapies yet exist, though drug cocktails, as they are known, can slow down the progression of the disease.[57] In addition to AIDS, viruses are responsible for smallpox, influenza, polio, chickenpox, and measles, as well as newly emerging and well-publicized hemorrhagic diseases such as Lassa fever, Ebola fever, and Hantavirus.

Other threats loom on the world's horizon. An outbreak of disease in one spot can affect persons thousands of miles away, as was demonstrated so dramatically in 2002–3 by the appearance in China of SARS (severe acute respiratory disease). This mysterious new type of pneumonia was first documented in Guangdong Province (adjacent to Hong Kong), where a businessman was hospitalized. That case and others that followed went unreported by the authorities for four months until February 2003, when the World Health Organization was first informed of a menacing outbreak throughout the province. The rapid spread astonished epidemiologists. In February one infected man traveled to seven countries before being hospitalized after returning to Hong Kong. By mid-March twenty countries listed cases, and the World Health Organization issued temporary travel advisories warning against visiting countries and cities as far from China as Toronto, Canada. The spread of infection among hospital workers in Beijing and other major Chinese centers was especially alarming, causing the quarantining of hospital wards that had a high level of infection among health practitioners and the closing of two entire hospitals. Mortality among infected persons rose from 3 percent initially to 10 percent within a few weeks and to more than 50 percent among patients older than sixty-five years in places such as Hong Kong.

As had been the case with plague in 1665, the authorities in 2003 had to rely on bodily signs and symptoms to identify SARS-infected individuals. The Centers for Disease Control developed a diagnostic blood test, but it could not detect the antibodies that the human genome forms against SARS corona-type virus until three weeks after infection. In Beijing in 2003, as in London in 1665, preservatives and cures appeared like magic in the medical marketplace, with anti-SARS herbal brews and disinfectant bleaches selling briskly on the word of government officials, popular newssheets, or neighborhood gossip, even as vendors acknowledged that the public "knew" there was no cure for SARS. Probably of greatest concern to medical professionals at the outset of the epidemic was the possibility that the SARS coronavirus would mutate, thereby hampering treatments. As of this writing, the silver lining is that the first major study of the virus's genome revealed little mutation during its spread to different countries.[58]

Some epidemics have originated in the heart of the most advanced nations. In the United States infectious diseases are the third greatest cause of death, following heart disease and cancer. In the world at large, infectious diseases remain the leading cause of death.

There have been victories, to be sure. The first "conquest of infectious disease" came with the much-heralded eradication of smallpox twenty-five years ago. Many epidemiologists hold out hope of eliminating measles by 2013. And some medical experts aim at eradicating yellow fever by the middle of the century.

Polio's recent history, however, raises alarm bells about the efficacy of eradicating infectious diseases. The World Health Organization itself keeps pushing back the target date for eliminating this dreaded disease of the young, despite polio's confinement in 2001 to 10 countries, a sharp drop from 125 in 1988. (The last case in the United States occurred in 1979.) A far more alarmist word comes from the head of the successful campaign against small-pox, Dr. D. A. Henderson. In October 2002, he shocked the medical world by asserting that elimination of polio would never succeed. Rogue polio, he argued, could always be possible, either by chance or by design. As proof, he gave three examples: (1) individuals with impaired immunity can per-manently harbor and transmit the polio virus; (2) a weakened polio virus used as a vaccine in the Dominican Republic mysteriously mutated, trigger-ing a polio outbreak in 2001; (3) in 2002, researchers at a New York lab-oratory synthesized a virile polio specimen from mail-order materials. The only way to fight polio (and presumably other infectious diseases), Hender-son concluded, was a return to routine vaccination.[59]

Known and unknown diseases recognize no boundaries. The Centers for Disease Control and Prevention in Atlanta, Georgia, has an entire depart-ment devoted to a project entitled "Unexplained Illness and Deaths Surveil-lance." Hospital-acquired diseases, or nosocomials, infect an estimated two million patients in the United States each year, killing about ninety thou-sand. At the beginning of this millennium, drug-resistant infections alone accounted for more than fourteen thousand of these deaths.[60]

Scientists and pharmaceutical companies are hard-pressed to develop new medicines fast enough to keep up with new pathogens or resistant strains. In wealthier countries, antibiotics are overprescribed, causing the development of drug resistance in microbes. In poorer countries, according to the World Health Organization, sick persons take cheaper, weaker drugs and fail to complete the treatment. We are reaping the bitter dual harvest of the im-proper application of drug therapies and the cost-effective concentration of the pharmaceutical companies on developing drugs for long-term use rather than against potential epidemic threats.[61]

The prospects and perils of the future cause us to grapple with a previously unthinkable dilemma: should we completely eliminate all traces of microor-ganisms that once caused such scourges as smallpox? Threats of bioterrorism have given us pause. Keeping our laboratory cultures of smallpox, along with other microbial pathogens, might prove essential for reconfiguring vaccines against biologically engineered or accidentally mutated rogue microbes.

The "microbe hunters" did not vanish after the appearance of Paul De-Kruf's classic book with that alluring title. We do live in a smaller world, and human encroachment on virgin forests and jungles keeps supplying us with new toxic diseases in company with exotic plants and animals. Microbes and their toxins may be just a breath or bite away. The challenge for future microbe hunters is to accelerate the discovery of new healing herbs and medicines and new medical understandings. From the past we can learn of other human resources that sustained men and women who fought against their own great plagues. The medical, religious, and administrative attempts at containment by Londoners in 1665, including the physicians' sweatings and purgatives, plague waters, and cauterizing of buboes, may not have saved many lives, but perhaps they offered a placebo-like relief. The refusal of some medical professionals to flee from the path of the disease and their struggle to carry on raise a standard for us to emulate as we face our own medical challenges with new uncertainties.

APPENDIX A

Bills of Mortality for Greater London

Table A.1. Greater London Bills of Mortality: Nonplague Burials in April and May 1665 and the Annual Average of Nonplague Burials for April and May 1655–1664

	Number of Burials					
	Consumption	*Dropsy*	*Contagious*	*Enteric*	*Birthing*	*Teething*
Annual average (1655–64)	507	137	418	173	31	140
1665	680	227	490	287	145	189

SOURCE: Bodleian Library, Gough Additional MSS London 4° 95–97.

NOTE: The averaging for April and May in 1655–64 is based on the only surviving run of weekly Greater London Bills of Mortality, which covers May 1655 and April and May for 1657, 1659, 1660, 1662, 1663, and 1664. Records are missing for the rest of the ten-year sequence. In the Bills of Mortality, "consumption" includes tissick and consumption. "Dropsy" was a health condition involving swelling of the limbs, especially at the ankles. "Contagious" includes the nonplague infectious diseases smallpox, spotted fever, (simple) fever, measles, and French pox (syphilis). "Enteric" includes griping of the guts, stopping of the stomach, surfeit, flux, and scouring. "Birthing" represents birth-related mortality such as death in childbed, stillborn infants, abortive rejection of the fetus, and chrisoms. "Teething" refers to early childhood death (before the age of three), mainly from "teeth" (eruption of teeth through the gums), "worms," and "thrush."

Table A.2. Greater London Bills of Mortality: Total Burials and
Plague Burials, December 27, 1664–December 26, 1665

Week	No. of Burials		Week	No. of Burials	
	Total	Plague		Total	Plague
12/27–1/3	349	0	5/30–6/6	405	43
1/3–1/10	394	0	6/6–6/13	558	112
1/10–1/17	415	0	6/13–6/20	615	168
1/17–1/24	474	0	6/20–6/27	684	267
1/24–1/31	409	0	**Subtotal**	**2,262**	**590**
Subtotal	**2,041**	**0**	6/27–7/4	1,006	470
1/31–2/7	393	0	7/4–7/11	1,268	725
2/7–2/14	462	1	7/11–7/18	1,761	1,089
2/14–2/21	393	0	7/18–7/25	2,785	1,843
2/21–2/28	396	0	**Subtotal**	**6,820**	**4,127**
Subtotal	**1,644**	**1**	7/25–8/1	3,014	2,010
2/28–3/7	441	0	8/1–8/8	4,030	2,817
3/7–3/14	433	0	8/8–8/15	5,310	3,880
3/14–3/21	363	0	8/15–8/22	5,568	4,237
3/21–3/28	353	0	8/22–8/29	7,496	6,102
Subtotal	**1,590**	**0**	**Subtotal**	**25,418**	**19,046**
3/28–4/4	344	0	8/29–9/5	8,252	6,988
4/4–4/11	382	0	9/5–9/12	7,690	6,544
4/11–4/18	344	0	9/12–9/19	8,297	7,165
4/18–4/25	398	2	9/19–9/26	6,460	5,533
Subtotal	**1,468**	**2**	**Subtotal**	**30,699**	**26,230**
4/25–5/2	388	0	9/26–10/3	5,720	4,929
5/2–5/9	347	9	10/3–10/10	5,068	4,327
5/9–5/16	353	3	10/10–10/17	3,219	2,665
5/16–5/23	385	14	10/17–10/24	1,806	1,421
5/23–5/30	400	17	10/24–10/31	1,388	1,031
Subtotal	**1,873**	**43**	**Subtotal**	**17,201**	**14,373**

Table A.2. *(continued)*

Week	No. of Burials		Week	No. of Burials	
	Total	*Plague*		*Total*	*Plague*
10/31–11/7	1,787	1,414	11/28–12/5	428	210
11/7–11/14	1,359	1,050	12/5–12/12	442	243
11/14–11/21	905	652	12/12–12/19	525	281
11/21–11/28	544	333	12/19–12/26	330	152
Subtotal	**4,595**	**3,449**	**Subtotal**	**1,725**	**886**
			Total for Year	**97,336**	**68,747**

SOURCES: *London's Dreadful Visitation;* GL, MS 3604/1/1. These figures reflect the plague toll in 1665 better than the printed annual bill, which begins with December 20–27, 1664 (1 plague burial), and omits December 19–26, 1665 (152 plague burials).

NOTE: The weekly Bill of Mortality in London was listed as being from Tuesday to Tuesday, but it covered the seven days from Tuesday to Monday, with the second Tuesday being a day of tallying the counts for the previous seven days.

To the official totals for the year must be added 156 burials at the Westminster pesthouse. These are tallied in the pesthouse column of the weekly bills and the General Bill of 1665 but are inexplicably omitted from the tally of total burials and plague burials in both the weekly bills and the General Bill. The General Bill's plague burial figures for each of the 97 parishes within the walls seem to include some incorrect numbers, since they add up to 77 more than the 9,887 given in this bill as the year's total of plague burials for these parishes, a sum derived by adding the 97 parishes' plague burial totals from the 52 weekly bills. Other arithmetic or printing errors in the General Bill are inconsequential.

Parish Records of Saint Margaret Westminster

Table B.1. Saint Margaret Westminster Churchwarden
Plague Accounts, Weeks of May 29–December 28, 1665

Week Beginning:	Warders	Nurses	Examiners	Widows	Pesthouse Patients
May 29	1	0	0	0	3
June 5	0	0	0	0	4
June 12	2	0	0	0	6
June 19	3	1	1	0	24
June 26	5	1	1	1	17
July 2	6	2	1	0	27
July 10	7	6	1	0	34
July 17	8	3	0	0	29
July 24	22	8	1	5	39
July 31	32	12	4	3	42
August 7	20	12	4	0	48
August 14	26	24	4	7	33
August 21	22	31	8	13	37
August 28	21	53	6	13	37
September 4	21	52	6	28	51
September 11	17	28	6	28	49
September 18	18	44	6	78	52
September 25	17	66	5	66	49
October 5	12	54	5	48	53
October 12	16	37	6	56	*
October 19	8	34	6	97	19

Table B.1. (continued)

Week Beginning:	Warders	Nurses	Examiners	Widows	Pesthouse Patients
October 26	8	21	6	55	19
November 2	5	20	6	52	*
November 9	5	12	4	37	11
November 16	5	15	6	45	13
November 23	5	11	6	46	9
November 27	2	7	6	32	7
December 7	1	5	6	32	7
December 14	1	4	6	32	4
December 21	1	3	6	32	4
December 28	1	2	6	20	4

SOURCE: Westminster City Library WL E47.

NOTE: For the week of September 18, there were 1,700 people receiving relief.

The weeks in this table, running from Monday to Sunday, follow the financial records of the parish's churchwardens, thereby differing from the Tuesday–Monday tabulation of the Greater London Bills of Mortality (listed as Tuesday–Tuesday).

*No record for these weeks.

APPENDIX C

Parish Records of Saint Giles Cripplegate

Table C.1. Saint Giles Cripplegate Parish Records:
Total Burials and Plague Burials in 1665

	No. of Burials			No. of Burials	
Week of:	Total	Plague	Week of:	Total	Plague
Jan. 1	25	0	Jun. 8	38	0
Jan. 8	25	0	Jun. 16	37	5
Jan. 16	32	0	Jun. 23	39	20
Jan. 23	23	0	Jul. 1	100	33
Feb. 1	18	0	Jul. 8	163	110
Feb. 8	36	0	Jul. 16	373	174
Feb. 16	38	0	Jul. 23	649	373
Feb. 23	32	0	Aug. 1	682	355
Mar. 1	35	0	Aug. 8	945	610
Mar. 8	34	0	Aug. 16	897	668
Mar. 16	20	0	Aug. 23	1,121	668
Mar. 23	45	0	Sep. 1	596	528
Apr. 1	31	0	Sep. 8	558	470
Apr. 8	25	0	Sep. 16	372	263
Apr. 16	21	0	Sep. 23	191	182
Apr. 23	19	0	Oct. 1	180	151
May 1	24	0	Oct. 8	123	100
May 8	21	0	Oct. 16	62	38
May 15	30	0	Oct. 23	48	23
May 23	27	0	Nov. 1	45	32
Jun. 1	29	4	Nov. 8	39	27

Table C.1. *(continued)*

Week of:	No. of Burials		Week of:	No. of Burials	
	Total	*Plague*		*Total*	*Plague*
Nov. 16	18	10	Dec. 8	19	8
Nov. 23	14	4	Dec. 16	14	4
Dec. 1	10	1	Dec. 23	13	1
			Total	7,936	5,604

SOURCE: Saint Giles Cripplegate Register, GL, MS 6419/7.

NOTE: The weeks tabulated here are composed of seven or eight days to accommodate months of twenty-eight, thirty, or thirty-one days. This is done to standardize four units of time each month, making comparisons of seasonal cycles more understandable. The parish register for the year listed burials daily beginning on January 1, a Sunday. This tabulation differs from the Greater London Bills of Mortality, which tabulated the week from Tuesday to Monday (listed as Tuesday–Tuesday).

Table C.2. Saint Giles Cripplegate Parish Records: Nonplague Burials in 1665 and the Previous Ten-Year Annual Average

Cause of Death	Jan.	Feb.	Mar.	Apr.	May	June	July	Aug.	Sept.	Oct.	Nov.	Dec.
Consumption												
1665	34	27	39	32	24	29	87	107	44	20	12	13
Annual average	24	21	26	24	21	14	17	19	22	19	22	21
Dropsy												
1665	10	15	15	14	6	8	20	40	10	12	6	4
Annual average	8	5	6	8	5	5	4	4	4	5	6	4
Enteric												
1665	16	15	8	8	11	30	120	163	19	17	5	4
Annual average	24	21	26	24	21	14	9	11	11	9	5	3
Contagious												
1665	7	11	11	25	20	32	182	498	91	12	11	4
Annual average	18	14	17	16	17	18	24	23	19	19	11	4

SOURCE: Saint Giles Cripplegate Register, GL, MS 6419/5–7.
See note to table A.1.

Table C.3. Saint Giles Cripplegate Parish Records: Occupations of Those Buried of the Plague in August 1665

	Number Buried	
Occupation	Subtotal	Total
Servant		289
Cloth worker		215
Weaver	90	
Cordwinder	52	
Glover	28	
Buttonmaker	18	
Tailor	17	
Pin and needleman	10	
Laborer		33
Porter		32
Foodhandler		25
Victualer	17	
Butcher	5	
Cook	3	
Building trades		24
Joiner	9	
Carpenter	6	
Bricklayer	4	
Nailer	2	
Plumber	2	
Plasterer	1	
Metalworker		21
Wiredrawer	11	
Twister	5	
Cooper	5	
Lawyer		15
Religious (churchwardens, sextons, priests, ministers)		11
Health worker		10
Barber	3	
Nurse	3	
Apothecary	2	
Burier	2	
All occupations		667

SOURCE: Saint Giles Cripplegate Register, GL, MS 6419/7.

APPENDIX D

The Three Plague Pandemics

Table D.1. Biovars of the Three Plague Pandemics Based on rRNA

	Biovar O *Antiqua* First Pandemic	Biovar O *Medievalis* Second Pandemic	Biovar B *Orientalis* Third Pandemic
Chemical Rx			
Ferment glycerol	+	+	−
Reduce nitrates	+	−	+
Where 70 specimens found	Kenya Belgian Congo	Kenya Kurdistan, Turkey	Asia, N. & S. America Madagascar

NOTES

Preface

1. Marilyn Chase, *The Barbary Plague: The Black Death in Victorian San Francisco* (New York, 2003).

2. *The Portable Voltaire*, ed. Ray Redmond (New York, 1949), 524–30, 560.

3. Two recent contributions are Laurie Garrett, *The Coming Plague: Newly Emerging Diseases in a World out of Balance* (New York, 1994), and Gina Kolata, *Flu: The Story of the Great Influenza Pandemic of 1918 and the Search for the Virus That Caused It* (New York, 1999).

4. A work of fiction drawn around the Great Plague's devastation of the remote Derbyshire village of Eyam has recently been published: Geraldine Brooks, *Year of Wonders: A Novel of the Plague* (London, 2001). The documentary film *The Great Plague* features poor residents of a London alley in 1665; it was produced for television by Juniper Communications, U.K., and edited by John Toba and Justin Hardy.

5. In summing up the structural side of responses to plague, Paul Slack notes hopefully: "It is only by looking more closely at the realities on the ground, at the reactions of the governed as well as of the governors, that we can fully appreciate the obstacles" to order and relief during a plague epidemic. Paul Slack, "Metropolitan Government in Crisis: The Response to Plague," in A. L. Beier and Roger Finlay, eds., *The Making of the Metropolis: London, 1500–1700* (London, 1986), 73. However, in his magisterial study of the subject, Slack is cautious about the prospect of such an inquiry: "How then did those who were infected and those who were left behind cope? The historical record only hints at the range of possible answers." Slack, *The Impact of Plague in Tudor and Stuart England* (Oxford, 1985; reprint with corrections, 1990), 20.

6. James S. Amelang, trans. and ed., *A Journal of the Plague Year: The Diary of the Barcelona Tanner Miguel Parets, 1651* (Oxford, 1991), 7, 111n. 21, calling on historians to shift their focus from "more objective themes and sources . . . to personal chronicles, autobiographies, and emotions of citizens of bygone times."

Prologue

1. Hodges' and Boghurst's medical accounts of the Great Plague of 1665 have been published: Nathaniel Hodges, *Loimologia: Or, an Historical Account of the Plague in London* (London, 1720); William Boghurst, *Loimographia: Or an Experimentall Relation of the Plague*, ed. Joseph Payne (London, 1894). Turner's account books and letters are at

the London Guildhall Library (hereafter GL), and his role in the city's government is recorded in the Court of Aldermen's Journal at the Corporation of London Record Office (hereafter CLRO). Patrick's correspondence, printed sermons, and short life history are in *The Works of Symon Patrick DD, including his Autobiography*, ed. Alexander Taylor, 9 vols. (London, 1858). The best guide to Pepys is his diary: Samuel Pepys, *Diary*, ed. R. C. Latham and W. Matthews, 11 vols. (London, 1970–83; reprint, 1995), esp. vol. 6 on the year 1665 and vol. 10, *Companion*, which contains scholarly entries on Pepys' personal, governmental, and financial doings. Claire Tomalin, *Samuel Pepys: The Unequalled Self* (London, 2002), brilliantly analyzes the complexities of Pepys' character.

2. On Pepys diary, see the introduction to Pepys, *Diary*. John Evelyn's voluminous correspondence, along with his wife's letters, now at the British Library (hereafter BL), are a better guide to his life during the Great Plague than is his well-known diary, cited by us in the edition by William Bray: John Evelyn, *Diary*, 2 vols. (London, 1952). We thank Frances Harris for her kind assistance in the use of the Evelyn papers and Joseph Levine for telling us of their acquisition by the library.

3. See Henry Roseveare, "Finances," in Pepys, *Diary*, 10:130–37, and Vincent Brome, *The Other Pepys* (London, 1992), using the index headings for Pepys' residences and employment.

4. The prime source for Josselin is *The Diary of Ralph Josselin, 1616–1683*, ed. Alan MacFarlane (London, 1976).

5. Gervase Jacques' correspondence with the countess of Huntingdon is in the Hastings papers at the Huntington Library (hereafter HL), San Marino, Calif.

6. John Allin's extensive correspondence with his country friends is in the Frewin Archive at the East Sussex Record Office (hereafter ESRO FRE). Extracts from some of his letters were published by William Durrant Cooper, *Notices of the Last Great Plague 1665–6 from the Letters of John Allin, formerly vicar of Rye, Sussex, to Philip Fryth and Samuel Jeake* (London, 1856), and drawn on by Walter George Bell, "John Allin's Letters," in *The Great Plague of London* (London, 1924; revised 1951; reprint, 1994), ch. 11. We thank Justin Champion for telling us where the original letters are kept and the archivists for photocopying all those relevant to the Great Plague.

7. The most comprehensive work on the history of plague is Jean-Noël Biraben, *Les hommes et la peste en France et dans les pays européens et méditeranéens*, vol. 1, *La peste dans l'histoire*; vol. 2, *Les hommes face à la peste* (Paris, 1975, 1976).

8. The term *pandemic* has also been used to describe a single epidemic that affects a wide geographic area.

9. We thank Dennis Twichett for information on the Chinese epidemics, whose sources note repeated episodes of great mortality without detailed description.

10. The most helpful version for general readers interested in the broader setting is the Norton Critical Edition: Daniel Defoe, *A Journal of the Plague Year: Authoritative Text, Backgrounds, Contexts, Criticisms*, ed. Paula R. Backscheider (New York, 1992).

11. On the Black Death's enormous literature, see Rosemary Horrox, trans. and ed., *The Black Death* (Manchester, 1994), an excellent, recent critical analysis with documents.

12. There are interesting comparisons of Venetian responses with those at Milan in William Naphy and Andrew Spicer, *The Black Death: A History of Plagues, 1345–1730* (Gloucestershire, 2000), 35–36.

13. Ann G. Carmichael, "Plague Legislation in the Italian Renaissance," *Bulletin of the History of Medicine* 57 (1983): 511.

14. Horrox, *The Black Death*, 234–35.

15. An excellent analysis of Italian evidence for plague, along with a discussion of other diseases like smallpox, influenza, and dysentery that may also have appeared in epidemic form, sometimes with plague, is Ann G. Carmichael, *Plague and the Poor in Renaissance Florence* (New York, 1986), esp. ch. 1, "Recurrent Epidemic Diseases: Plague and Other Plagues." For northern Europe, see Edward A. Eckert, "Plague and Other Pestilences," in *The Structure of Plagues and Pestilences in Early Modern Europe: Central Europe, 1560–1640* (Basel, 1996), ch. 6, and A. Lynn Martin, *Plague? Jesuit Accounts of Epidemic Disease in the Sixteenth Century* (Kirksville, Mo., 1996), 1–20.

16. Horrox, *The Black Death*, 13.

17. Samuel K. Cohn Jr., *The Black Death Transformed: Disease and Culture in Early Renaissance Europe* (London, 2002), and Cohn, "The Black Death: End of a Paradigm," *American Historical Review* 107 (2002): 715–35, emphasize alterations in the nature of plague during this pandemic. See epilogue, "Of Once and Future Plagues," this volume.

18. Rosemary Horrox poses the question "whether the regularity of subsequent outbreaks [after the Black Death] allowed familiarity to breed contempt, or whether (as most modern writers seem to assume) plague remained uniquely terrifying." She concludes: "In the cultural arena it is now more widely recognized that people under pressure are likely to articulate their anxieties in ways which are already familiar to them, and that cultural continuities spanning the plague cannot therefore be taken as evidence for the insignificance of those anxieties, or of the upheaval which triggered them." Horrox, *The Black Death*, 13, 236. Paul Slack, while contrasting the effects of plague in 1347 as a new disease with its later visitations, notes that these events were "important landmarks in the annals of local societies . . . Their effects were recorded in diaries and chronicles, and each successive 'great plague' or 'great pestilence' was used as a natural point of reference until its place was usurped by the next epidemic year." Slack, "Mortality Crises and Epidemic Disease in England, 1485–1610," in Charles Webster, ed., *Health, Medicine, and Mortality in the Sixteenth Century* (Cambridge, 1979), 9. For a contrary view that European culture became optimistic about living with plague, rather than traumatized by its repeated epidemics, see Cohn, "The Black Death," 705–10.

19. Vivian Nutton, "Medieval Western Europe, 1000–1500," in Lawrence I. Conrad, Michael Neve, Vivian Nutton, Roy Porter, and Andrew Wear, eds., *The Western Medical Tradition, 800 BC to AD 1800* (Cambridge, 1995), 191. A superb assessment of the demographic and economic effects in England is John Hatcher, *Plague, Population, and the English Economy, 1348–1530* (London, 1977), including his "Introduction to the Controversy," 11–20.

20. For the entire scope of the second pandemic, see Biraben, *Les hommes et la peste,*

306 · NOTES TO PAGES 9–13

supplemented on England by J. F. D. Shrewsbury, *A History of Bubonic Plague in the British Isles* (Cambridge, 1970), which tends to leap to diagnostic conclusions in distinguishing between plague and alternative diseases.

21. Amelang, *Journal of the Plague Year.*

22. Biraben, *Les hommes et la peste,* 1:186–87, 213–18, including table 3 on Barcelona.

23. Slack, *The Impact of Plague,* 150–51, 376nn. 20–21. See also Ian Sutherland, "When Was the Great Plague? Mortality in London, 1563 to 1665," in *Population and Social Change,* ed. D. V. Glass and Roger Revelle (London, 1972), 287–320.

24. "As about one fifth of the whole people died in the great Plague-years, so two other fifth parts fled." John Graunt, *Natural and Political Observations made upon the Bills of Mortality* (Oxford, 1665), 44.

25. There is a superb volume of relevant essays on early modern diseases by specialists in a variety of disciplines. We have used the French edition: *Histoire de la pensée médicale en Occident,* ed. Mirko D. Grmek, vol. 2, *De la Renaissance aux Lumières* (Paris, 1999). See esp. the essay by Henri Mollaret, "Les grands fléaux," 253–78. See also the excellent multinational collection of conference essays *Maladies et société (XIIe–XVIIIe siècles),* ed. Neithard Bulst and Robert Delort (Paris, 1989).

26. Carmichael, *Plague and the Poor,* 90–93, summarizes different findings by historians.

27. Henri Mollaret and his late colleague at the Pasteur Institute in Paris, Jacqueline Brossolet, pioneered the exploration of plague through the prism of art from the time of past epidemics. Their trailblazing work, *La peste: Source méconnue d'inspiration artistique,* was published as an offprint from *Annuaire du Musée royal des Beaux-Arts d'Anvers* (1965), 3–112. Brossolet's fascinating retrospective on this innovative venture and the ensuing battle with skeptics within the medical profession is in the preface of Christine M. Boeckl, *Images of Plague and Pestilence: Iconography and Iconology* (Kirksville, Mo., 2000), x–xiv.

28. Luke 16:19–31.

29. See Slack, *The Impact of Plague,* 299.

30. Giulia Calvi, *Histories of a Plague Year: The Social and the Imaginary in Baroque Florence,* trans. Dario Biocca and Bryant T. Ragan Jr. (Berkeley and Los Angeles, 1989), 195–96.

31. A rare exception was the ritual execution of a health official and a barber during Milan's 1630 epidemic. Confessing under torture of smearing plague poison around the city, the two men were executed, their bodies burned, the ashes thrown into the river, and the house where they had "plotted" replaced by a "column of infamy." This incident and a contemporary engraving were part of an exhibit at the Wellcome Institute for the History of Medicine in 1985. The Wellcome Library's guide, *The Pest Anatomized: Five Centuries of Plague in Western Europe,* is a superb introduction to the history of plague, including public health measures.

32. John Henderson, "Epidemics in Renaissance Florence: Medical Theory and Government Response," in Bulst and Delort, *Maladies et société,* 175–86. A useful guide to Italian plague facilities and measures is Brian Pullan, "Support and Redeem: Charity

and Poor Relief in Italian Cities from the Fourteenth to the Seventeenth Century," *Continuity and Change* 3 (1988): 177–208.

33. Biraben, *Les hommes et la peste*, 1:186.

34. *Journal d'Antoine Denesde, marchand ferron à Poitiers et de Marie Barré sa femme (1628–1687)*, ed. E. Bricauld de Verneuil (Poitiers, 1885), 226. We thank Nicole Pellegrin for sharing this account and others with us.

35. *The Pest Anatomized*, 13.

36. See Carlo M. Cipolla, *Miasmas and Disease: Public Health and the Environment in the Pre-industrial Age*, trans. Elizabeth Potter (New Haven, 1992).

37. The outstanding authority on this subject is Carlo Cipolla, whose relevant books include *Faith, Reason, and the Plague in Seventeenth-Century Tuscany*, trans. Muriel Kittel (New York, 1979).

38. Brian Pullan, "Support and Redeem," 184, 186.

39. Amelang, *Journal of the Plague Year*. Jeremy Boulton begins his remarkable microstudy of the early modern London neighborhood of St. Saviour Southwark by acknowledging the "little [that] is yet known of how the capital's inhabitants actually lived." Jeremy Boulton, *Neighborhood and Society: A London Suburb in the Seventeenth Century* (Cambridge, 1987), 5. Calvi, *Histories of a Plague Year*, uses criminal trials recorded by Florence's Public Health Magistracy to uncover some ways of coping by working people—notably illegal use of dead persons' clothes and other possessions and the transfer of the male members of a shopkeeper's family from the infected house to the shop, where they continued to make and sell their goods. But most adaptation techniques escaped the eyes and ears of the authorities.

40. Giovanni Boccaccio, *The Decameron* (written 1348–53), quoted in Defoe, *Journal of the Plague Year*, Norton ed., 235, 237.

41. On the literary tradition, see "Contexts," in Defoe, *Journal of the Plague Year*, Norton ed., 231–64. Among historians of the Great Plague, see Bell, *The Great Plague*, ix–x, 124–29, 247, 253. "The Great Plague of London," he concludes, "was a tragedy of errors. If only those fated people could have known." Stephen Porter, *The Great Plague* (Stroud, Gloucestershire, 1999), 133–45, continues the tradition with a focus on economic difficulties and weaknesses in the public safety net. Françoise Hildesheimer expresses a similar stark view of early modern plague epidemics in France: "The plague constituted an undermining of life, a crisis of the economy, a temporary undoing of the social order, a profound psychological trauma." Hildesheimer, *La terreur et la pitié: L'ancien régime à l'épreuve de la peste* (Paris, 1990), 154. Cf. Hildesheimer, *Fléaux et société: De la Grande Peste au choléra* (Paris, 1993). The twin themes of the unraveling of society and the abandonment of the poor by the authorities are prominent in the documentary film by Toba and Hardy, cited in our preface, n. 4.

42. Pullan, "Support and Redeem," 117.

43. Roger Finlay, *Population and Metropolis: The Demography of London, 1580–1650* (London, 1981), 17–18, 130. There is a brilliant analysis of an English community's postplague reconstitution by Roger Schofield, "An Anatomy of an Epidemic: Colyton, November 1645 to November 1646," in *The Plague Reconsidered: A New Look at Its Origins*

and Effects in Sixteenth and Seventeenth Century England (Matlock, Derbyshire, 1977), 115–21.

44. Daniel Defoe, *Journal of the Plague Year,* ed. Louis Landa (London, 1969), xvi. We thank George Rousseau for discussing the work of Landa with us.

45. Charles Mullett, *The Bubonic Plague and England* (Lexington, Ky., 1956), 215.

46. Josselin, *Diary,* 524.

Chapter 1. Winter, 1664–1665

1. Holborn Local History Library (London), St. Giles in the Fields Churchwardens' Accounts, 1640–1723: P/GF/C/1–2.

2. There is a helpful price list for items of food and clothes in Liza Picard, *Restoration London* (New York, 1997), 146–47.

3. Hodges, *Loimologia,* 5.

4. The weekly bills for 1665, from December 27, 1664, to December 19, 1665, were printed as *London's Dreadful Visitation: Or, A Collection of the Bills of Mortality for this present year* (London, 1665). We are using a facsimile reprint, ca. 1800, in our possession.

5. John Gadbury, *De Cometis: or a Discourse of the Natures and Effects of Comets* (London, 1665), 47.

6. Pepys, *Diary,* 5:348.

7. Gadbury, *De Cometis,* 47.

8. William Andrews, *News from the Stars or an Ephemeris for 1665* (London, 1665), 34. Curiously, very few of these "ephemerides" for 1665 have turned up at the British Library. There are several at the Bodleian Library in Oxford, some of them in the original manuscript versions by the authors. Editions for 1664 and 1666 are plentiful. For a typical astrological reading on 1665, see *The Prophecies and Predictions for London's Deliverance, with Conjunctions, Effects and Influences of the Superior Planets* (London, 1665).

9. Thomas Rugge, *"Mercurius Politicus Redivivus" or "Diurnal,"* BL, Addit. MSS 10,117, fols. 125, 130v.

10. Charles II personally leaned toward Catholicism, the religion of his mother, but he did not declare himself a Catholic until on his deathbed. His brother, the duke of York and future James II, was an avowed Catholic.

11. Thomas Salisbury to the earl of Huntingdon, Jan. 9, 1665, HL, Hastings Correspondence (HA), 10663.

12. Josselin, *Diary,* 516–17.

13. John Allin to Philip Fryth, Jan. 13 and Mar. 31, 1665, ESRO FRE 5429, 5444.

14. Pepys, *Diary,* 6:20, 32 (Feb. 6–7, 1665).

15. Early modern English carnivalesque celebrations have not been studied as deeply as have continental European Catholic practices. See Peter Burke, "The World of Carnival," in *Popular Culture in Early Modern Europe* (New York, 1978), 178–204, and Michael D. Bristol, "Carnival and Plebeian Culture," in *Carnival and Theater: Plebeian Culture and the Structure of Authority in Renaissance England* (New York, 1989), 40–53.

16. *Intelligencer,* Jan. 1, 1665.

17. We are using the modern reckoning of the beginning of the year at January 1. The

calendar year in Restoration England changed formally on Lady Day, March 25, despite the celebration of New Year's on the first of January, so 1665 began officially on the twenty-fifth of March. Ritual and other observances of the calendar are richly documented in David Cressy, *Bonfires and Bells: National Memory and the Protestant Calendar in Elizabethan and Stuart England* (Berkeley and Los Angeles, 1989).

18. On Pepys' status, see Pepys, *Diary*, 10:131, 295 (on "Finances" and "The Clerk of the Acts").

19. Translated as "everything I could wish with her."

20. Pepys, *Diary*, 6:1–2.

21. The average size of the ninety-seven parishes has been calculated as more than four acres, but this figure is misleading, since a few larger parishes along the wall and others that spiked northward from the Thames have to be averaged with dozens that were each only a fraction of an acre. See A. L. Beier, "Engine of Manufacture: The Trades of London," in Beier and Finlay, *The Making of the Metropolis*, 157.

22. On the trades and crafts of London, see ibid., 141–67.

23. The starting point for scholarly discussions of the early modern city is Gideon Sjoberg, *The Preindustrial City* (New York, 1960). Modifications of his model include Anthony Wrigley, "A Simple Model of London's Importance in Changing English Society, 1650–1750," *Past and Present* 37 (1967): 52–55, and M. J. Power, "The Social Topography of Restoration London," in Beier and Finlay, *The Making of the Metropolis*, 199–206.

24. A superb overview of London's social-economic contours is Charles Wilson, *England's Apprenticeship, 1603–1763* (Oxford, 1965), 45–52, 81–87.

25. The essays in Beier and Finlay, *The Making of the Metropolis*, analyze various aspects of London's growth in the sixteenth and seventeenth centuries. See also Paul Griffiths and Mark S. R. Jenner, eds., *Essays in the Cultural and Social History of Early Modern London* (Manchester, 2000); Lena Cowen Orlson, ed., *Material London, ca. 1600* (Philadelphia, 2000); and Craig Spence, *London in the 1690s: A Social Atlas* (London, 2000).

26. On population, see Vanessa Harding's survey of opinion, "The Population of London, 1500–1700," *London Journal* 15 (1990): 111–28; Roger Finlay, *Population and Metropolis: The Demography of London, 1580–1660* (Cambridge, 1981), 51–52; Peter Clark and Paul Slack, eds., *English Towns in Transition, 1500–1700* (London, 1976), 83.

27. We have adjusted the figures given for 1650 as 2.5% for Paris (Wrigley, "Simple Model of London's Importance," 45) and as 7.7% for London (Anthony Wrigley and Roger Schofield, *The Population History of England, 1541–1871* [London, 1981], 528–29).

28. This is an exceedingly complex subject. See Peter Clark and David Souden, ed., *Migration and Society in Early Modern England* (Towota, N.J., 1988), and M. J. Kitch, "Capital and Kingdom: Migration to Later Stuart London," in Beier and Finlay, *The Making of the Metropolis*, 224–51. On wages, see ibid., 171, table 16, comparing wage rates for building craftsmen and laborers in London and southern England, 1590s–1750.

29. Graunt, *Natural and Political Observations*, 131.

30. See Wrigley, "Simple Model of London's Importance," 49, and Jeremy Boulton, "Neighborhood Migration in Early Modern London," in Clark and Souden, *Migration and Society*, 108–10.

31. See J. A. Chartres, "Food Consumption and Internal Trade," in Beier and Finlay, *The Making of the Metropolis,* esp. 184–91.

32. Graunt, *Natural and Political Observations,* 3, 74.

33. Margaret Pelling, "Appearance and Reality: Barber-surgeons, the Body and Disease," in Beier and Finlay, *The Making of the Metropolis,* 86.

34. See J. R. Woodhead, *The Rulers of London, 1660–1689: A Biographical Record of the Aldermen and Common Councilmen of the City of London* (London, 1955), and Wilson, *England's Apprenticeship,* 49.

35. On Turner, see CLRO, Biographical Notes File, "Sir William Turner," and Alfred Baldwin, "A Short History of the Turner Family," typescript CLRO ref. P.D. 112.7.

36. GL, MS 5101/3, Sir William Turner Factory Book 1664/5.

37. See Pepys, *Diary,* 10:32–33, 16–17, 464 (on "Finances," "Backwell," and "Vyner").

38. Paraphrasing Wilson, *England's Apprenticeship,* 45.

39. On the Royal Exchange, see Harold Priestley, *London: The Years of Change* (London, 1966), 68.

40. On London Bridge, see ibid., 69, and John Hearsey, *London and the Great Fire* (London, 1965), 95.

41. There is no adequate study of Restoration London, but Norman Brett-James, *The Growth of Stuart London* (London, 1935), is worth consulting. The databases of Derek Keene's Center for Metropolitan History are invaluable for the Cheapside area. Cf. Keene, *Cheapside before the Great Fire* (London, 1985). It is estimated that one-third of the residents of the inner city lived along a street, one-third on the narrower lanes, and one-third in cul-de-sac yards or blind alleys. Power, "Social Topography of Restoration London," 209.

42. John Allin's correspondence, ESRO FRE 5429.

43. CLRO, Ex Guildhall Library MS 359, "Miscellaneous entries as to entertainments, military affairs, plague, fire of London . . . "

44. Pepys, *Diary,* 2:82–83.

45. For a good description and map, see ibid., 10:477–84.

46. There are brief descriptions of these places, under their separate names, in Pepys, *Diary,* 10:14, 122, 127–28, 400, 490–92.

47. Roy Porter, *London: A Social History* (London, 1995), 69.

48. Ibid., 70–71; Pepys, *Diary,* 10:235.

49. Pepys, *Diary,* 6:10. On Restoration theater and its audience, 10:337–42 ("Plays") and 431–45 ("Theatre").

50. Picard, *Restoration London,* 92–93.

Chapter 2. The Other London

1. For Patrick's early life and career, see "A Brief Account of My Life," in *Works,* 9:407, 410, 415–16, 426, 438–39. Cf. the entry "Simon Patrick" in the *Dictionary of National Biography,* ed. Sir Leslie Stephen, 21 vols. (London, 1885–90), 15:490–92.

2. These figures are from the hearth tax records for 1662, 1664, and 1666, as interpreted by M. J. Power, "The Social Topography of Restoration London," in Beier and

Finlay, *The Making of the Metropolis,* 208. On Restoration taxes, see C. D. Chandaman, *The English Public Revenue, 1660–1688* (Oxford, 1975).

3. Roger Finlay, *Population and Metropolis: The Demography of London, 1580–1650* (Cambridge, 1981), 76.

4. The classic study on the evolution of relief in medieval and early modern England is still useful, although its categories of help are weighted against religious motives and the financial figures ignore inflation. W. D. Jordan, *Philanthropy in England, 1480–1660* (London, 1959), esp. tables 1 and 2, 368–69.

5. On the Poor Law, including the Amendment Act of 1662, see the classic account by Sidney and Beatrice Webb, *English Local Government: English Poor Law History. Part 1: The Old Poor Law* (London, 1927); for the application of the Poor Law in the countryside, see F. G. Emmison, ed., "Introduction: The Overseers of the Poor," in *Catalogue of Essex Parish Records, 1260–1894* (Chelmsford, Essex, 1966), which was brought to our attention by Jane Bedford. A useful summary on poverty is Liza Picard, *Restoration London* (New York, 1997), 250–57.

6. For excellent studies of poor relief in London parishes, see Andrew Wear, "Caring for the Sick Poor in St. Bartholomew's Exchange: 1580–1676," in W. F. Bynum and Roy Porter, eds., *Living and Dying in London* (*Medical History,* suppl. 11) (London, 1991), 41–60, and two articles by Ronald W. Herlan: "Poor Relief in the London Parish of Antholin's Bridge Row, 1638–1664," *Guildhall Studies in London History* 2 (1997): 179–99, and "Aspects of Population History in the London Parish of St. Olave, Old Jewry, 1646–1667," *Guildhall Studies* 4 (1980): 133–40.

7. The St. Paul Covent Garden Overseers of the Poor records are in Westminster Record Office (WRO), H 446 (1664–66), H 448 (1666–67). The Harleian Society has published the *Register* in vol. 36, ed. Rev. William H. Hunt (London, 1908).

8. St. Paul Covent Garden Churchwardens' account, 1664–66, in WRO MS H 446, Overseers of the Poor, 1664–65.

9. *The Vestry of the United Parish of St. Margaret and St. John the Evangelist, Westminster* (London, 1889), 90–91.

10. Rugge, *Diurnal,* fols. 136, 138.

11. CLRO Common Council Journal (CC) 46, fols. 25–26.

12. Ibid., fols. 26, 59.

13. Ibid., fol. 25.

14. See Slack, *The Impact of Plague,* 154–57; Edwin Freshfield, *Some Remarks Upon the Book of Records of the Parish of St. Stephen, Coleman Street* (Westminster, 1887), xxxiv.

15. A good survey of public health in early modern England is in Slack, *The Impact of Plague,* 44–47, 199–226. For a new appraisal of the assumptions that hindered medical shaping of public policy on health in England, see Andrew Wear, *Knowledge and Practice in English Medicine* (Cambridge, 2000), esp. 16–18, 16n. 20, 314–20, 314n. 2. George Rosen, "Mercantilism, Absolutism, and the Health of the People (1500–1750)," in *A History of Public Health* (expanded ed., Baltimore, 1993), ch. 4, while dated, provides a broad European perspective on the subject.

16. On the St. Michels, see Pepys, *Diary,* 10:374–75.

17. Ibid., 76–77.

18. Brett-James, *Growth of Stuart London*, 116, 160–65.

19. Pepys, *Diary*, 6:93, 92.

20. John Allin, London, to Philip Fryth, Rye, Sussex, Apr. 27, 1665, ESRO FRE 5447.

21. Brett-James, *Growth of Stuart London*, 143–44; Pepys, *Diary*, 10:416–28, on "Taverns, Inns and Eating Houses."

22. On plague facilities at Milan and elsewhere, including a print of the Amsterdam pesthouse, see Porter, *The Great Plague*, 10–12.

23. John Evelyn, *Fumifugium, or the Inconveniences of the Aer and Smoak of London Dissipated* (London, 1661); Pepys, *Diary*, 10:122–24.

24. Bell, *The Great Plague*, 47; St. Andrew Holborn Vestry Minutes, 1624–1714, GL MS 4251/1, 83–84.

25. Caroline Gordon and Wilfrid Dewhirst, *The Ward of Cripplegate in the City of London* (London, 1985), 110, 114; Bell, *The Great Plague*, 9, 146.

26. Bell, *The Great Plague*, 250–52, provides an overview of the situation. For specific regulations, see CLRO CC 46 and CLRO Court of Aldermen Repertory (CA) 70.

27. On external quarantining, see Public Record Office (PRO), Privy Council Records (PC) 2/56, 592; 2/57, 23.

28. PRO State Papers (SP) 29/105.

29. St. Paul Covent Garden *Register*, 32.

30. On Charles II's interest in astrology, see Keith Thomas, *Religion and the Decline of Magic* (New York, 1971), 291, 312–13, 329.

31. PRO PC 2/58, 114.

32. Knowledge of the pre-1665 pesthouses is sketchy. There are scattered references in Slack, *The Impact of Plague*, and Bell, *The Great Plague*.

33. On the royal government's actions, see PRO PC 2/58, 114, 118.

34. Bell, *The Great Plague*, citing the Quaker George Whitehead's *Christian Progress*.

35. Boghurst, *Loimographia*, 26, 90; Thomas Cocke, *A Plain and Practical Discourse . . . for the Preservation of People in this Time of Sickness* (London, 1665), 10; Hodges, *Loimologia*, 2, 30.

36. Defoe, *Journal of the Plague Year*, Norton ed., 5, 9. Cf. Boghurst, *Loimographia*, xi.

37. See *An Historical Narrative of the Great Plague . . . and . . . other Remarkable Plagues* (London, 1769) and *History of the Plague in London in 1665 with Suitable Reflections* (London, 1795), 297–98. Peter Kennedy, *Discourse on Pestilence* (London, 1721), cites a Captain Floyd as having lived through the ordeal and attributing its beginning to sick Dutch prisoners of war and cotton from Holland. Cf. Thomas Hancock, *Research into the Law and Phenomena of the Pestilence . . . and Remarks on Quarantine* (London, 1821), 200.

38. Today's vicar of St. Giles in the Fields has written more specifically about the first half of this story, speculating that Flemish weavers contracted the plague from goods imported from Holland, which were opened "in a house in an alley off the west side of the upper end of Drury Lane." Gordon Taylor, *St. Giles in the Field: Its Part in History* (London, 1988). We thank Reverend Taylor for sharing this pamphlet and opening the parish archival records for our use.

39. CLRO CC 46, fol. 59; BL, Addit. MSS 4182 (newsletters), fol. 15; Bell, *The Great Plague,* 23.

40. CLRO CC 46, fol. 60.

Chapter 3. Signs and Sources

1. Boghurst, *Loimographia,* 19.

2. George Wither was typical. He wrote two dramatic representations of the Great Plague of 1625, *History of the Pestilence* (1625) and *Britains Remembrancer* (1628), and returned to the theme while in residence during the 1665 epidemic with *A Memorandum to London, Occasioned by the Pestilence there begun this present year* (London, 1665).

3. John Quarles, *The Citizens Flight* (London, 1665).

4. Pepys, *Diary,* 10:49.

5. Boghurst, *Loimographia,* 27.

6. The statistics come from *London's Dreadful Visitation.*

7. On fever as symptom, see Don G. Bates, "Thomas Willis and the Fevers Literature of the Seventeenth Century," in W. F. Bynum and V. Nutton, eds., *Theories of Fever from Antiquity to the Enlightenment* (*Medical History,* suppl. 1) (London, 1981), 45–70. On the identification of spotted fever during this time, we thank Andrew Wear.

8. The figures come from Ian Sutherland, "A Summary Tabulation of Annual Totals of Burials, Plague Deaths, and Christenings in London Prior to 1666," typescript (Medical Research Council Statistical Research and Service Unit, London, 1972, rev. 1986), 20–21.

9. On Garencières, see Wear, *Knowledge and Practice,* 295.

10. Historians of medicine disagree on the originality of early modern observations of plague. Nancy Siraisi suggests wholesale copying of earlier texts, as it was "more acceptable to stretch existing categories of disease to encompass plague (often assimilating it to various types of fever) than to allow for the existence of a disease not described in authoritative medical textbooks and not susceptible of rational explanation." Biraben argues for greater firsthand knowledge: "First of all, let us be very precise in saying that the specificity of the illness was recognized everywhere . . . From the fifteenth to the seventeenth century, when people spoke of plague, they knew what they were talking about and did not confuse it with any other complaint." Regrettably, he divides his description of plague into two, a modern clinical discussion and a culling of historical accounts spread over the long history of the disease, so it is difficult to see how specifically firsthand the analyses were for any single epidemic. Nancy Siraisi, *Medieval and Renaissance Medicine: An Introduction to Knowledge and Practice* (Chicago, 1990), 128; Biraben, *Les hommes et la peste,* 2:41.

For the Great Plague of London in 1665, there is little analysis of medical observations beyond the brief descriptive chapter, "The Plague of 1665 in Literature," in Mullett, *The Bubonic Plague and England,* 223–50. Bell, *The Great Plague,* 340, calls the medical literature "small." Slack, *The Impact of Plague,* 244, finds the number of plague tracts in 1665 impressive by comparison with earlier epidemics, with almost two-thirds of the forty-six treatises focusing on medical information as opposed to the religious focus in the others.

11. See Boghurst, *Loimographia*. Historical discussions of plague tract literature include Karl Sudhoff, "Pestschriften aus den ersten 150 jahren der Epidemie des 'Schwarzen Todes,'" *Archiv für Geschichte der Medizin*, 1911–25. On the tracts from the Black Death, see Anna Montgomery Campbell, *The Black Death and Men of Learning* (New York, 1931).

12. "The plague began first at the west end of the city, as at St Giles and St Martins Westminster. Afterwards it gradually insinuated, and crept down Holborne and the Strand, and then into the city and at last to the east end of the Suburbs." Boghurst, *Loimographia*, 26.

13. The term *sign* was also used in 1665 to denote portents and forerunners of plague. On the changing meaning of signs and symptoms over time, see Lester S. King, "Signs and Symptoms," in *Medical Thinking: A Historical Preface* (Princeton, 1982), ch. 3.

14. For premodern classifications of disease, see Vivian Nutton, "Medicine in the Greek World, 800–50 BC," in Conrad et al., *The Western Medical Tradition*, 26–28.

15. Boghurst, *Loimographia*, 31.

16. Ibid., 32.

17. Pepys, *Diary*, 6:165; Theophilus Garencières, *A Mite Cast into the Treasury of the Famous City of London; A Discourse on the Plague* (London, 1665), 1.

18. Gideon Harvey, *A Discourse of the Plague* (London, 1665). Sydenham's celebrated paper on plague was published in his *Observationes Medicae civea Morborum acutorum historiam et curationem* (London, 1676). There is a useful guide to Willis and Sydenham on fevers in L. J. Rather, "Pathology at Mid-century: A Reassessment of Thomas Willis and Thomas Sydenham," in *Medicine in Seventeenth-Century England*, ed. Allen G. Debus (Berkeley, 1974), 75–84.

19. Boghurst, *Loimographia*, 1.

20. *The Diary of Bulstrode Whitelocke*, ed. Ruth Spalding (Oxford, 1990), 687–90.

21. *London's Dreadful Visitation*.

22. [John Bell], *Londons Remembrancer. Or a true Account of every particular weeks christenings and mortality in all the years of pestilence within the cognizance of the Bills of mortality* (London, 1665).

23. Graunt, *Observations*, 19–20, 23–27.

24. Hodges, *Loimologia*, 139.

25. A historical epidemiologist has identified, during outbreaks of plague in early modern German communities, what he believes to be dysentery (which would appear as flux, stopping of the stomach, or griping of the guts in the London Bills of Mortality). However, the mortality peak for this malady of the summer season is not nearly as high as for plague, and its peak lasts much longer. In the German towns in this study, the peak of mortality lasted for up to eight weeks. By contrast, in the parishes of London with the best records for 1665, the epidemic's peak lasted for a single week at St. Margaret Westminster and two weeks at St. Giles Cripplegate. See Edward Eckert, *The Structure of Plagues and Pestilences in Early Modern Europe: Central Europe, 1560–1640* (Basel, 1996), 52–53.

26. In mid-seventeenth-century England, infant mortality claimed 150–200 per 1,000 live births. Conrad et al., *The Western Medical Tradition*, 215. Ann G. Carmichael, *Plague and the Poor in Renaissance Florence* (New York, 1986), discusses the mix of other diseases along with plague in Florence's plague epidemics. The question of whether plague and another illness struck the same individuals and how this affected mortality rates remains to be examined. The Bills of Mortality and other sources in 1665 list only one cause of death.

27. Josselin, *Diary*, 516–17, Mar. 12, Apr. 19, 1665; Boghurst, *Loimographia*, 29; Hodges, *Loimologia*, 14–15.

28. The various views of the causes of plague can be followed most easily in Wear, *Knowledge and Practice*, 281–313. The distinction between "religious" and "medical" views of plague in early modern England and France is made clear in the work of Paul Slack and Colin Jones, respectively. The sharpest drawing of the lines is found in Carlo Cipolla's little classic, *Faith, Reason, and the Plague in Seventeenth-Century Tuscany*, trans. Muriel Kittel (New York, 1979), where the magistrates are pitted against clerical hostility to public health measures that interfere with religious sensibilities. However, Cipolla shows some blurring of the lines by a few individuals. Vivian Nutton, by contrast, has demonstrated a remarkable agreement on medical understanding of plague across post-Reformation confessional lines. Nutton, "Religion and Medicine in Reformation Europe" (paper presented to the Rutgers, Princeton and Philadelphia Early Modern Historians, Princeton, N.J., Apr. 2000).

It is possible that there was more fluidity in Protestant-dominated English culture than in some continental Catholic cultures, but considerable flexibility in French Catholic circles, including borrowing from Protestant writers, has been detected by Alison Klairmont, "The Problem of the Plague: New Challenges to Healing in Sixteenth-Century France," *Proceedings of the Western Society for French History* 5 (1977): 119–27.

29. Patrick, *Works*, 3:669–72.

30. Hodges concludes, logically: "In this Contagion before us . . . it is sufficient for the purpose of the physician to assigne natural and obvious Causes; and where such is discoverable it is unworthy of him and the divine Art he possesses, as well as an Affront to good sense, to have recourse to any other." Hodges, *Loimologia*, 30–31.

31. John Gadbury, *Londons Deliverance Predicted, showing the Causes of Plagues . . . and when the present PEST may abate* (London, 1665), A6; Bernard Capp, *English Almanacs, 1500–1800: Astrology and the Popular Press* (Ithaca, N.Y., 1979), 36.

32. John Allin to Philip Fryth, Sept. 20, 1665, ESRO FRE 5468.

33. Lady Ranelagh's handwritten treatise is at the Royal Society Library (RSL), Boyle Papers 14, fols. 28–42. Robert Boyle's views on plague are revealed in correspondence with the secretary of the Royal Society, Henry Oldenburg. RSL Letter Book Supplement, 1663–93, 2:36–56. On the Boyle family, see Barbara Beigun Kaplan, *"Divulging Useful Truths in Physick": The Medical Agenda of Robert Boyle* (Baltimore, 1993), 9–16.

34. Much of Richard Kephale's *Medela Pestilentiae* (London, 1665) was lifted from a work by Stephen Bradwell, published in 1636. On Bradwell, see Slack, *The Impact of Plague*, 27–28.

35. Boghurst, *Loimographia*, 20–26; Symon Patrick to Elizabeth Gauden, Sept. 30, 1665, in Patrick, *Works*, 9:584.

36. The historical literature is enormous, but the evolution of these concepts can be followed in Leonard F. Hirst, *The Conquest of Plague: A Study of the Evolution of Epidemiology* (Oxford, England, 1953), chs. 2 and 3. Cipolla, *Miasmas and Disease*, brings the subject up to date for Italian medical culture. The Wellcome Trust symposium on "Contagion: Perspectives from Pre-modern Societies" in September 1994 included very informative discussions. We thank the presenters and discussants, esp. Vivian Nutton. On theories of early modern hygiene, see Heikki Mikkeli, *Hygiene in the Early Modern Medical Tradition* (Helsinki, 1999). Mary J. Dobson, *Contours of Death and Disease in Early Modern England* (Cambridge, 1997), is definitive on the role of the environment.

37. Girolamo Fracastoro, *De Contagione et Contagionis Morbis*, trans. Wilbur Cave Wright (Los Angeles, 1992), 151–57.

38. For the continuing intellectual ferment over plague on the medical frontier, see ch. 7 (this volume), "The Doctors Stumble."

39. The most searching and balanced analysis of Fracastoro's understanding of infectious disease and his influence on modern interpretations is Vivian Nutton, "The Reception of Fracastoro's Theory of Contagion," *Osiris*, 2d ser., 6 (1990): 196–234.

Chapter 4. Fleeing or Staying?

1. M. J. Power, "The Social Topography of Restoration London," in Beier and Finlay, *The Making of the Metropolis*, 211, table 26.

2. On the Davies family, see Esther S. Cope, *Handmaid of the Holy Spirit: Dame Eleanor Davies, "Never Soe Mad a Ladie"* (Ann Arbor, 1992). We thank Phyllis Mack for bringing this informative study to our attention.

3. The Hastings papers at the Huntington Library in San Marino, Calif., are an extraordinary family trove, to be supplemented by Cope, *Handmaid of the Holy Spirit*. We thank the curator of manuscripts, Mary Robertson, for assisting us.

4. Gervase Jacques to the countess and earl of Huntingdon, Apr. 25, 1665, HL HA 7649.

5. Beatrix Clarke to the countess of Huntingdon, Oct. 28, 1666, HL HA 1466.

6. Jacques to the countess and earl, May 9, 1665, HL HA 7650.

7. John Allin to Philip Fryth, May 26, 1665, ESRO FRE 5450; Josselin, *Diary*, 518–19.

8. See the metropolitan bill for May 9–16; St. Paul Covent Garden *Register*, 33; Patrick, *Works*, 9:442; and Bell, *The Great Plague*, 19–20.

9. In the east end, poor Whitechapel and St. Botolph Bishopsgate averaged only 2.4 and 2.6 hearths per residence. But in the west end's courtier area, St. Martin in the Fields had a moderately wealthy median of 5 hearths, and across the river John Allin's St. Olave Southwark was just below that figure at 4.3 hearths. North of the wall, the immense parish of St. Giles Cripplegate had only 3 hearths on average, while western suburbs of St. Dunstan in the West, St. Clement Danes, and St. Andrew Holborn had the highly respectable figures of 5.3, 5.9, and 6.3 hearths. These figures from M. J.

Power's data are compiled in J. A. I. Champion, *London's Dreaded Visitation: The Social Geography of the Great Plague in 1665* (London, 1995), 104–7, app. 1.

10. Gervase Jacques to the countess and earl of Huntingdon, June 1665, HL HA 7561. The letter mentions the naval battle of Lowestoft on June 3 and relates information scaling down early reports of an overwhelming victory over the Dutch.

11. Sir William Petty, "Of Lessening ye Plagues of London" (written in 1667). See *The Economic Writings of Sir William Petty*, ed. Charles Henry Hull, 2 vols. (Cambridge, 1899), 1:109n. 1.

12. Defoe, *Journal of the Plague Year*, Norton ed., 11–16. Defoe humanizes the formulaic arguments of the plague tracts of 1665, but the people's actual struggles have not been brought out in historians' accounts, partly because the documents are difficult to uncover.

Our discussion is framed in part by two quite different pieces of evidence. First, the emotional ups and downs before flight are mapped in medical astrologer William Lilly's copy of his almanac for 1665, which we discovered at the Bodleian Library. His marginal notes include mention of going from his London quarters to his country home in Surrey in March. In April: "Came to London" and "Woe to the Dut[ch]. Now we fight." Then, beside his almanac prediction ("The pestilence may now be feared in France"), he scribbles in: "Lord deliver England from fear yt a pestilential summer." Finally: "Reports of Loss to his Maj[est]y. Its hoped otherwise," and in June, an allusion to the English naval victory off Lowestoft: "Fight with the Dutch and they routed." We surmise that his flight, discussed in ch. 5, took place a short time later, when visits by plague patients to Lilly's rented quarters terrified his landlord. William Lilly, *Merlini Anglici Ephemeris, or Astrological Judgments for the year 1665* (London, 1665), Bodleian Library, Ashmole MS 264.

A second insight into flight is exemplified by a letter written in distant Westmoreland telling of a London friend's ambitious plans: "Mr Dugdale . . . was resolved to remove out of London (on account of the sicknesse) sometime ye last week, into Warwickshire; and from thence in August he intends for Yorkeshire." Thomas Smith to Daniel Fleming at Rydall from Cockermouth, June 28, 1665. Original letter, London Museum, Walter George Bell Great Plague Collection 1/122.

13. Defoe's simple view of Muslim reactions to plague echoes the opinions held in 1665. For the more complex and ever-debated reality of Muslim culture on disease and pestilence, see Michael W. Dols, *The Black Death in the Middle East* (Princeton, 1977), 109–21, under "Religious Interpretation." We also thank Lawrence Conrad for discussions on this fascinating topic.

14. Dr. Hall, bishop of Chester, *A Discourse of Fleeing or Staying in the Time of Pestilence. Whether Lawful for Ministers or People* (London, 1666).

15. Differences of opinion among religious denominations on who might flee, which were often distinct in the early Reformation, including between Lutherans and Calvinists, seem to have become considerably nuanced in England by the time of the Restoration. While individuals differed, it is hard to pin down the religious persuasion of the

pamphleteers of the Great Plague. Apart from sectarians, readers were probably most interested in the arguments per se (though reader opinion is virtually impossible to verify from the extant sources). The work of Ole Peter Grell on Protestant views on caring is relevant, e.g.: "The Protestant Imperative of Christian Care and Neighborly Love," in *Health Care and Poor Relief in Protestant Europe, 1500–1700*, ed. Ole Peter Grell and Andrew Cunningham (London, 1997), 43–65, and "Conflicting Duties: Plague and the Obligations of Early Modern Physicians towards Patients and Commonwealth in England and the Netherlands," in *Doctors and Ethics: The Earlier Historical Setting of Professional Ethics*, ed. Andrew Wear, Johanna Geyer-Kordesch, and Roger French (Amsterdam, 1993), 131–52. For a thorough discussion of religious, magisterial, and medical views in Catholic France, see Colin Jones, "Plague and Its Metaphors in Early Modern France," *Representations* 53 (1996): 97–127. We are grateful to the author for showing us his essay before it was published.

16. Tracts relating to London (e.g., *Londons Lord Have Mercy Upon Us. A True Relation of Seven Modern Plagues* [London, 1665]) are located by BL pressmark 816, m. 24–26.

17. *The Shepherd's Lash Lash'd Or a Confutation of the Fugitives Vindication* (London, 1665).

18. *The Life and Times of Anthony Wood, Antiquary, of Oxford, 1632–1695*, ed. Andrew Clark (Oxford, 1892), 2:39–40, 40n. 6, 43n. 3.

19. See Pepys, *Diary*, 10:192–97, "[Pepys] Household: Domestic Servants."

20. Josselin, *Diary*, 518–19.

21. Pepys, *Diary*, 6:116, 122–23, 123n. 1; Evelyn, *Diary*, 1:398–401.

22. PRO PC 2/57, 178; Pepys, *Diary*, 6:128.

23. Pepys, *Diary*, 6:130–31.

24. Ibid., 141–42.

25. Hodges, *Loimologia*, 12.

26. Graunt, *Observations*, 44.

27. Porter, *London*, 69.

28. Patrick, *Works*, 9:446.

29. Sir William Petty, *Verbum Sapienti* (published 1691, written 1665); Hull, *Writings of Sir William Petty*, 1:108.

30. Bridget Croft to Lady Mary Hastings, Mar. 27 [1664?], HL HA 1754.

31. Pepys, *Diary*, 10:452; Petty, "Of Lessening ye Plagues."

32. Benjamin Rush, *Thomas Sydenham, MD, on Acute and Chronic Diseases* (Philadelphia, 1809), 52; Wear, *Knowledge and Practice*, 334.

33. On Busby's character and action, see Bell, *The Great Plague*, 49, and James Anderson Winn, *John Dryden and His World* (New Haven, 1987), 36–42. The effect of the Great Plague on the upstream area is chronicled in an unpaginated manuscript by Charles Hailstone, "If on a Sudden: The Great Plague in Richmond and Neighborhood," Barnes and Mortlake Local Historical Society Library, Greater London. We greatly appreciate the kindness of Mr. Iain Radford of Barnes for bringing this much-overlooked work to our attention and making it available for our personal use.

34. All this information is from Hailstone, "If on a Sudden."

35. Richard Baxter, *Reliquiae Baxterianae* (London, 1696), 3:2.

36. Anne Stavely to the countess of Huntingdon, Aug. 7, 1665, HL HA 12673.

37. Sir James Langham to the countess of Huntingdon, Aug. 16, 1665, HL HA 8126.

38. On Dryden, see Bell, *The Great Plague,* 255, and Winn, *John Dryden and His World,* 158–59.

39. Don M. Wolfe, *Milton and His England* (Princeton, 1971), 108.

40. *Surrey Quarter Sessions Records: The Order Books and Session Rolls, Easter 1663–Epiphany 1666,* ed. Dorothy L. Powell and Hilary Jenkison (Surrey Record Society), 16:70.

41. Peter Barwick to William Sancroft, Aug. 5, 1665; John Tillison to Sancroft, Aug. 15, 1665; BL Harleian MS 3845, esp. fols. 25–26, 31.

42. John Moore, London, to Charles Moore at Little Appleby, Leicestershire, June 19, 1665, Wellcome Institute Library (WIL) MS 7382/3. We thank Richard Aspin for making this extraordinary document available to us on its acquisition in 1994 and Christopher Hilton for his kind assistance in deciphering the letter. The other John Moore papers, at the Guildhall Library of London, contain no other letters by him among the correspondence and financial accounts. On his death, Biographical Notes File on Sir John Moore, CLRO.

43. Patrick, *Works,* 9:442–43.

44. Pepys, *Diary,* 6:133–34, 149.

Chapter 5. The Medical Marketplace

1. A mountebank is literally someone on a mounted bench; colloquially, a seller of quack medicines from a platform, attracting a crowd with tricks and tales.

2. Roy Porter, *Quacks* (Charleston, S.C., 1989, 2001), 11. For Catholic European views on this subject, see Alison Klairmont Lingo, "Empirics and Charlatans in Early Modern France: The Genesis of the Classification of the 'Other' in Medical Practice," *Journal of Social History* 19 (1986): 583–603.

3. Wear, *Knowledge and Practice,* 37, 38, 23.

4. Porter, *Quacks,* 35; Wear, *Knowledge and Practice,* 210–13; Pepys, *Diary,* 4:59–60.

5. Wear, *Knowledge and Practice,* 23–24.

6. On the training of unlicensed health-care providers, see Margaret Pelling, "Knowledge Common and Acquired: The Education of Unlicensed Medical Practitioners in Early Modern London," in *The History of Medical Education in Britain,* ed. Vivian Nutton and Roy Porter (Amsterdam, 1995), 250–79. Quotation from Hodges, *Loimologia,* 21.

7. The breadth of Willis's medical perspective is reexamined by Wear, *Knowledge and Practice,* 469–72.

8. Thomas Cocke, *Kitchin Physick: Or, Advice to the Poor* (London, 1676), 18–19.

9. On Lady Mary Luckyn, daughter of the keeper of the seals, Sir Harbottle Grimston, see J. H. Round, "Some Essex Family Correspondence in the Seventeenth Cen-

tury," *Transactions of the Essex Archaeological Society*, n.s., 6 (1896–98): 207–21. Her plague recipe is described below, n. 20.

10. Today's doctors very likely have medicines with roots in the distant past. At Los Angeles County Hospital, there are boxes of live leeches for "fevers of unknown origin."

11. Cocke, *Kitchin Physick*, 33. In 1660, the nephew of a prominent London physician excused his late repayment of a loan by saying: "I have transgressed in not doeing it sooner, but desire your pardon. It hath pleased God to visit me with sickness." The nephew and uncle assumed that God's presence had played a role in the illness and in the young city man's return to health and prosperity. Edmund Thomas to Francis Glisson, Feb. 27, 1660, BL, Sloane MS 2251, fol. 88. On the connections between religion and medicine, see Peter Elmer, "Medicine, Religion, and the Puritan Revolution," in Roger French and Andrew Wear, eds., *The Medical Revolution of the Seventeenth Century* (Cambridge, 1989), 10–45, and above, ch. 3, n. 28.

12. Josselin, *Diary*, 519, entry for July 2. Josselin's medical views are summarized in Lucinda McCray Beier, *Sufferers and Healers: The Experience of Illness in Seventeenth-Century England* (London, 1987).

13. Symon Patrick to Elizabeth Gauden at Burntwood [Brentwood], Essex, Aug. 9, 1665, in Patrick, *Works*, 9:571–73; *A Consolatory Discourse Persuading to a Cheerful trust in God in these times of Trouble and Danger* and "Brief Account of My Life," in ibid., 3:671, 9:443.

14. S. Patrick to E. Gauden, Sept. 22, 28, 30, in ibid., 9:576–78, 582–85.

15. See Dr. Edmund King, "Medical receipts and cases, 1664–1686," BL, Sloane MS 1588, esp. fols. 99, 275, 285, including notes against the plague and against the pestilence and prevention against the contagion.

16. William Kemp, *A Brief Treatise of the Pestilence* (London, 1665), quoted in *The Pest Anatomized*, 6.

17. London College of Physicians, *Certain Necessary Directions for the Prevention and Cure of the Plague* (London, 1665), 49. See Lester S. King, "Reflections on Blood-Letting," in *Medical Thinking: A Historical Preface* (Princeton, 1982), ch. 11. Reducing the blood volume can temporarily relieve a variety of conditions, ranging from the strain on the heart in lobar pneumonia to high blood pressure accompanied by a severe headache.

18. An excellent overview of drugs for plague is "Remedies," in Wear, *Knowledge and Practice*, ch. 2. On the history of theriac as adapted for plague, see *The Pest Anatomized*, 8–9.

19. See the *Newes*, June 3, July 5.

20. "A Booke of Divers Receipts," WIL Western MS 1322, fol. 30. Cf. the comment by Lady Luckyn on her family's plague recipe, which she deemed good also against "the swetting sicknes, surffits, mesels and small poxe. Kepe this above all medsons and use as follows: If you think your self infected, each morning and evening take a large sponfull at a time luke warm. If not infected, each morning take one sponfull of itt. Nex[t] under God, trust to this remedy, if the hart be not clere mortyfid[e] and drowned with ye poison so long before the drink." Her recipe reads: "Take 3 pints of the best Malmsey ore Sake [wine], Boyle therin one handful of Rue, as much Sage till one pint is boyled away.

Then strayn it and ad to that liquer long pepper ginger nuttmege of each thre[e] drames bruised. Boyle itt a while, yn [then] take it of[f] ye ffyer and dissolve in itt 1 ounce of Mitridate and 2 ounces of yr best Treacel and a quarter of a pint of Angelica Watter or strong Aqua Vita." ERO MS D/DRg 1/141.

21. Pepys, *Diary*, 6:161, 163, 108, 120; Bell, *The Great Plague*, 47, 155–56.

22. A modern psychoanalyst has offered a clue to this tightrope-balancing act, describing Pepys' behavior as a fear-of-death syndrome. Martin Howard Stein, "[Pepys'] Health—A Psychoanalyst's View," in Pepys, *Diary*, 10:177.

23. Pepys, *Diary*, 6:154–55.

24. Peter Laslett, *The World We Have Lost—Further Explored* (London, 1983), 232–33, suggests that 60% of women and 40% of men could not write a century after the Great Plague. Unlike writing, reading left no records, but it is assumed that reading on its own was more widely practiced than the combination of reading and writing. See Wear, *Knowledge and Practice*, 40n. 74.

25. See Thomas Cocke, *Advice for the Poor by Way of Cure and Caution* (London, 1665), 1, 5.

26. [William Winstanley], *Poor Robin. The Yea and Nay Almanack* for 1666 but dated June 11, 1665.

27. Biographical details for William Lilly are in Capp, *English Almanacs*, esp. 57–59.

28. See above, ch. 4, n. 12.

29. *The Lives of those Eminent Antiquaries Elias Ashmole, Esquire, and Mr William Lilly, written by themselves* (London, 1774), 139–40; Slack, *The Impact of Plague*, 34.

30. On Lilly's clientele, see Thomas, *Religion and the Decline of Magic*, 319. The section on "Medicine and Magic" in Capp, *English Almanacs*, 204–14, is less suggestive than Thomas's reflections. The entire area of early modern medical astrology deserves a fresh reading; the English almanacs are plentiful, though there are lamentably very few for 1665, mainly in their original manuscript form, with L'Estrange's censorship alterations added. See Bodleian Library, Oxford, Ashmole MSS 158, 180, 264, 347.

31. Robert Neve, *A New Almanack* (London, 1666), is a good example: "Spring is the most temperate time of the year. Therefore the humours are fit to be emptied, whether by bloodletting, purging, or otherwise, as the learned physitian shall advise." In July: "Use cold herbs and meats, abstain from physick [purging], let the sun be set before you walk about in the time of any pestilence or plague, keep your windows shut." After surviving the pestilential summer, you were advised to "finish your physick" in November and ease off other treatment until March, "unless out of necessity." This was written while the Great Plague was still around London and the countryside, and the reference to the infection may have been added to the normal regime. We have been unable to find Neve's almanac for 1665.

32. Andrew Wear, "Early Modern Europe, 1500–1700," in Conrad et al., *The Western Medical Tradition*, 243; Thomas, *Religion and the Decline of Magic*, 668.

33. Alan Macfarlane, *Witchcraft in Tudor and Stuart England* (London, 1970), 117–18, 179, 184.

34. See George Thomson, *Loimotomia, or the Pest Anatomized* (London, 1666), 166–70.

35. John Allin to Philip Fryth at Rye, Aug. 24, Sept. 14, 1665, ESRO FRE 5462, 5466. Cf. Bell, *The Great Plague*, 159–60, which dismisses Allin as delusional and wrong-headed in his quest.

36. The great popularizer of academic herbal recipes during the Puritan era, Nicholas Culpeper, had tried his hand with this potable gold. And Lilly's mentor in astrology had offered patients a month's free supply of the magical liquid—bringing down on his head the wrath of the archbishop of Canterbury and the College of Physicians for this affront to true religion and medicine. See Capp, *English Almanacs*, 204–8.

37. *Newes*, July 13; *Intelligencer*, Nov. 7.

38. Allin to Fryth, Aug. 24, ESRO FRE 5462.

39. The herbalist was Nicholas Culpeper (1616–54). His *Complete Herbal*, Wordsworth Reference ed. (Ware, Hertfordshire, 1995) is still in print in paperback editions, touting his remedies "for all ills known to Seventeenth century society."

40. See *The Pest Anatomized*, 8–10.

41. Bell, *The Great Plague*, 156.

42. Thomas Cocke, *Hygiene, or a Plain and Practical Discourse upon the First of the Six Non-Naturals, viz: Air* (London, 1665), 14; John Allin to Fryth, Aug. 1665, ESRO FRE 5462.

Chapter 6. Plague's Progress

1. Pepys, *Diary*, 6:160, July 16; Josselin, *Diary*, 519, July 9, 28, Aug. 6.

2. Perhaps the best study of normal urban dynamics in London is Beier and Finlay, *The Making of the Metropolis*.

3. A. L. Beier, "Engine of Manufacture: The Trades of London," in ibid., 145, 147.

4. We thank John Burkhalter for information on the king's musicians traveling with the king during the Great Plague. Pepys, *Diary*, 6:154, July 10.

5. See Richard Deering's *Fancy of London Cries*, BL, Addit. MSS 29372–7.

6. CLRO, CA 70: fol. 136v; CLRO, CC 46: fol. 60r.

7. BL, Addit. MSS 4182, fol. 21v, June 23 newsletter.

8. The city regulations can be traced in CLRO CA 70; BL, Guildhall Proclamations 21.h.5; and London Museum's Walter George Bell broadside collection. On Bartholomew's fair, see Bell, *The Great Plague*, 195.

9. Sir William Turner to Pocquelin of Paris, June 29, GL MS 5106/1.

10. The fullest records are from St. Bride's parish at the London Guildhall Library.

11. *London's Dreadful Visitation*.

12. See St. Margaret Poor Law Assessments and Payments, Westminster City Library (WL), E47; Slack, *The Impact of Plague*, 278; Champion, *London's Dreaded Visitation*, 106.

13. The long-lost thick black volume was recovered after surviving bombs and fire-hose watering in World War II.

14. "The Account of Richard Arnold and Nicholas Upham Churchwardens of ye Parish of St. Margaret Westminster of all their Receipts and Disbursements in Relation to ye Poore Visited of ye Plague within the sayd Parish in the Years 1665 and 1666" (WL E47).

15. The register has been printed for 1665 and 1666. See *The Registers of St. Margaret's Westminster,* London Harleian Society, vols. 88 and 89 (London, 1977).

16. WL E47.

17. Bell, *The Great Plague,* 44.

18. "Benevolence upon the Buryall of the several Persons next following towards the reliefe of the poor visited of ye Plague within this parish" (WL E47).

19. For a very different view of poor relief during the Great Plague, see Bell, *The Great Plague,* 112, where he sums up his negative assessment: "There was a Poor Law well adapted to damping down the claims of the helpless . . . No charge of inhumanity lies against the ruling class at the Restoration. They acted according to the light at that time. The parsimony of the parochial authorities almost defied belief . . . It was perhaps just possible to maintain life on [the plaguetime] dole."

20. Stephen Bing, London, to William Sancroft at the Rose and Crown, Tunbridge Wells, Kent, July 24, 1665, BL, Harleian MS 3785, fol. 19.

21. St. Olave Hart Street *Register,* Harleian Society, vol. 36.

22. Pepys, *Diary,* 6:163–64, July 18–22.

23. Ibid., 165, July 22.

24. Ibid., 6:157, 175, 10:409.

25. See above, ch. 5, n. 22, for Martin Howard Stein's "fear-of-death" psychoanalytical explanation of Pepys' dalliances. Somewhat similarly, Claire Tomalin's brief account of Pepys' life during the Great Plague concludes, "The parallel [to Pepys' overall behavior] is obvious with men and women at war or bombardment who have found themselves living on an adrenalin high that gives extra intensity to every experience." While noting Pepys' fears, Tomalin tends to downplay his attention to the havoc caused by the epidemic: "The year was so packed with events that the plague was largely relegated to the background in [his] *Diary* as Pepys pursued his activities with triumphant energy." Tomalin, *Samuel Pepys,* 168.

26. Pepys, *Diary,* 6:156, 162.

27. Ibid., 157, 171, 173, 175.

28. Ibid., 177.

29. Ibid., 174, 176.

30. Samuel Herne, London, to Samuel Blithe at Clare College, Cambridge, July 18, 1665, in J. R. Wardale, ed., *Clare College Letters and Documents* (Cambridge, 1903), as quoted by Bell, *The Great Plague,* 80–81. The spread of the plague in Hertfordshire was very uneven, but the toll was enormous in places like Ware on the main roads. Hertfordshire Record Office, parish registers.

31. *London's Dreadful Visitation.*

32. Patrick, *Works,* 9:571.

33. Evelyn, *Diary,* 1:403; Pepys, *Diary,* 6:179; George Boddington Family Commonplace Book, GL, MS 10823/1, 35, 39–40; GL, St. Margaret Lothbury parish records.

34. Thomas Vincent, *God's Terrible Voice in the City* (London, 1667), 31–32. The parts of this tract on the Great Plague blend his sermons with later reflections.

35. St. Olave Hart Street *Register;* Pepys, *Diary,* 6:189, 206–7, Aug. 12, 30.

36. Pepys, *Diary*, 6:187, Aug. 11–12; 200, Aug. 20.

37. Ibid., 200–201.

38. Ibid., 204, 207–8, Aug. 26, 30, 31.

39. Sir William Turner, London, to Pocquelin père et fils at Paris, Aug. 8, GL, MS 5106/1.

40. BL, Addit. MS 4182, fol. 29r.

41. One explanation for the name *cripple gate* is that it is where disabled travelers, hoping for cures, left relics, icons, and statues. More likely, the name comes from the Anglo-Saxon word *crepel*, a covered way, as seen in the cantilevered placements of horizontal boards forming the gate. There are two historical guides to Cripplegate: John James Baddeley, *An Account of the Church and Parish of St. Giles Cripplegate* (London, 1880), and Caroline Gordon and Wilfred Dewhirst, *The Ward of Cripplegate in the City of London* (Oxford, 1985).

42. Hertfordshire Record Office, Bridgewater correspondence, AH 109 and 1100. On Bridgewater's life, see the *Dictionary of National Biography* entry for John Egerton, second earl of Bridgewater (1622–86).

43. St. Giles Cripplegate Parish Register, GL, MS 6419/7. Cf. Bell, *The Great Plague*, 144–52.

44. George Boddington Family Commonplace Book, GL, MS 10,823/1, 40. For a statistical breakdown by occupation of fatalities at Cripplegate, see ch. 8 and app. C, this volume.

45. St. Giles Cripplegate Vestry Minutes, May 23, 1665, GL, 6048/1, fol. 18v.

46. Samuel Foster to Dean Sancroft, Redgrave Hall, Cambridge, Jan. 22, 1666, BL, Harleian MS 3785, fol. 81.

47. Bell, *The Great Plague*, 149.

48. Baddeley, *St. Giles Cripplegate*, 22; *The Obituary of Richard Smyth . . . being a catalogue of all such persons as he knew, 1627–1674*, ed. Henry Ellis (London, 1849), 63–65.

49. St. Giles Cripplegate Parish Register, GL, MS 6419/7.

50. St. Paul Covent Garden *Register*, 34.

Chapter 7. The Doctors Stumble

1. We thank Graham Twigg for these figures.

2. Hodges, *Loimologia*, 14.

3. Wear, *Knowledge and Practice*, 309, offers a revisionist view of Hodges as a forward-looking "modern Galenist."

4. On the pamphlet war between the Galenist and chemical physicians, see Henry Thomas, "The Society of Chymical Physicians: An Echo of the Great Plague of London, 1665," in *Science, Medicine, and History*, ed. Edgar Ashworth Underwood (New York, 1953), 2:56–64, and Harold J. Cook, *The Decline of the Old Medical Regime in Stuart London* (Ithaca, N.Y., 1986), 150, 159–60.

5. Cf. Andrew Wear's observation for the entire early modern period in England: "Medical practitioners faced a supreme test of their art, their knowledge, procedures and remedies; plague posed the ultimate challenge." Wear's study is the most probing

work we have seen on the intellectual milieu of medicine throughout the early modern world and on plague. His analysis features a crucial issue neglected in historical literature: "whether it was thought possible that plague could be treated." His answer, a "qualified yes," can be compared with our view of the doctors "stumbling" but striving. Wear, *Knowledge and Practice*, 275, 277.

6. Dekker had kinder words for the doctors' performance in the epidemics of 1625 and 1630, at least by comparison with empirics, whom he rated outright quacks. "Is sickness [plague] come to thy doore?" he asked. "A Physitian is Gods second, and in a duell or single fight (of this nature) will stand bravely to thee." Thomas Dekker, *London Looke back at that Yeare of Yeares 1625, and Looke Forward upon this Yeare 1630* (London, 1630); quotation in Wear, *Knowledge and Practice*, 33.

7. Hodges, *Loimologia*, 227.

8. Peter Barwick, London, to William Sancroft at the Rose and Crown, Tunbridge Wells, Aug. 5, 9, 1665, BL, Harleian MS 3785, fols. 23, 25.

9. *Intelligencer*, July 31, 1665.

10. Boghurst, *Loimographia*, 30.

11. In addition to older estimates, the reader can read with profit what Andrew Wear says about medical professionals fleeing and staying in 1665. Wear, *Knowledge and Practice*, 337–38. T. D. Whittet, *The Apothecaries in the Great Plague of London in 1665* (London, 1965), 29, estimated that about two hundred apothecaries were present at the peak of the epidemic, half of them being mentioned "on numerous occasions." His count may be high, since some are mentioned in June and are heard of no more during the epidemic, suggesting that they fled.

12. John Allin to Philip Fryth, Sept. 14, 1665, ESRO FRE 6566; Pepys, *Diary*, 6:268, Oct. 16, 1665.

13. Royal College of Physicians, MS 2298, *Annals* 4:131; *Certain Necessary Directions*, item 1; CLRO, CA, *Repertory*, 70, fols. 144–45; Ex GH, MS 270, fol. 58.

14. See CLRO CA Repertory 7, fol. 147.

15. CLRO, Ex GH, MS 270, fol. 58.

16. Ibid.

17. Bell, *The Great Plague*, 88; *Resolution of those Physicians presented by the College to the ... Mayor and Court of Aldermen ... for the Prevention and Cure of the Plague, 2 August* (London, 1665), quoted by Cook, *Decline of the Old Medical Regime*, 157.

18. Boghurst, *Loimographia*, 60, quoted by Wear, *Knowledge and Practice*, 338.

19. On the above appointments, see CLRO CA Repertory 70, fol. 152; CLRO, Ex GH, MS 270, fol. 58; and the records of St. Margaret Westminster parish.

20. See Wear, *Knowledge and Practice*, 337, and Bell, *The Great Plague*, using the index listing of "Physicians who stayed in London."

21. Slack, *The Impact of Plague*, 246.

22. Boghurst, *Loimographia*, 4.

23. Despite Charles II's suspension of the London doctors' "watch and ward" obligations, most of them failed to take the hint to use their free time for plague service. College of Physicians, MS 2298, *Annals*, 4:132, dated June 28, 1665.

24. Whittet, *Apothecaries in the Great Plague*, 18–19.

25. See Sir Edward Charles Dodds, "A Physician in the Plague Year: Thomas Wharton (and Some of His Contemporaries)" (1965), RCP MS 3118, 16–19; William Johnson, *Agurto-Mastix, or Some Brief Animadversions Upon Two Late Treatises* (licensed, May 10, 1665), 12, 129–33.

26. Nathaniel Hodges, *Vindiciae Medicinae et Medicorum: Or an Apology for the Profession and Professors of Physick* (London, 1666), 54–55.

27. RCP MS 2073, 11; Whittet, *Apothecaries in the Great Plague*, 6, 11.

28. Hodges, *Vindiciae Medicinae*, 4–6, 47; Cook, *Decline of the Old Medical Regime*, 152.

29. George Thomson, *Galeno-pale: or a Chymical Trial of the Galenists, that their Dross in Physick may be discovered*, printed by R. Wood for Edward Thomas, at the Adam and Eve in Little Brittain (London, 1665), 3–8, 99–101, 103; Thomson, "Apology against the Calumnies of the Galenists" and "A work to Mr. Nath Hodges, concerning his late Vindiciae Medicinae," in *Loimotomia*, 172–89. Cf. Cook, *Decline of the Old Medical Regime*, 159–60.

30. Johannes Nohl, *The Black Death: A Chronicle of the Plague* (New York, 1924), 75.

31. Thomson's language on the archeus is striking to us moderns. "The Archeus which is an instrument of sanity is likewise the Author of Maladies," he wrote. When it recognized a poisonous seed and let it pass, the battle within the body began. "The vital spirit . . . cowardly running from the poison [betrays] that trust that was reposed in it . . . The archeus becomes a vassal to perpetuate those things that tend to Ruin and Destruction." Thomson, *Loimotomia*, 33–35, 40–41.

32. On Helmontian medicine, see Wear, *Knowledge and Practice*, chs. 8 and 9. For the Paracelsian-Helmontian idea of the archeus, see also Walter Pagel, "From Paracelsus to van Helmont," in *Studies in Renaissance Medicine and Science* (London, 1986), 421, 429, 453–54.

33. Thomson, *Loimotomia*, 83–84, 100–104.

34. John Tillison to William Sancroft, Sept. 14, 1665, BL, Harleian MS 3785, fol. 36.

35. Allin to Fryth in Rye, Sussex, Sept. 14, 1665, ESRO FRE 5466.

36. Thomson, "An Historical Account of the Dissection of a Pestilential Body," in *Loimotomia*, pt. 5, 113–14.

37. Thomson saw his dissection as the climax of a twenty-year quest to understand "malignant" diseases, "giving medicines of my own preparation and observing from one [patient] what might be useful to another," yet being restless in the search for "therapeutic truth . . . until I had the full view of the inward parts of a pestilential body. This [conformed to] some of my judgment." Thomson, preface to *Loimotomia*.

38. Francis Bacon, *The Advancement of Learning* (1605).

39. A good introduction to the broader intellectual-scientific currents is Charles Webster, *The Great Instauration: Science, Medicine, and Reform, 1626–1660* (New York, 1975). Wear superbly places these currents in their medical context. See "Conflict and Revolution in Medicine—the Helmontians," in *Knowledge and Practice*, ch. 8, 353–98.

40. Wear, *Knowledge and Practice*, 325n. 35.

41. Sydenham denied the relevance of the microscope, was unenthusiastic about Harvey's theory of the circulation of blood, and refused to consider the practice of dissecting, not seeing its applicability to the cause or treatment of disease. His observations, he proudly said, stopped at the "outer husk of things." See Kaplan, *"Divulging Useful Truths in Physick,"* 146–49, and Rather, "Pathology at Mid-century," 73–75.

42. Pepys, *Diary,* 6:95. Traditional surveys of the history of medicine pay scant attention to the effect of the virtuosi on medicine. A good corrective is Wear, "Early Modern Europe," in Conrad et al., *The Western Medical Tradition,* 340–59. One of the best introductions, focusing on Boyle, is Kaplan, *"Divulging Useful Truths in Physick."*

43. Wear, *Knowledge and Practice,* 442–43.

44. Robert Boyle to Henry Oldenburg, Sept. 30, 1665, RSL, Letter Book Supplement, 2:37–38.

45. Boghurst, *Loimographia,* 98.

46. See Kaplan, *"Divulging of Useful Truths in Physick,"* 1–4, 128–30; Wear, "Early Modern Europe," 341–42; and Lester S. King, "Robert Boyle as an Amateur Physician," in *Medical Investigation in Seventeenth Century England,* William Andrews Clark Library Papers (Los Angeles, 1968), 23–41.

47. D. Coxe to Robert Boyle, Mar. 5, 1665/6, RSL, Letter Book Supplement, 2:64–65; Kaplan, *"Divulging Useful Truths in Physick,"* 129–30.

48. Boyle to Oldenburg, Aug. 27, 1665, RSL, Letter Book Supplement, 2:29–31. However, Boyle was very cautious about plague antidotes whose advocates failed to spell out "which way the medicine works." And he was scathing in his denunciation of conventional Galenic therapies in times of plague, "there being several Examples of those who in infectious times have fallen into pestilential Fevers upon their having purged or bled to prevent them . . . having excited and by degrees brought inwards those latent seeds of contagion, which Nature might else have by degrees discharged by Transpiration." Boyle to Oldenburg, Sept. 30, 1665, RSL, Letter Book Supplement, 2:36–37.

49. Before 1665 Willis had published innovative treatises on fermentation and fevers, muscular motion, and transmission by nerves. He is credited as the first to recognize scarlet fever, and he detected sweetness in a patient's urine, connecting it to diabetes. In 1664, his crowning achievement came with *Anatomy of the Brain,* describing the vascular system at the base of the brain. Anatomical textbooks still refer to the "circle of Willis" circuit.

50. See Thomas Willis, *A Plain and Easie Method for preserving those that are well from the infection of the Plague* (written in 1666; London, 1691), and Rather, "Pathology at Mid-century." Wear, *Knowledge and Practice,* 342–43, offers a balanced evaluation of Willis's mix of innovation and traditionalism.

51. *The City Remembrancer: Being Historical Narratives of the Great Plague at London* (London, 1769), 130–31.

52. Marchamont Nedham, *Medella Medicinae. A Plea for the free Profession, and a Renovation of the Art of Physic Tending to the Rescue of Mankind from the Tyranny of Diseases* (London, 1665), 193–94; Cook, *Decline of the Old Medical Regime,* 200.

53. Wear, "Early Modern Europe," 352.

54. "But for the shape and figure of these Atomes or small bodyes which . . . alter and change the motion of these corpuscles or particles which compose the spirits and blood, wee can say nothing to satisfaction . . . The seedes of the Pestilence are soe hidden and removed from sense that wee can see them better in their effects than we can in themselves." Boghurst, *Loimographia,* 10.

55. Hodges, *Loimologia,* 14–15, 17.

56. The reexamination of plague reached the households of great persons, including the literary and scientific writer Margaret Cavendish, duchess of Newcastle. In 1665 she was hard at work on her forthcoming *Observations upon Experimental Philosophy* and *The Blazing World* and decided to incorporate her thoughts about this invasive disease. An Italian gentleman, she knew, had used his microscope "to see Atoms through it, and could also perceive the Plague; which he affirmed to be a swarm of living Animals, as little as Atoms, which entered into mens bodies, through their mouths, nostrils, ears." Lady Margaret had her doubts because contagion, while undiscriminating, was not universal, as this learned man proposed; otherwise, these atoms would enter beasts and birds as well as humans. Drawing on Galenic notions of individual constitutions, Paracelsian belief that a human could catch the plague by imagining it, and Boyle's corpuscular theory of motion, she offered her own explanation. "Since it is often observed that all Bodies are not infected, even in a great plague," she averred, "it proves that the Infection is made by imitation; and as one and the same Agent cannot occasion the like effects in every Patient, as . . . some Wood takes fire sooner . . . so it is also with the Plague." See Margaret Cavendish, *Observations upon Experimental Philosophy* (London, 1668). We thank John T. O'Connor for bringing her work, including the quotations, to our attention.

Chapter 8. Business Not as Usual

1. There has never been a serious examination of the economic impact of the Great Plague of 1665, perhaps in the belief that documents on business and vital services do not exist. Historians' generalizations on the subject range from the consensus of a bleak reality to a few suggestions that Londoners coped better than one would have expected. On the former side, Walter George Bell and J. D. Shrewsbury are typical. For the latter, revisionist view, we can cite Charles Mullett and to an extent Stephen Porter, though he stresses the weaknesses of the public safety net and the economic and financial difficulties. Richard Grassby's work is central to an understanding of merchant capital and credit flexibility during normal times. See his "English Merchant Capitalism in the Late Seventeenth Century: The Composition of Business Fortunes," *Past and Present* 46 (1970): 93–94. We made some preliminary suggestions in A. Lloyd Moote, "Did Grass Grow in London's Streets? Personal Wealth, Commercial Activity, and Public Culture during the Great Plague of 1665," in *Trading Cultures: The Worlds of Western Merchants,* ed. Jeremy Adelman and Stephen Aron (Turnhout, Belgium, 2001), 35–57.

2. Sir William Turner, London, to Pocquelin père et fils at Paris, Aug. 8, Aug. 28, Oct. 16, 1665.

3. For Gauden, Vyner, and Colvill, see their biographical entries in Pepys, *Diary*, 10.

4. Pepys, *Diary*, 6:165, 10:16–17.

5. Ibid., 6:162–64. A succinct description of the system is by Henry Roseveare, "The Exchequer," in Pepys, *Diary*, 10:124–27.

6. Pepys, *Diary*, 6:165–66.

7. Boghurst, *Loimographia*, 53–54; Allin to Fryth, London, Sept. 14, ESRO FRE 5466; James Hickes to Joseph Williamson, Oct. 4, cited by Bell, *The Great Plague*, 299.

8. *The Economic Writings of Sir William Petty*, ed. Charles Henry Hull, 2 vols. (Cambridge, 1899), 1:103–13. A similar appreciation of the worth of workers was triggered by the Great Plague in the mind of Sir Josiah Child, a future titan in London's financial circles. See Charles Wilson, *England's Apprenticeship, 1603–1763* (New York, 1965), 233, quoting Child's *Brief Observations*.

9. John Graunt, *Reflections on the Bills of Mortality . . . from the year 1592 to the Great Plague in 1665* (London, 1665), reprinted in *A Collection of Very Valuable and Scarce Pieces relating to the last Plague in the year 1665* (London, 1721), 53–82. *Economic Writings of Sir William Petty*, 1:109–10.

10. St. Giles Cripplegate Parish Register, GL, MS 6419/7.

11. Bell, *The Great Plague*, 59.

12. Pepys, *Diary*, 6:165, 174–79, July 22, 29, 30.

13. Bell, *The Great Plague*, 216–17.

14. Symon Patrick to Elizabeth Gauden, Sept. 21, 1665, in *Works*, 9:579.

15. The ebb and flow of coastal and overseas trade can be followed partly in the port tax records for London and Colchester. PRO 190/50/4, 5; E 190/607/1, 3.

16. Symon Patrick to Elizabeth Gauden, Dec. 16, 1665, in *Works*, 9:602–3.

17. Patrick to Gauden, Sept. 19, in *Works*, 9:577–78.

18. See Chandaman, *English Public Revenue*, 55–56, and Pepys, *Diary*, 10:48.

19. Pepys, *Diary*, 6:186.

20. The accounts in Hodges, *Loimologia*, and Boghurst, *Loimographia*, are similar.

21. See the weekly Bills of Mortality and the Middlesex and Surrey Quarter Session judicial records.

22. *The Victoria History of the County of Middlesex*, vol. 5, ed. T. F. T. Baker (London, 1976), 164–65; Masie Brown, *The Market Gardens of Barnes and Mortlake* (Barnes and Mortlake, 1985); Ronald Webber, *Covent Garden* (London, 1969), 26, 31. We thank Masie Brown for sharing her insights.

23. St. Katherine Creechurch Churchwarden account, GL, MS 1198/1.

24. The guilds' records are in the Guildhall Library. These companies had closed down most of their activities in July, but their vital services continued.

25. See Richard Grassby, *The English Gentleman in Trade* (Oxford, 1994), 94, 94n. 3.

26. William Turner to the Pocquelins, Sept. 4, 1665, GL, MS 5106/1.

27. Factory Booke Merchandise, two-thirds for Msrs. Pocquelin Accompt of Paris and one-third for Sir William Turner in London, GL, MS 5101/3.

28. Turner to the Pocquelins, July 20, 27, 1665, GL, MS 5106/1.

29. In July Turner had persuaded Lord Berkeley, who was a major player in overseas

trade, to work for him on a continental trip by coming up with an advance of £9,000. In September he added two-thirds of a joint credit line of £2,026, secured by a complicated four-party involvement. Ibid., July 10, 12, Sept. 7.

30. Ibid., Aug. 8.

31. Ibid., Aug. 10, 28, Sept. 28.

32. Holborn Local History Library, St. Giles in the Fields Churchwarden Account for 1665.

33. John Tillison to William Sancroft, Aug. 10, 23, Sept. 14, Oct. 13, 1665, BL, Harleian MS 3785, fols. 30, 34–35, 38.

34. On Sandwich, see "Edward Mountagu, Earl of Sandwich," in Pepys, *Diary*, 10:252–55. On Pepys' finances, in addition to the superb essay by Henry Roseveare on "Finances" in ibid., 130–37, see Vincent Brome, *The Other Pepys* (London, 1992), using the index headings for Pepys' residences and employment.

35. See Brome, *The Other Pepys*, 100; Pepys, *Diary*, 6:341.

36. Roy Porter places Pepys in the mainstream of contemporary practice; Vincent Brome believes he skirted the line and could be called corrupt. Personal conversations with the authors. A quick guide to Pepys' financial practices is Tomalin, *Samuel Pepys*, under the index subcategory "Pepys, Samuel: finances" (twenty entries).

37. Pepys, *Diary*, 5:267; 6:88–89.

38. Ibid., 6:224.

39. Ibid., 224–26, Sept. 14 and 15, 1665.

40. Ibid., 225.

41. *Obituary of Richard Smyth*, 67–70.

42. Bell, *The Great Plague*, 214. Dr. Kay Redfield Jamison, a specialist on manic depression and suicide, has made a similar suggestion in conversations with us.

43. Pepys, *Diary*, 6:266.

44. Ibid., 251.

Chapter 9. Requiem for London

1. Pepys, *Diary*, 6:233–34.

2. The total fatalities in St. Botolph Bishopsgate for 1655–64, tabulated by Graham Twigg from the parish register, were 4,324, with an average of 432.4 per year. Using the demographers' method, called the Crisis Mortality Ratio, but dividing the 3,464 total for 1665 in the Bills of Mortality (their figure) by the average of 432.4 during the previous decade in the parish register (our substitution for the average from the bills, used by the demographers), we calculate an increase of 8.0. For the demographers' calculation of a 6.7 increase, see Champion, *London's Dreaded Visitation*, app. 1, 106, using M. J. Power's data.

3. St. Botolph Bishopsgate *Register*, ed. A. W. C. Hallen (1889–95), vol. 1 (marriages); vol. 2 (burials, baptisms).

4. Hodges, *Loimologia*, 8.

5. See Millard Meiss, *Painting in Florence and Siena after the Black Death* (Princeton,

N.J., 1951), and Christine M. Boeckl, *Images of Plague and Pestilence: Iconography and Iconology* (Kirksville, Mo., 2000).

6. Pepys, *Diary,* 6:213–14.

7. Ibid., 204, 207.

8. Stephen Bing to Dean Sancroft, Aug. 7, 10; John Tillison to Sancroft, Aug. 15, Sept. 14; BL, Harleian MS 3785, fols. 27, 29, 31, 35–36.

9. Samuel Pepys to Lady Carteret, Sept. 4, quoted in Pepys, *Diary,* 10:332; John Allin to Philip Fryth, Aug. 24, ESRO FRE 5462.

10. Symon Patrick to Elizabeth Gauden, Sept. 19, in Patrick, *Works,* 9:576; St. Paul Covent Garden *Register,* 3:37; Rugge, *Diurnal,* fol. 147r.

11. Pepys, *Diary,* 6:207–8.

12. St. Giles Cripplegate Vestry Book, GL, MS 6048/1, fol. 19v. Similar words were used when the vestry met the following January after the worst was over.

13. St. Giles Cripplegate Churchwardens Accounts, GL, 6047/1.

14. See A. Povah, *Annals of St. Olave Hart Street* (London, 1894); *St. Olave Hart Street and All Hallows Staining* (London, 1908).

15. Pepys, *Diary,* 7:6–7, Jan. 7, 30, 1666.

16. *Newes,* July 20, Aug. 9. Cf. Bell, *The Great Plague,* 95–96.

17. On these families' economic situations, see London Poor Rate Books, 1664–65, GL, MS 872/9.

18. St. Olave Hart Street *Register,* 200–202.

19. Hodges, *Loimologia,* 14.

20. See ch. 11, this volume.

21. Rugge, *Diurnal,* fol. 147v.

22. See Vanessa Harding, *"And One More May Be Laid There':* The Location of Burials in Early Modern London," *London Journal* 14 (1989): esp. 120; Bell, *The Great Plague,* 152–53, 178, 258–59, 282–83; Mrs. Basil Holmes, *London's Burial Grounds* (London, 1906); and the Archives of St. Bartholomew's Hospital, HE 10/3, "Burials."

23. St. Bride's Vestry meetings on June 16, July 3 and 7, Aug. 12 and 29, GL, MS 6554/1.

24. St. Giles Cripplegate Vestry meeting, May 23, GL, MS 6049/1, fol. 18v.

25. St. Bride's Churchwardens Accounts, GL, MS 6552/1; St. Bride's Register, 1653–72, GL, MS 6540/1.

26. St. Paul Covent Garden *Register,* entries for July–September 1665.

27. CLRO CA 70, fols. 153, 155; CA 71, fol. 5, Sept. 5, Oct. 19, Dec. 12.

28. PRO PC Register 58, fol. 171; Bell, *The Great Plague,* 38.

29. *The Petition of Charles Wilcox* (London, 1667). Cf. Bell, *The Great Plague,* 165–66.

30. CLRO CA 70, fol. 136, June 17; Baddeley, *St. Giles Cripplegate,* 24.

31. St. Margaret Westminster Churchwarden Accounts, WL E 47.

32. Mabel Richmond Brailsford, *The Making of William Penn* (London, 1930), 195. The Friends' burial records list the first plague fatality as Henry Stokes of Stepney, buried on June 24. They were extremely reluctant to list plague in this tally, however, with the second acknowledgment—Katherine Stokes of Stepney—coming on July 10.

33. George Whitehead, *The Christian Progress*, quoted in the *Select Series of Biographical Narratives . . . of Early Members of the Society of Friends*, ed. John Barclay (London, 1841), 118–19; Society of Friends London Burials, PRO RG 449.

34. There is a helpful discussion by Porter, *The Great Plague*, 73–74.

35. Morgan Watkins to Mary Pennington, Sept. 18, 1665, in Barclay, *Select Series of Biographical Narratives*, 148–49.

36. Oleg Peter Grell, "Plague in Elizabethan and Stuart London: The Dutch Response," *Medical History* 38 (1990): 424–39.

37. Wilfred S. Samuel, "The Jews of London and the Great Plague (1665)," in *Jewish Historical Society Miscellanies* 3 (1937): 11–12. Cf. Bell, *The Great Plague*, 180–82.

38. John Tillison to Dean Sancroft, Sept. 14, BL, Harleian MS 3785, fol. 35.

39. Lambeth Palace Library, Archbishop Sheldon Papers, 1664–67. We thank Richard Palmer and his staff for locating for our use these and other papers relevant to the Great Plague.

40. St. Giles Cripplegate Vestry Book, GL, MS 6048/1, fol. 20v, Sept. 28. Similar burials in churches were recorded at St. Christopher le Stocks and St. Margaret Lothbury inside the wall. The latter's minister was buried in a vault under the communion table. Pepys, *Diary*, 6:21, Sept. 3.

41. Bell, *The Great Plague*, 134–35; J. J. Cartwright, ed., *The Memoirs of Sir John Reresby* (London, 1875). Photos of the piper are on the cover of the Norton edition of Defoe's *Journal of the Plague Year*, as well as in Bell.

42. Albert Camus, *The Plague* (1947), quoted in Defoe, *Journal of the Plague Year*, Norton ed., 242.

Chapter 10. Contagion in the Countryside

1. F. J. Fisher's essays on the London economy are still of importance, especially "London as an 'Engine of Economic Growth,'" reprinted in *London and the English Economy, 1500–1700: F. J. Fisher*, ed. P. J. Corfield and N. B. Harte (London, 1990), 185–98. Also useful is a trenchant review by James Alexander, "The Economic Structure of the City of London at the End of the Seventeenth Century," in Richard Roger, ed., *Urban History Yearbook* 16 (Leicester, 1989), 47–62.

2. William Lilly, *Merlini Angelici Ephemeris* (London, 1666), dated Oct. 5, 1665; John Tanner, *Angelicus Britannicus* (London, 1666); Thomas Trigge, *Calendrium Astrologicum* (London, 1666).

3. Colchester's Port Books for 1665 and 1666 are an exceptional source for tracking provincial trade with London. They list each ship, its captain, cargo, date of arrival and/or departure, and destination. PRO E 190/607: 1 (coastal), 3 (overseas).

4. Defoe, *Journal of the Plague Year*, Norton ed., 113–15.

5. Symon Patrick to Elizabeth Gauden, Sept. 30, 1665, in Patrick, *Works*, 9:582.

6. Patrick to Gauden, Aug. 9, Sept. 2, 19, 23, ibid., 571, 575, 577, 580–81.

7. Essex Record Office (ERO), D/P268/1/2 (Bocking), QS Ba 2/105–6 (Braintree); H. J. Cunnington, *An Account of the Charities and Charitable Benefactions of Braintree*

(London, 1904), 60–65; Slack, *The Impact of Plague,* 106–7; W. F. Quin, *A History of Braintree and Bocking* (Lavenham, 1981), 91–99.

8. Elizabeth Gauden to Symon Patrick, Oct. 5, 1665, in Patrick, *Works,* 9:585. Patrick's letters continually reflected his anxiety about Elizabeth's health. On September 23 he had written, "I am sorry you speak so faintly of your own condition and tell me only that you are presently well in health. I pray study to be better, and I wish your mind and body may both recover together" (581).

9. Josselin, *Diary,* 519–20.

10. John Evelyn, Sayes Court, to the duke of Albemarle, Deptford, Sept. 8, 1665; Evelyn to Lord Viscount Corniberry, Lord Chamberlain to Her Majesty, Sept. 9; BL, John Evelyn Book of Letters, 3:250, 3:251.

11. F. H. Dinnis, ed., *Paddington in 1665: The Year of the Great Plague, being Extracts . . . from Old Parish Registers* (London, 1814), 20 (Paddington parish register entry for July 24, 1665); Sir Thomas Peynton to Sir Joseph Williamson, Under-Secretary of State, Knowlton, Kent, Aug. 7, quoted by William Durrant Cooper, *Letters of John Allin . . . to Philip Fryth and Samuel Jeake* (London, 1856), 3n. a.

12. Josselin, *Diary,* 519–20.

13. BL, Stowe MS 840, fol. 44r. Copy by the Colchester historian Phillip Morant.

14. "Ye sickness increase at Norwich. 42 there last weeke. And at Colchester having bene at nere 200 weekly there it is this last weeke risen to nere 300." John Allin to Philip Fryth, Nov. 8, 1665, ESRO FRE 5479; Josselin, *Diary,* 520.

15. There is a good description of Colchester in Diary of Edward Browne, fol. 40v, BL, Sloane MS 1906; Peter Clark and Paul Slack, ed., *English Towns in Transition, 1500–1700* (Oxford, 1976), 9.

16. The best account of Colchester's economy is the *Victoria History of the Counties of England: Essex,* vol. 9, *Colchester,* ed. Janet Cooper (London, 1994), 81–99. Quotation from ibid., 68. Similarly, Paul Slack concluded that "the great city of Colchester suffered most of all" during the Great Plague. Slack, *The Impact of Plague,* 107. The most sweeping assessment remains that of Charles Creighton: "The plague at Colchester in 1665–66 was the greatest of all provincial plagues since the Black Death. It reproduced the mortality of the Great Plague of London on a scale more than proportionate to its size." Charles Creighton, *A History of Epidemics in Britain* (London, 1891), 688. See PRO E 179/246/20, Colchester Hearth Taxes, 1666. The best short guide to the epidemic in Colchester is Rosalyn Barker's pamphlet on Essex plague epidemics, in the Colchester Record Office.

17. ERO SR 406/104.

18. William Doyly to John Evelyn, Colchester, July 10, BL, Addit. MSS 4182, fol. 37r; BL, Evelyn Papers SXW 1 1665. The Quakers had especially strong contacts with London and the Netherlands. ERO (Colchester branch) Microfilm T/A 424/6/3, "A Collection of Letters Written by Many of the People called Quakers from the Year 1662 to 1777," esp. the letters by William Caton from Amsterdam (original at the University of Essex Library).

19. In St. Botolph parish, 502 died from the plague and 47 of other diseases. At St. Giles, there were 581 plague victims, plus 47 others. St. Peters on North Street lost 691 to the distemper and 81 from other causes (a gross overcount from other years). During the two-year epidemic, the mortality from all causes in these three parishes stood roughly at 1,950. The overall total for the entire sixteen parishes was about five thousand.

20. Timothy C. Glines, "Politics and Government in the Borough of Colchester, 1660–1693" (Ph.D. diss., University of Wisconsin-Madison, 1974), 7–8; Doyly to Evelyn, Aug. 17, BL, Evelyn Papers SXW 1 1665.

21. Slack, *The Impact of Plague,* 281, concludes that money raised inside the town could have maintained the sick and poor during one-third to two-fifths of the plague epidemic. A rare plague book from one of the poorest parishes reveals the contours of plaguetime financing. St. Leonard's Parish Book, 61–63, ERO (Colchester) D/P/ 245//8/2.

22. We thank Linda Dunnett for showing us this mound.

23. Revisionist studies have stressed a quick demographic and economic rebound after Colchester's Great Plague, pointing to the surge in fines on cloth that did not meet strict standards. See I. G. Doolittle, "The Effects of the Plague on a Provincial Town in the Sixteenth and Seventeenth Centuries," *Medical History* 19 (1975): 333–41. The effect of loss of life and livelihood at the time cannot be ignored, however. There has also been some misreading of hearth tax assessments before and after the local epidemic (confusing assessments, nonpayments, and empty houses), resulting in understating the economic and financial difficulties of rebounding.

24. See esp. Leslie Bradley, "The Most Famous of All English Plagues: A Detailed Analysis of the Plague at Eyam, 1665–6," in *The Plague Reconsidered,* 63–94.

25. On the plague's path up the Thames, see Hailstone, "If on a Sudden." On Portsmouth's pesthouse, see Rugge, *Diurnal,* fol. 143.

26. *Newes,* Aug. 3, 1665.

27. BL, Addit. MSS 4182, fols. 30, 32, 34: PRO PC 2/58, fol. 246; Bell, *The Great Plague,* 170–71.

28. Pepys, *Diary,* 6:218, Sept. 9, 1665.

29. John Evelyn to Lord Viscount Cornibery, Sept. 9, Evelyn Letter Book 3:251.

30. Albemarle to Evelyn, Sept. 25, Oct. 3, 4, 22, BL, Evelyn Papers SXW 1 1665.

31. Evelyn, *Diary,* 1:404–5; Albemarle to Evelyn, Oct. 9, BL, Evelyn Papers SXW 1 1665.

32. Evelyn to Sir William Coventry, a privy councilor, Oct. 2, BL, Evelyn Letter Book 3, no. 257.

33. Rugge, *Diurnal,* fol. 151r.

34. Slack, *The Impact of Plague,* 224.

35. BL, Addit. MSS 4182, fols. 44–48.

36. Elizabeth Gauden, Hutton Hall, Burntwood [Brentwood], Essex, to Symon Patrick, Oct. 5, 1665, in Patrick, *Works,* 9:585.

37. Symon Patrick to Elizabeth Gauden, Oct. 14, in ibid., 588–89.

38. Patrick to Gauden, Oct. 12, 26, in ibid., 590.

39. Mary Evelyn to Sir Richard Browne, Oct. 8, 1665, BL, Mrs. Evelyn Correspondence, 2.

40. John Allin to Philip Fryth, Aug. 11, Nov. 23, ESRO FRE 5459, 5483.

41. Evelyn, *Diary*, 1:406, 2:1–2.

42. Josselin, *Diary*, 522–24; *Records of an English Village, Earls Colne, 1400–1750*, ed. Alan Macfarlane (microfilm at Colchester Public Library); Slack, *The Impact of Plague*, 108.

Chapter 11. The Web of Authority

1. Pepys, *Diary*, 6:213, Sept. 6, 1665; BL, Addit. MSS 4182, fol. 43r.

2. Evelyn, *Diary*, 1:404, Sept. 7.

3. Newsletter, ca. Sept. 23, BL, Addit. MSS 4182, fol. 43r.

4. Bell, *The Great Plague*, 236–38. For the proclamation, see BL, Pressmark 21.4.5, no. 35.

5. Hodges, *Loimologia*, 19–20.

6. Josselin, *Diary*, 520, 527; Rugge, *Diurnal*, fol. 144v.

7. On the location of the fires, see Shrewsbury, *A History of Bubonic Plague*, 466, citing Noorthouck, *London*.

8. Bell, *The Great Plague*, 237–38.

9. CLRO CC 46, fol. 60.

10. Peter Barwick to Dean Sancroft, Aug. 9, 1665, BL, Harleian MS 3785, fol. 23.

11. CLRO CA 70, fols. 143, 152; CLRO CC 46, fol. 60.

12. CLRO CA 70, fol. 152.

13. [Bell], *Londons Remembrancer*; Bell, *The Great Plague*, 83, 278.

14. Bell, *The Great Plague*, 26, 82–83; J. R. Woodhead, *The Rulers of London, 1660–1689* (London, 1955), 106; *Newes*, Nov. 1, 1665.

15. CLRO CA 70, fol. 150v, July 27.

16. Ibid., fol. 152v, Sept. 5; *Obituary of Richard Smyth*, 68.

17. *The Petition of Charles Wilcox* (London, 1667); Bell, *The Great Plague*, 165–66.

18. Quotation: "La Contagion s'est augmenté, la semaine passé, ce qui augmente le crainte de ceux qui ont peur de se retourner en la ville." See Turner to the Pocquelins, Aug. 10, Sept. 4, Oct. 4, 6, Dec. 15, GL, MS 5106/1.

19. Rugge, *Diurnal*, fol. 147v, BL, Addit. MSS 10,117.

20. Based on Craven's exhaustive report on public health after the plague. See Slack, *The Impact of Plague*, 317–18.

21. This subject is rich in materials, but most of what has been studied comes from the 1640s and 1650s, not the 1660s. A reappraisal is in A. Lloyd Moote, "Conversion and Backsliding in Seventeenth Century England: From Puritan Millenarianism to the Great Plague," Princeton University Davis Center paper, Sept. 2000. For a published overview, see Michael McKeon, *Politics and Poetry in Restoration England: The Case of Dryden's Annus Mirabilis* (Cambridge, Mass., 1975).

22. Peter Barwick and Stephen Bing to William Sancroft, Aug. 5, 10, 1665, BL, Harleian MS 3785, fols. 25, 29r.

23. BL, Addit. MSS 4182, fols. 29, 31; Pepys, *Diary*, 6:184.

24. Albemarle to Evelyn, July 25, Sept. 6, Oct. 3 (I); Thomas Forster to Evelyn, Nov. 27, 1665 (VII); Edward Mason to Evelyn, n.d. (IX), BL, Letters to John Evelyn.

25. Fifteen percent of St. Margaret's widows receiving regular stipends are listed separately by name for nursing services paid.

26. St. Martin Orgar Register, GL, MS 959/1.

27. The most dramatic example is Reverend Pearson's signature on page after page of St. Bride's burial register during the epidemic.

28. St. Bride's records are immense and detailed: GL, MS 6554/1 Vestry; MS 6552/1 Churchwardens Accounts; MS 6570/1 Parish Papers (burials and rough relief account); and MS 6540/1 Register, 1653–72.

29. CLRO Ex GL MS 359, Miscellaneous entries on entertainments, military affairs, plague, fire of London, "Sicknes and Pesthouse."

30. See GL Ex GL MS 270: "Monies Rec'd for ye reliefe of the Poore Visited with ye plague in London and liberties" and "Paid to parishes"; GL, MS 6552/1, St. Bride's Churchwardens Accounts.

31. CLRO CA 70, fol. 156v; Ex GL MS 270, "Moneys rec'd on Account of the Second Years Rate for ye visited Poore."

32. CLRO CC 46, fol. 61.

Chapter 12. Not by Bread Alone

1. There are glimpses of George Boddington Sr.'s character in his son's commonplace book writings; his offices at St. Margaret Lothbury are listed in the parish records at the Guildhall Library. On Hannah Boddington, see GL, MS 10823/1 Boddington Commonplace Book, 36, 42.

2. George Boddington Jr.'s account of the Great Plague is on one packed page of his commonplace book, ibid., 40.

3. John Bunyan, *Grace Abounding to the Chief of Sinners*, first published in 1666. See Owen C. Watkins, *The Puritan Experience: Studies in Spiritual Autobiography* (New York, 1972), 101–20.

4. Deuteronomy 8:3; Matthew 4:4. We thank Judith Lee for locating these passages.

5. William Caton to Friends and Brethren in England, Sept. 8, ERO T/A 424/6/3, "Collection of Letters."

6. Vincent, *God's Terrible Voice*, 28, 39–40.

7. See "A Brief Account of My Life," in Patrick, *Works*, 9:443–44; Pickering's *Christmas Classics* (1847), cited by Cooper, *Letters of John Allin*, 10; Patrick, *Works*, 3:655–74.

8. Mary Evelyn to John Evelyn, Sept. 2, 1665, BL, Letters to Evelyn, VII; Evelyn, *Diary*, 1:350–54.

9. Evelyn, *Diary*, 1:394, 406.

10. John Evelyn to Mary Evelyn, Sept. 17, 1665, BL, Evelyn Papers, Mrs. Evelyn I.

11. Pepys, *Diary*, 6:189–90, Aug. 13, 1665.

12. Slack, *The Impact of Plague*, 356n. 95.

13. A sermon is printed verbatim in Patrick, *Works*, 3:65–74.

14. Bishop Humphrey Henchman to Dean William Sancroft, June 11, 17, 29, July 9, 1665, BL, Harleian MS 3784, fols. 281, 285, 296; MS 3785, fol. 10.

15. *A Form of Common Prayer for the Averting of God's Heavy Visitation to be Read on Wednesday in Every Week* (London, 1665); John Evelyn to Sir Richard Browne, Sept. 23, 1665, BL, Evelyn Letters, XIII.

16. Dinnis, *Paddington in 1665,* 22; Josselin, *Diary,* 520.

17. Symon Patrick to Elizabeth Gauden, Sept. 30, 1665, in Patrick, *Works,* 9:583–84.

18. John Allin to Philip Fryth, Sept. 5, 7, 1665, ESRO FRE 5464, 5465.

19. Allin to Fryth, Sept. 14, 1665, ibid., 5466.

20. John Allin to Samuel Jeake, Sept. 20, 1665, ibid., 5467.

21. Patrick, *Works,* 9:443, 576.

22. Patrick, "Brief Account of My Life," ibid., 439–46; letter of Dec. 21, 1665, ibid., 579.

23. Some dissenters felt remorse for leaving their secret congregations. An anguished Owen Stockton of Colchester wanted to stay but told himself that staying would risk arrest for his worshipers, whom the town authorities would suspect of plotting an uprising under cover of the plague. After much prayer and scripture reading, his mind was made up by a passage in Isaiah: "Hide thy selfe for a little moment till ye indignation be past." But as he and his wife and children passed through the Essex countryside from conventicle to conventicle, he kept seeing "signs" of God's displeasure, culminating in the death of one of his children. Scripture again came to his relief, at least temporarily, with the passage: "The Lord is all I have; therefore I will wait for him patiently." See Dr. Williams' Library, MS 24.7, fols. 17–18, 28, Owen Stockton papers, and MS 24.8, Eleanor Stockton's diary. We thank David Harley for bringing these sources to our attention.

24. Samuel Foster to Dean Sancroft, Jan. 22, 1666, BL, Harleian MS 3785, fol. 81; Francis Lewys, from the parsonage of St. Botolph without Bishopsgate, to Dean Sancroft, Oct. 25, 1665, fol. 37r; Bishop Henchman to Dean Sancroft, Fulham, Feb. 9, 1666, fol. 96.

Chapter 13. The Awakening

1. Thomas Cocke, *Rules for Returning Citizens and Such as are Already Returned,* in his *Plain Discourse upon the First of the Six Non-Naturals, viz, Air* (London, 1665).

2. Rugge, *Diurnal,* fol. 148; *Newes,* Nov. 1, 1665.

3. Turner to the Pocquelins, Oct. 26, Nov. 2, 13, 14, 27, 1665, GL, MS 5106/1.

4. Pepys, *Diary,* 6:285 (Nov. 1), 201.

5. Pepys suggested a gatekeeper for the inefficient victualing system and was appointed Surveyor General at three hundred pounds per annum. Pepys to Albemarle, Oct. 6, PRO SP 29/134/46; Pepys, *Diary,* 6:254n. 2, 264, 306–7.

6. Pepys, *Diary,* 6:332; PRO SP 29/134/46.

7. Symon Patrick to Elizabeth Gauden, Nov. 4, 7, 1665, in Patrick, *Works,* 9:594–95.

8. John Allin to Samuel Jeake, Nov. 14, ESRO FRE 5481; Allin to Philip Fryth, Dec. 14, FRE 5489.

9. Pepys, *Diary,* 6:328–29, 335, 339.

10. Turner to the Pocquelins, Dec. 14, GL, MS 5106/1.

11. Symon Patrick to Elizabeth Gauden, Dec. 14, 16, 19, 21, in Patrick, *Works*, 9:599, 601–4.

12. Elizabeth Gauden to Symon Patrick, Dec. 27, 1665, ibid., 607.

13. Symon Patrick to Elizabeth Gauden, Dec. 26, 28, 1665; Jan. 6, 11, 1666, ibid., 605, 607–9.

14. Symon Patrick to Elizabeth Gauden, Jan. 18, 1666, ibid., 612–13; Hodges, *Loimologia*, 27; Boghurst, *Loimographia*, 70; Bell, *The Great Plague*, 285–86, citing a letter by the teller of the Exchequer, Sir George Downing, to Undersecretary of State Joseph Williamson, Dec. 14.

15. After Dec. 19, 1665, the weekly bills, which for 1665 are printed in *London's Dreadful Visitation*, are available in GL, MS 3604/1/1, "The Parish Clerks Company Weekly Bills of Mortality, December 1664–October 1669."

16. Pepys, *Diary*, 7:35. See also Bell, *The Great Plague*, 292–93.

17. Guildhall payments to infected parishes during the last half of the year came to £7,663. Another city account, largely for medical services, came to £2,784. A third account, which included expenses for the city pesthouse and burial grounds, as well as the medical team and the dog killer, totaled £2,025. CLRO Ex GL MSS 270, 295, 359.

18. See Bell, *The Great Plague*, 286–89.

19. For some typical costs for rebuilding after the Great Fire, see CLRO Ex GL MS 359: "Paid for the Great Fire," £2,673; "paid more," £3,462; "common sewer cleansing, etc.," £2,210; "conduit and pipes," £4,564. The cost of maintaining 37,000 navy men, 20,000 Dutch prisoners, and the royal fleet from April 1 to September 30, 1665, totaled £1,006,075. *Further Correspondence of Samuel Pepys, 1662–1679*, ed. J. R. Tanner (London, 1929), 58.

20. In 1665, Londoners also paid thousands of pounds for their new navy ship, and the Crown had not repaid a £200,000 city loan.

21. On Pepys, see his *Diary*, 6:340–42. Turner's assets in 1665 must have been considerably more than the two thousand pounds he had been worth in 1660. J. R. Woodward, *The Rulers of London, 1660–1689* (London, 1955), 166.

22. Steven Pincus has told us of later crises when London found money despite insolvency.

23. Mayoral Proclamation, Dec. 7, 1665, as cited in Bell, *The Great Plague*, 285.

24. Ibid., 313–16.

25. *The Economic Writings of Sir William Petty*, ed. Charles Henry Hull, 2 vols. (Cambridge, 1899), 1:108–10; Porter, *The Great Plague*, 126.

26. Hodges, *Loimologia*, 7–11; Boghurst, *Loimographia*, 25–27, 57, 99, 123; CLRO Lord Mayor's Waiting Book, 2, Sept. 22, 1665, cited by Porter, *The Great Plague*, 123. Cf. Slack, *The Impact of Plague*, 251.

27. *Middlesex Sessions Rolls*, 3:373–75; Bell, *The Great Plague*, 315–16.

28. PRO SP 149/88, Feb. 19, 1665/6; Bell, *The Great Plague*, 315–16.

29. Bell, *The Great Plague*, 317–18; PRO PC 2/59, fols. 44–45.

30. The Plague Orders are reprinted in Bell, *The Great Plague*, 333–35.

31. Evelyn, *Diary,* 2:2, Jan. 29, Feb. 6, 1666; Mary Evelyn to Sir Richard Browne, Dec. 6, 1665; Browne to Mary Evelyn, Dec. 17, 1665, Jan. 8, 1666, BL, Mrs. Evelyn Papers 2.

32. Evelyn, *Diary,* 2:4–6, 9, Apr. 15, June 6, Aug. 26, 1666.

33. Josselin, *Diary,* 527, May 20, 1666; Earls Colne burial register, *Records of an English Village,* microfilm, ed. Alan MacFarlane, Apr. 28, May 15, 24, June 3, 1666; PRO PC2/59, fol. 5, May 9, 1666.

34. BL, Stowe MS 840, fols. 44–45; cf. ERO D/P 200/1/6.

35. *VHC Essex, Colchester,* 9:68.

36. Pepys, *Diary,* 6:340–42.

37. See Patrick's "Brief Account of My Life" and letter of Jan. 18, 1666, in *Works,* 3:445–47, 9:612–13.

38. ERO Colchester, D/B 5 Gb 4, Colchester Assembly Book, fol. 360.

39. London Parish Clerks Company Weekly Bills of Mortality, GL, MS 3604/1/1.

40. See Slack, *The Impact of Plague,* 154.

41. Letter by Dr. Grumble in Leonard W. Cowie, *Plague and Fire: London, 1665–66* (New York, 1970), 56.

Epilogue. Of Once and Future Plagues

1. Sir William Petty, *Verbum Sapienti,* published in 1691, and *Political Arithmetick,* which appeared in 1690. See Hull, *Writings of Sir William Petty,* 1:108–10, 243, 2:475–76; Porter, *The Great Plague,* 154.

2. See Porter, *London,* 90–91.

3. Whittet, *Apothecaries in the Great Plague,* 22.

4. Bell, *The Great Plague,* 161–62, and the article on Hodges in the *Dictionary of National Biography,* 9:953–54.

5. Roseveare, "Finances," in Pepys, *Diary,* 10:136–37.

6. Pepys, *Diary,* 10:64–65, on "Christ's Hospital."

7. Frances Harris, curator of the Evelyn papers at the British Library, provided us with this information during our visit with her in March 2000.

8. See Stein, "Health," in Pepys, *Diary,* 10:177–78.

9. The history of the diary is recounted in Pepys, *Diary,* 1:xli and 10:89, "The Diary and Related Manuscripts."

10. Baldwin, "History of the Turner Family," 8, 42.

11. *A Sermon Preached on the Fast Day,* Apr. 11, 1679, in Patrick, *Works,* 8:71–79.

12. See Porter, *The Great Plague,* 158–59.

13. Joseph Browne, *A Practical Treatise of the Plague* (London, 1720), 6–8, 12; Richard Bradley, *The Plague of Marseilles* (London, 1721), 48–49.

14. There are several of these bogus works in the British Library and Wellcome Institute Library, masquerading as true accounts of 1665 for the unwary modern researcher eager to find a new source!

15. For example, J. Lyons, *A preventive of the Plague, being a discovery of a method to hinder its propagation by destroying the pestiferous atoms* (London, 1743); T. Lobb, *Letters Related to the Plague* (London, 1745).

16. See John T. Alexander, *Bubonic Plague in Early Modern Russia: Public Health and Urban Disaster* (Baltimore, 1980).

17. *House of Commons Report from the Select Committee appointed to consider the validity of the doctrine of contagion in the Plague* (London, 1819); G. Milroy, *Quarantine and Plague; being a summary of the report on these subjects recently addressed to the Royal Academy of Medicine of France* (London, 1846). Cf. Hirst, *The Conquest of Plague*, 63–64, 72.

18. See Norman Howard-Jones, *The Scientific Background of the International Sanitary Conferences, 1851–1938* (Geneva, 1975), introduction, 9–11. The summaries of the early conferences in 1851, 1859, 1866, and 1874 make fascinating reading.

19. Charles E. Rosenberg, *Explaining Epidemics and Other Studies in Medicine* (Cambridge, 1992), 112.

20. The U.S. National Library of Medicine has a fascinating list of British and American publications: *Index Catalogue of the Library of the Surgeon General's Office.*

21. See George Rosen, *A History of Public Health,* expanded edition with an introduction by Elizabeth Fee and a bibliographical essay by Edward T. Morman (Baltimore, 1993), 290.

22. The foremost authority on Yersin remains Henri Mollaret. See Henri Mollaret and Jacqueline Brossolet, *Alexandre Yersin, le vainqueur de la peste* (Paris, 1985). For documentation of this phase of Yersin's life, see Jack Moseley, "Travels of Alexandre Yersin: Letters of a Pastorian in Indochina, 1890–1894," *Perspectives in Biology and Medicine* 24 (1981): 607–18.

23. E. Lagrange, "Concerning the Discovery of the Plague Bacillus," *Journal of Tropical Medicine and Hygiene* 29 (1926): 299.

24. Shibasaburo Kitasato, "The Bacillus of Bubonic Plague," *Lancet,* July–December 1894, 2:428. Cf. *The Collected Papers of Shibasaburo Kitasato* (Tokyo, 1977).

25. Andrew Cunningham, "Transforming Plague," in *The Laboratory Revolution in Medicine,* ed. Andrew Cunningham and Perry Williams (Cambridge, 1992), 233, 235; Tom Solomon, "Alexandre Yersin and the Plague Bacillus," *Journal of Tropical Medicine and Hygiene* 98 (1995): 210; Thomas Butler, *Plague and Other Yersinia Infections* (New York, 1983), 23.

26. Solomon, "Yersin and the Plague Bacillus," 210–11.

27. For a lay formulation, see Emmanuel Le Roy Ladurie, "A Concept: The Unification of the Globe by Disease (Fourteenth to Seventeenth Centuries)," reprinted in his *The Mind and Method of the Historian,* trans. S. and B. Reynolds (Chicago, 1981), 31.

28. Cunningham, "Transforming Plague," 234.

29. Rosen, *A History of Public Health,* 306.

30. Solomon, "Yersin and the Plague Bacillus," 211; Pasteur Institute *Annales,* vol. 8.

31. It is a daunting undertaking to summarize current findings in the fast-moving fields of epidemiology and micro- and molecular biology. We thank Elisabeth Carniel and Henri Mollaret, of the Institut Pasteur in Paris, and Elizabeth Fee, at the National Library of Medicine in Bethesda, Maryland, for their generous assistance. Martin Nowak and his guest lecturers in the Program of Theoretical Biology at the Institute for Advanced Study have kept us current with an exciting, fast-moving area of research.

New general works on the history of epidemic disease continue to roll off the presses, along with studies on individual infective diseases. The *New England Journal of Medicine* is an invaluable source of new findings.

32. Institut Pasteur, *Activity Report of the Research Departments* (Paris, 1996); Annie Guiyoule, Francine Grimont, Isabelle Iteman, et al., "Plague Pandemics Investigated by Ribotyping of *Yersinia pestis* Strains," *Journal of Clinical Microbiology* 32 (1994): 634–41; Annie Guiyoule, B. Rasoamanana, C. Buchrieser, et al., "Recent Emergence of New Variants of *Yersinia pestis* in Madagascar," *Journal of Clinical Microbiology* 35 (1997): 2826.

33. Guiyoule et al., "*Yersinia pestis* in Madagascar," 2826; Guiyoule et al., "Plague Pandemics," 634.

34. Frédérique Audoin-Rouzeau, "La peste et les rats: La réponse de l'archéozoologie," in *Maladies et société (XVIIe–XVIIIe siècles): Actes du colloque de Bielefeld, Novembre 1986,* ed. Neithard Bulst and Robert Delort (Paris, 1989), 65–71; Graham I. Twigg, *The Black Death: A Biological Appraisal* (London, 1984); Mark Derr, "New Theories Link Black Death to Ebola-like Virus," *New York Times,* Oct. 2, 2001.

35. "An Empire's Epidemic," *Los Angeles Times,* May 6, 2002.

36. Ibid.

37. See the summary in Graham I. Twigg, "The Black Death in England: An Epidemiological Dilemma," in Bulst and Delort, *Maladies et société,* 84–86.

38. See Slack, *The Impact of Plague,* 7–15; Biraben, *Les hommes et la peste,* vol. 1, ch. 1, emphasizing the role of the human flea; Jean-Claude Beaucournu, "Diversité des puces vectrices en fonction des foyers pesteux," *Bulletin de la Société de Pathologie Exotique* 92 (1999): 419–21; Beaucournu, "Actualité de la conquête de L'Afrique intertropicale par *pulex irritans* Linné, 1758," *Bulletin de la Société de Pathologie Exotique* 86 (1993): 290–94; Beaucournu, "A propos du vecteur de la peste en Europe occidentale au cours de la deuxième pandémie," *Bulletin de la Société Française de Parasitologie* 13 (1995): 233–52. An excellent medical description is in B. Joseph Hinnebusch, "Bubonic Plague: A Molecular Genetic Case History of the Emergence of an Infectious Disease," *Journal of Molecular Medicine* 75 (1997): 646–48.

39. Champion, *London's Dreaded Visitation,* 2–3, 6–10; Graham Twigg, "Plague in London: Spatial and Temporal Aspects of Mortality," in Justin Champion, ed., *Epidemics in London* (London, 1993), 1–19.

40. Abraham Braude, Charles Davis, and Joshua Fierer, eds., *Infectious Diseases and Medical Microbiology* (Philadelphia, 1986), 338.

41. Thomas Brock, *Biology of Microorganisms* (Englewood Cliffs, N.J., 1984), 607.

42. Hinnebusch, "Bubonic Plague," 648.

43. Marc Galimand, M. Guiyoule, G. Cernaud, et al., "Multidrug Resistance in *Yersinia pestis* Mediated by a Transferable Plastid," *New England Journal of Medicine* 337 (1997): 677.

44. On the disappearance of plague from Europe, see Slack, *The Impact of Plague,* 313–26; the classic early exploration of this fascinating subject by Andrew Appleby, "The Disappearance of Plague: A Continuing Puzzle," *Economic History Review,* 2nd series, 33 (1980); Hirst, *The Conquest of Plague;* and R. Politzer, *Plague* (Geneva, 1954).

45. Personal communications by Dr. Mollaret to the authors, 1998–99.

46. Andrew Wear, Wellcome Institute, personal communication to the authors. A measured support of this view is in Slack, *The Impact of Plague*, 323–26. Slack points out that the return of plague to Britain in Liverpool, Glasgow, and Suffolk in the early twentieth century was probably via steamships that bypassed the quarantines. He suggests that the outbreaks were contained because of hygienic and environmental improvements and the absence of the black rat by that time.

47. Braude et al., *Infectious Diseases*, 334.

48. It is possible that there was an additional adjustment between the plague microbes and fleas. Joseph Hinnebusch reports from the Laboratory of Microbial Structure and Function in Montana: "Proventricular blockage by *Y. pestis* is an inefficient process in all fleas that have been examined, which may reflect a recent adaptation to the insect host. Unless they ingest a large number of bacteria, most fleas clear themselves of infection without ever becoming blocked." Hinnebusch, "Bubonic Plague," 648.

49. Guiyoule et al., "Plague Pandemics," 634–41.

50. The reservations are summarized by Samuel K. Cohn Jr., "The Black Death: End of a Paradigm," *American Historical Review* 107 (2002): 735n. 133. Andrew Wear, after noting Cohn's skepticism of the accuracy of the DNA findings, concludes, "However, if further positive DNA findings are produced, we will have to begin to consider that plague was after all one disease, but bearing Cohn's research in mind, an extremely protean one." Andrew Wear, review of Cohn, *The Black Death Transformed: Disease and Culture in Early Renaissance Europe* (London, 2002), in *Times Literary Supplement*, Nov. 5, 2002.

51. For research on dental pulp from Montpellier dated to the Black Death period, see Didier Raoult, Gérard Aboulharen, Eric Crubézy, et al., "Molecular Identification by Suicide PCR of *Yersinia pestis* as the Agent of Medieval Black Death," *Proceedings of the National Academy of Science* 97 (2000): 12800–3. For similar identification on dental pulp in southern France in charnel houses dating to 1590 and 1720, see G. Aboudharam, M. Signoli, E. Crubézy, et al., "La mémoire des dentes: le cas de la peste," in *Peste: Entre épidémies et sociétés*, International Congresses on the Evolution and Paleoepidemiology of Infectious Diseases (Marseille, 2001), 70.

52. Thomas, *Religion and the Decline of Magic*, 7.

53. Hinnebusch, "Bubonic Plague," 645–52.

54. Mirko Grmek, *Diseases in the Ancient Greek World*, trans. Mireille Muellner and Leonard Muellner (Baltimore, 1989), 277.

55. See Tim Radford, "Chinese Malaria Remedy Tested," *Guardian*, April 25, 2001. We thank Audrey B. Wright for locating this reference.

56. Thomas Daniel, *Captain of Death: The Story of Tuberculosis* (Rochester, N.Y., 1997), 1, 52.

57. A good introduction on AIDS is Garrett, *The Coming Plague*, 281–389.

58. This summary of the early stages of the SARS epidemic is based on major newspaper reports, including Lawrence K. Altman and Denise Grady, "Study Says [SARS]

Virus Has Remained Stable," *New York Times,* May 9, 2003, and Elizabeth Rosenthal, "Herbs? Bull Thymus? Beijing Leaps at Anti-SARS Potions," *New York Times,* May 10, 2003.

59. "Polio Eradication Called Impossible," *Times,* Trenton, N.J., Oct. 27, 2002. Dr. Henderson addressed the Infectious Diseases Society of America.

60. See Garrett, *The Coming Plague,* esp. 411–622, and an update: "Doctors Are Told Alcohol Gels Are Better than Soap and Water," *New York Times,* Oct. 26, 2002.

61. The WHO report is summarized in the lead editorial of the *New York Times,* June 18, 2000.

ACKNOWLEDGMENTS

While working on this book, we began many conversations with the warning: "We take the plague everywhere with us." This never seemed to stop inquiries; indeed, it drew us into many lively exchanges, clarified our ideas, and sharpened our story telling. There is a certain time when authors must stop talking, finish writing, and simply thank those who have helped the process. Our preface mentions individuals who played major supporting roles. Endnotes are a guide to source materials and historical scholarship underlying our work. Here we add our thanks to individuals who helped along the way—often with quite different perspectives on plague.

In the United Kingdom, Justin Champion, Larry Conrad, Mary Dobson, Derek Keene, Vivian Nutton, Margaret Pelling, Paul Slack, and Graham Twigg enriched our study with suggestions and support. Among European specialists on present and past plague and other diseases, we warmly thank Elisabeth Carniel and Henri and Martine Mollaret of the Pasteur Institute as well as Neithard Bulst and Thomas Rütten. In the United States, Gert Brieger placed the facilities of the Johns Hopkins Institute for the History of Medicine at our disposal, as did Elizabeth Fee at the National Library of Medicine and Mary Robertson at the Henry Huntington Library. At the Institute for Advanced Study, Martin Novak's outstanding lecture series on theoretical biology and Robert, Lord May helped with current biomedical knowledge.

Several persons read parts or all of our book at some stage of its development, and each helped make it better: Mary Fissell, Maurice D. Lee, Salley May, Lawrence Stone, Harriet Trueblood, Andrew Wear, Susan Whyman, and Roy Porter, who read the entire manuscript shortly before his untimely death, giving us a very welcome endorsement. We had lively discussions of our presentations at the Colchester Castle's Social History Series, the Rutgers Center for Historical Analysis, the Davis Center of Princeton University, and New Jersey's Peapack-Gladstone Library. Archival and library staffs in London, Colchester, Chelmsford, Oxford, East Sussex, and Hartford helped at various stages of our research. Our research in England was aided by grants by the Wellcome Trust, U.K., the Burroughs-Wellcome fund, U.S.A., and the Rutgers Center for Historical Analysis.

We have benefited greatly from editorial assistance and suggestions by Heather McCollum, Kirk Jensen, and Angela von der Lippe. Hilary Hinzmann played an even stronger role. By challenging us to let our protagonists speak for themselves, to probe the pragmatic relations between rich and poor, and to develop chapters fully, Hilary greatly improved our book. Linda Forlifer not only added her expert touch and helpful suggestions at the copyediting stage but also fortified us with her encouragement. The most important editorial decisions and support have come from Jacqueline Wehmueller at the Johns Hopkins University Press. Jackie's enthusiasm, judgment, and good sense are models for the publishing profession and a delight that all authors should enjoy. When we encountered computer breakdowns, Chris Beyer and his colleagues at the Princeton Workstation quickly came to our rescue. Finally, we thank Katherine Lima for her enthusiastic response to all our requests for help, including creating the graphs.

INDEX

advertisements, 81, 96, 105, 142

AIDS, xvii, 284, 288–89

Albemarle, duke of, 88, 124–25, 127, 180, 201, 218–19, 225–28, 255–56

Aldermen, Court of, 27, 56, 88, 94, 131, 188, 220–23, 231, 251. *See also* Turner, Sir William

alchemists. *See* Allin, John

Allin, John: alchemy and astrology of, 5, 21, 96, 110–11, 248; faith and fear of, 188, 213, 242; family needs and resources, 4, 166, 213, 242; and flight, 80, 90, 94; medical practice of, 4–5, 94, 213, 242, 270; new quarters required by, 213, 270; on plague, 5, 47, 68, 110, 112, 151, 162; and religious dissenters, 4, 94, 213, 240, 243

almanacs, 10, 21, 62, 101, 108, 321n. 31. *See also* astrology

Amsterdam, 13, 36–37, 51, 205

Anglican church: abolition and restoration of, 4, 9, 10; and licensing of doctors, 97; plague services of, 86–87, 92, 103, 117, 128–29, 240–41; role in Great Plague, 231. *See also* parishes; religious responses to plague

anthrax, xvii, 272–73, 279

antibiotics, 278, 284, 289, 291

antidotes. *See* preventive measures; treatments

apothecaries, 95, 98, 104, 140, 143–44, 146, 148–49, 251, 325n. 11. *See also* Boghurst, William

archeus, 150–52, 282, 326n. 31

astrology, 20–21, 53, 68, 96, 108–9, 159, 198. *See also* almanacs

Athens, Plague of, 5

Backwell, Edward, 29, 125, 159, 163

Barwick, Dr. Peter, 92, 123, 141–42, 277

Battersea, 39, 200, 212. *See also* Patrick, Rev. Symon

beadles, 56, 115

bearers, 118, 225–26; pay of, 189

Bedford, dukes of, 35, 39, 44

Bethlehem (Bedlam) hospital, 77, 132, 190, 253, 269

Bible: ancient plague in, 5; consolatory passages in, 68, 70, 91, 83, 103, 129, 237, 240–41, 337n. 23; and the year 1666, 21

bills of exchange, 170–71, 176, 245

Bills of Mortality: compiling of, 32, 45, 64–65, 118, 128; locations of, 14, 202. *See also* burial practices; Great Plague chronology; mortality and vulnerability

Bing, Stephen, 123, 127, 231

Black Death, 5–9, 15, 50, 150, 182, 281; meaning of term, 7

bleeding: criticized, 149, 327n. 48; Galenic medicine and, 97, 104, 140; leeches used for, 320n. 10; practical uses of, 320n. 17

Bludworth, Sir Thomas, 223, 244–45, 251, 253, 264

Bocking, 200, 208

Boddington, George, 233–35

Boghurst, William: character and interests of, 1, 60, 63, 266; criticisms by, 147, 249,